Psychological groupwork
with acute psychiatric inpatients

Psychological groupwork with acute psychiatric inpatients

Edited by

Jonathan Radcliffe, Katja Hajek
Jerome Carson, and Oded Manor

W&B

MMX

© Whiting & Birch Ltd, 2010
Published by Whiting & Birch Ltd,
Forest Hill, London SE23 3HZ

ISBN (hardback) 9781861771148
ISBN (paperback) 9781861771186
ISBN (electronic) 9781861771193

Printed in England and the United States by Lightning Source

Contents

Foreword

This book is a most important response to widespread concerns that the therapeutic capacities of inpatient mental health wards and similar facilities have been in considerable decline in recent decades and that some patients even undergo further damage or trauma during admissions.

The chapter authors are all therapists who bring patients (or patients and staff) together into groups in ward or day hospital settings. They share generously with the reader their experiences, knowledge and skills in demonstrating ways of assisting the potential of these groups to be a source of containment and to be a setting in which emotions and experiences can be processed or even 'recovered'. Perhaps most important of all, the authors demonstrate ways in which individual patients can recover a degree of hope and trust that suffering fellow human beings can play a part in their recovery and feel again that they want to be part of 'society'.

I am impressed with Radcliffe and Smith's historical perspective, which charts the waxing and waning of emphasis over the centuries on the centrality of human relationships and activities in recovery from mental disturbances. Some of the authors trained a few decades ago when a good number of hospitals and wards were run much more along therapeutic community approaches than now. They make clear how indebted they are to the training and experiences they received at that time. In the state of overall decline of our wards, a crucial factor in their recovery is whether there are sufficient staff remaining with skills and experiences to be able to transmit these to the new generation, so that its members have confidence in using them to create an early upturn in the waxing and waning cycle. This book, which collates a wide body of experience and 'know-how', should play an important part in the current concern, which has also been expressed by major bodies through the development of the AIMS and Star Wards projects referred to in the texts.

On reading through this book, two particular themes stood out for me. Although the aim of the book is to demonstrate how to create safe groups *for patients* to assist one another at an emotional level, many of the authors recognise the crucial role of *helping staff* without group experience to feel respected and safe enough to process their own experiences in a group setting. The corollary of this, is the profound respect of many of the authors for groups of human beings to harm one another and hence the considerable care and skill needed in forming and facilitating therapeutic groups. I could go as far as saying that the need for therapeutic groups is precisely because the group experience of these patients in society, in families and on the wards has not been sufficiently containing and sometimes actively harmful. Duggins's chapter is a profound illustration of the parallel negative experiences of a staff member and of patients with schizophrenia exposed to wards without any group setting in which either staff or patient can process and productively reflect on their emotional experience.

A particular strength of the book is that in many of the chapters there is a detailed account of group sessions that allows one to almost be in the group room as an active resonating participant. This aspect of the book should play an important part in making it meaningful to staff who work on wards. The vivid descriptions of groups at work complement the most useful summaries of healing factors of groups and the considerable amount of advice as to the work needed in creating and protecting such groups and in generating useful research into their effectiveness.

The fact that this a multi-author book gives it considerable further strength in that it describes therapeutic groups that have been set up in quite a wide variety of conditions and settings (e.g. in-patient units, adolescent units and day units). The adaptations that are necessary are made clear. For example: the spectrum of frequency of meetings ranges from those in which participants may only meet once, to those where patients may be attendees in multiple groups during a week, each with different purposes and lasting several months.

I would like to congratulate Jonathan Radcliffe, Katja Hajek, Jerome Carson, Oded Manor and their chapter authors on bringing together such a useful range of contributions to such an important topic. I would also congratulate Whiting and Birch on agreeing to publish this book. Together with this book, there are at least three other recent books (Gale et al., 2008; Hardcastle et al, 2007; Hinshelwood, 2004) that complement one another and if they can all find a way onto wards and day units for staff to read and study, together a significant contribution will have been made to improving the experience of the inpatient.

Brian Martindale

References

Gale, J., Realpe, A., and Pedriali, E. (2008) *Therapeutic Communities for Psychosis: Philosophy, History and Clinical Practice*. London: Routledge.

Hardcastle, M. Kennard, D., Grandison, S., and Fagin, L. (2007) *Experiences of Mental Health In-patient Care: Narratives from Service Users, Carers and Professionals*. London: Routledge.

Hinshelwood, R.D. (2004) *Suffering Insanity*. Hove: Brunner-Routledge.

Introduction

Jonathan Radcliffe

This book is an introductory guide to psychological groupwork with acute psychiatric inpatients. Its contributors come from a range of professional backgrounds and orientations. Part I sets the scene describing the context of acute inpatient care. The ten chapters in Part II each describe specific approaches to running groups. In this introduction I will discuss why there is a need for more psychological therapy groups on wards, make some general points about the differing aims, focus, time-frame, group membership and skills needed using different models. Finally there is a brief overview of each chapter.

The need for psychological groupwork with acute psychiatric inpatients

The difficulties confronting acute inpatient care have long been reported and there is ample evidence that many acute wards cannot be relied on to provide patients with a therapeutic experience. Research in the 1990s revealed a decline in the amount of patient-nurse contact and ward life that was both boring and unsafe (Quirk & Lelliott, 2008). Problems have included pressure on beds, staffing difficulties, lack of clarity about the purpose of admissions and an absence of psychological therapy. Most patients are unoccupied and spend much of their time alone in their bedroom (Chapter 1). The traditional emphasis of acute care is medication, case-management and nursing care (McCulloch et al, 2005) and many healthcare professionals hold the view that psychological therapy is irrelevant or not a priority. Although the NICE Guidelines (National Institute for Health and Clinical Excellence) recommend psychological therapy for severe mental health problems, the provision of psychological therapy on most acute psychiatric wards in the UK is poor (Sainsbury Centre, 2004) and the provision of talking groups on wards is also limited (see Chapter 1). Seeing patients for psychological work in groups enables therapists to work with more patients than would be possible otherwise. Numerous official publications refer to the need for groups (eg Department of Health, 2002). Star Wards (Janner, 2006) and the

Accreditation for Acute Inpatient Mental Health Services (AIMS) (Royal College of Psychiatrists, 2009), both promote groupwork. For example, AIMS standards include offering patients daily therapeutic group contact, regular psycho-educational groups, gender-sensitive groups, weekly community meetings and relapse-prevention groups. However, there are very few recent publications on how to run psychological therapy groups for inpatients, hence this book.

Working psychologically with groups of patients can help make wards become more therapeutic. They provide safe structures where patients can engage and talk with each other about their experiences and receive help in understanding them. Groups can also be used to address social aspects of mental health problems that individualistic approaches miss out (Farquharson, 2007). Positive interactions in a group will carry over into relationships on the ward. Several chapters show how groups can be used to help patients cope with being on the ward. Chapters 9 and 10, describe the contribution of groups to improving patients' interpersonal skills. Chapter 11 shows how groups can be used to improve patients' ability to deal with the types of conflict that typically arise on wards. Chapter 17 shows how groups can be used to help adolescent inpatients improve their social functioning and behavioural difficulties. Good experiences of engaging with others, feeling supported and being able to offer support to others can create a positive cycle. Patients who are helped to engage with psychological therapy in groups in hospital may be more likely to accept individual or group psychotherapy after discharge, especially if the hand-over is handled in a coordinated fashion. This is especially so for patients who would not normally think that therapy is for them. A psychiatric admission presents an important opportunity to engage patients from socio-cultural and ethnic groups who do not traditionally access psychological therapy and who are often not referred for psychological therapy in the community.

Adapting the group to the setting

Providing groups in the acute inpatient setting is a challenge. The aims and methods must be realistic and congruent with the ward setting, and in particular the acute nature of patients' problems, the short-term nature of the work and constantly changing ward population. There are both generic benefits to patients from having good experiences in groups as well as specific benefits accruing from the particular approach taken. Aims include spotting and dealing with problems, ameliorating the stresses and frustrations of ward life, and being able to help other patients. Some chapters include helping patients understand the nature of their symptoms (Chapters 12, 13 and 15). One aspect uniting the different approaches to running ward groups is the need for the therapist to take an active stance. Whilst in some outpatient groups the therapist avoids talking too much in order to discourage dependency, the inpatient group leader needs to actively manage the group rather than taking too much of a back-seat, although in such a way as to help the patients engage.

Types of focus

The degree to which the group focuses on what has been happening on the ward as opposed to individuals' difficulties and experiences varies according to the approach taken. Some groups focus more on the individual, others on interpersonal relations, and some emphasise group processes (matrix); and the group as a microcosm of the ward and hospital (the network). For example, the problem-solving approach (chapter 11) and CBT approaches (chapter 12) focus on individual skills and knowledge albeit usually in relation to a social situation. Interpersonal approaches (chapters 9 and 10) frame individuals' difficulties in terms of habitual patterns of conducting relationships. Psychodynamic and group analytic approaches (chapters 14, 15, 16 and 18) see internalised relationships that inhabit the mind being played out on an interpersonal stage. The systemic approach views what happens in the group as a biopsy of the ward and hospital (chapter 14). The relationship between ward and group are also addressed in most chapters and especially in chapters 2, 3, 6, 10 and 14. Chapters 17 and 18 describe highly specific ward settings where groups play a central role in the treatment. Some groups teach skills and knowledge (chapters 11 and 12), whilst group analytic and psychodynamic groups are insight-oriented. Approaches also vary in whether they use events and relationships that occur in the 'here-and-now' of the therapy room as opposed to the 'there-and-then' of life outside the group and in the past. Another difference is between groups where the therapist sets the content of the discussion, and more exploratory groups where the therapist leaves the content to emerge. The latter are often described as being unstructured, although in fact they have a structure but of a different kind. A fuller group programme would include a range of psychological groups, some which are more general and others more specific.

The time-frame

Outpatient therapy groups have a fixed membership for a set number of sessions (closed groups) or a slowly evolving membership (slow-open groups). The CBT groups described in chapter 12 are closed groups where the same patients attend a set number of sessions. This has the advantage of greater continuity and an increased 'dose' for those who attend. The other chapters in the second part of the book describe groups where patients can attend for varying numbers of sessions and the group membership changes from session to session. Some patients will only attend once or twice, others may attend for months and some will return to the group on successive stays. Although turnover is high, some therapists emphasise the value of working over several sessions. Others use a more single-frame approach that focuses purely on the session taking place with no assumptions about what has gone before, and this is described by Oded Manor in chapter 8. In general, patients who attend more often will benefit more and so they are encouraged to attend consistently. In terms of frequency, most groups described in this book are once-weekly, the exceptions being an adolescent ward (chapter 17), and groups described in Denmark (chapter 14) and Portugal (chapter 18). Weekly talking groups are one part of the ward activities programme and a programme that contains daily talking groups is more likely to create a culture of engagement on the ward as opposed to one of passivity and avoidance.

Group membership

Clinicians running one group often want to offer a group that is accessible to as many patients as possible. Such groups are described as heterogeneous and are described in chapters 9, 10, 11, 14, 15, 17 and 18. Mixing patients who have different problems and are functioning at different levels has the advantage of fostering links between them and giving them an opportunity to discuss shared ward experiences. Patients may have more in common with patients with different diagnoses from their own, for example, some patients may be more psychologically-minded, motivated and able to deal with interpersonal conflict than others regardless of diagnosis. The advantage of selective or homogenous groups is that they can focus more on specific problems such as those facing patients with psychosis, described in chapters 12, 13 and 16. Ideally both heterogeneous and homogenous groups are needed on wards.

Skills needed

The term 'group therapy' is not widely applied to talking groups on acute wards, as groups run on wards differ in many ways from groups run in specialist outpatient psychotherapy departments. Many staff working in psychotherapy departments have undertaken post-qualification training in group psychotherapy, whilst the staff running groups on wards come from backgrounds including psychology, nursing, occupational therapy, psychiatry, psychotherapy and social work, and have in most cases developed groupwork skills after professionally qualifying. Specific training for working with groups of inpatients is not widely available. The level of experience and training required to deliver groupwork varies according to approach. Staff such as qualified nurses and trained psychology graduates can run the groups described in chapters 9, 10 and 11, if trained and supported. A comprehensive group programme would encompass groups delivered by staff with differing levels of skills and training but with interest and aptitude.

Overview of the book

In *Chapter 1*, Roger Smith and I give a historical perspective on how patients spent their time in psychiatric hospitals in earlier centuries, followed by a description of our study of patient activity on 16 wards in south London in 2004. We measured social disengagement and passivity, and audited the types of groups provided and the numbers of patients attending.

In *Chapter 2*, Leonard Fagin describes engendering a therapeutic milieu on an acute ward. He gives a vivid description of running a twice-weekly therapy group. He suggests that ward groups can be unique and therapeutic, but that their potential benefits are widely ignored. He shows how the group can contribute to patients' welfare, to understanding of their difficulties, and to the atmosphere on the ward. He also describes the benefits of ward assemblies, crisis meetings and other opportunities for therapeutic interactions.

In *Chapter 3*, Bob Harris shares his experiences of running groups in a traditional large asylum in the 80s and later on a long-stay secure unit. He shows how patients with serious mental disorders can explore, reflect and achieve a measure of acceptance of their difficulties during group therapy. He emphasises the value of the involvement and support of doctors, nurses and hospital managers. He also considers the potential of groupwork for helping patients cope with societal issues.

In *Chapter 4*, Frank Holloway provides a contextual account of the state of inpatient care, beginning with a personal account of his 35 years of experience of working in psychiatry, and then going on to describe important changes including the move from large asylums to local care, and increased concentrations of detained patients on wards. He discusses the centrality of the acute ward to effective community mental health provision and speculates on future developments.

In Chapter 5, Richard Duggins gives an account of why inhumane and anti-therapeutic practices can become part of ward culture as a defence against contact with disturbed patients. Both patients and staff tend to avoid therapeutic activities as these provide a context for getting in touch with states of mind felt to be intolerable. He describes how therapeutic groups can help contain anxieties thereby countering defensive isolation and allowing patients to experience and bear some of their feelings.

In Chapter 6, Ian Simpson describes how staff support groups can provide the containment to enable staff to cope with daily pressures of being in contact with disturbed and disturbing patients, and from stresses deriving from institutional problems. He describes the types of issues that arise and how to take these up, and how staff support groups can help ensure that working practices remain therapeutic and reduce the risk of staff burnout.

In Chapter 7, Chris Evans, Nick Huband, Tom O'Reilly and Eleanor Overton, look at different types of research evidence for inpatient groups. Using an imaginary situation of a service manager and clinical director asking some therapists to provide evidence to justify their method of group therapy, they describe how the therapists might address this task given the complexities involved. The authors review the accepted hierarchy of research evidence, and the problems with applying randomised-control trials to ward groups and aggregating results in systematic reviews. They compare three very different kinds of research papers on inpatient group therapy.

In Chapter 8, the last chapter in Part I, Oded Manor identifies some important common features of inpatient groupwork from the literature with reference to chapters that follow in Part II. He emphasises the need for modest goals, the value of an active approach to running ward groups, and the value of fostering the working alliance in the group. He discusses the advantages of working within a single-session format and describes how to manage the beginning, middle and end phases of a session to facilitate maximum benefits to the patients.

Part II covers a range of models, including *interpersonal* (chapters 9 and 10), *problem-solving* (Chapter 11), *CBT* (Chapter 12), *Kanas' integrative* model for schizophrenia (chapter 13) and *psychodynamically informed approaches* (Chapters 14, 15 and 16) an *adolescent ward* (cChapter 17) and a *partial hospitalisation unit* in Portugal (chapter 18).

In Chapter 9, Katja Hajek describes how she and her psychology assistants conduct an adapted version of Yalom's interpersonal model of inpatient group therapy. She outlines the aims and principles of running a Yalom group. Hajek employs Yalom's approach for lower functioning patients but adapts it for use with the full range. The therapist starts each session by setting the patients an individual task, and then helps them focus and reflect on each other's contributions, give and receive feedback. Hajek describes the findings of her evaluation of patients' satisfaction with her group as compared with other ward activities.

In Chapter 10, Adam Jefford, Alistair Grandison and Bhupinderjit Kaur Pharwaha describe a group that is run by the ward nurses and doctors with the help of outside supervision from the first author. A sub-group of ward staff facilitate the group on a rotational basis with fortnightly supervision. This has enabled the staff to develop their skills and share ownership of the group. The authors describe how issues are taken up in supervision, and the impact of the group on staff.

In Chapter 11, Susan J. Grey describes how problem-solving approaches can be adapted for use on the acute psychiatric ward. She has developed 25 problem scenarios which can be used to help patients practise the three stages of problem-solving: identifying the problem, generating solutions and evaluating these solutions. The chapter provides guidance for staff on how to organise and run the group and a structure to help patients then learn the necessary skills. The group format is suitable for any patients and can be used by psychology graduates or qualified nursing staff.

In Chapter 12 Stephen Livingstone and Til Wykes describe a range of cognitive behaviour therapy groups for acute inpatients with psychosis. They emphasise the research evidence underpinning CBT approaches and delineate cognitive and behavioural techniques. The groups are closed and consist of a series of sessions with a focus on a specific problem and a pre-defined intended outcome. They give a detailed case example of a patient who benefited from this approach.

In Chapter 13, Ronan McIvor and Wil Pennycook describe how they used Kanas' integrative model of group therapy for inpatients with schizophrenia, which they extend to include other types of psychosis. The model combines systems, psychodynamic and educative theoretical approaches. The authors describe the social context in which the group takes place, how they worked with staff to embed the group into the ward, and the practicalities of running the group.

In Chapter 14, Torben Heinskou describes the application of Howard Kibel's model of inpatient group therapy. Kibel groups are run on all the unlocked acute psychiatric hospitals in a large area of Copenhagen. The approach is based on an integration of systems and object relations theories. The group is seen as a subgroup of the unit and is a meeting place between patients' internalised relationships and the dynamics operating on the ward and hospital. Patients can use the group to express, clarify and reality-test their reactions to hospital. The facilitators use feedback from the group to help others in the organisation consider organisational dynamics operating on the ward and hospital.

In Chapter 15, Debora Diamond and I describe a psychodynamic ward group based on the psychoanalytic view that symptoms are expressions of unconscious feelings. Patients are encouraged to talk about what has been happening to them and how they are feeling. The therapists aim to create a safe space where painful or conflictual thoughts and feelings can be expressed, using the group process to facilitate this aim. The authors explain how we use psychoanalytic thinking to understand symptoms including delusions, paranoia, depression and mania. We give a session transcription as an illustration.

In Chapter 16, Jack Nathan applies Fonagy and Bateman's theory of mentalisation in his group approach to inpatients with psychosis. He develops his own theoretical ideas of three levels of mentalisation; rudimentary, simple and complex. He goes on to delineate patients' emotional engagement with other people, outlining five levels of what he terms 'psychic states of engagement'. He describes working with patients operating on these two dimensions in a ward group that he co-facilitates with a consultant psychiatrist.

In Chapter 17, Dylan Griffiths describes the unique challenges posed in working on an adolescent ward where he is a consultant psychiatrist. The work of the unit is influenced by ideas from therapeutic communities. Rules and expectations provide the young people with containment with a balance between firmness and liberality. Participatory and user-led groups help the young people to develop independence and autonomy. They spend their week in a range of groups including teaching groups and structured therapy groups. Griffiths focuses on three groups that are used to structure the young people's week; the 'start of week group', the mid-week community meeting, and the 'end of week group'. The young people are helped to take responsibility for chairing the mid-week group.

In Chapter 18, Isaura Manso Neto describes a day hospital with partial hospitalisation in Portugal. The unit is in effect a therapeutic community for acute patients, who attend for about eight months. She describes the advantages of partial hospitalisation over full hospitalisation. She pays special attention to the three times a week psychotherapy group, a parents group and a multi-family group. She also describes the therapeutic culture that has been developed over the 30 years including the structures that staff use to supervise, support and train each other.

Where case examples are given patient details have been disguised to protect anonymity.

Concluding comments

I started this chapter by outlining the need for psychological groupwork with acute psychiatric inpatients. I then considered how inpatient groups need to be adapted to the unique nature of the inpatient setting. I looked at whether groups should have an individual or social focus, the time frame of groups, group membership and the skills needed to facilitate inpatient groups. Finally, I gave a brief overview of the book chapters.

There are a number of features which make this book unique. First, all of the chapters are written by experienced clinicians, most of whom are active groupwork practitioners. Second, the book has a multidisciplinary focus, with contributions from psychiatrists, psychologists, mental health nurses, social workers and group analysts. Third, apart from describing their specific theoretical orientation, each groupworker provide illustrative case material that brings the groupwork 'to life.' Fourth, the contributors bring with them a range of insights and observations from their work, which will hopefully inform and inspire other groupworkers. I would like to thank all our contributors as well as my co-editors, Katja Hajek, Jerome Carson and Oded Manor.

Jonathan Radcliffe
London September 2009

References

Department of Health (2002) *Mental Health Policy Implementation Guide: Adult Acute Inpatient Care Provision*. London: Department of Health.

Farquharson, G. (2007) 'How Good Staff become bad'. In P.Campling, S.Davies & G.Farquharson (Eds.) *From Toxic Institutions to Therapeutic Environments*. Glasgow: Royal College of Psychiatry, Gaskell.

Janner, M. (2006) *Star Wards Handbook 1*. London: Bright (and on-line).

McCulloch, A., Ryrie, I., Williamson, T. & St John, T. (2005) 'Has the medical model a future?' *Mental Health Review*, 10, 7-15.

Quirk, A. & Lelliott, P. (2008) 'Users' experiences of inpatient services'. In P.Campling, S.Davies & G.Farquharson (Eds.) *From toxic institutions to therapeutic environments.* Glasgow: Royal College of Psychiatry, Gaskell.

Royal College of Psychiatrists' Centre for Quality Improvement (2009) *Accreditation for Acute Inpatient Mental Health Services (AIMS).* Royal College of Psychiatry. http://www. rcpsych.ac.uk/clinicalservicestandards/centreforqualityimprovement/aims.aspx (accessed April 2009).

Sainsbury Centre for Mental Health (2004) *Briefing 28. Acute Care 2004: A National Survey of Adult Psychiatric Wards in England.* London: Sainsbury Centre for Mental Health.

I

What patients do in hospital

Activity and inactivity, social interaction and isolation

Jonathan Radcliffe and Roger Smith

Introduction

Visitors to acute psychiatric wards and patients on their first admission are often struck by the lack of purposeful activity. Patients are mostly sitting, wandering around, or in their rooms. Sizeable proportions complain that they are bored and do not have enough to do (Sainsbury Centre, 1998, 2002; Department of Health, 2002; Sundram, 1987). In 1953 the World Health Organization named the need for activity and a proper working day for all patients as one of the constituent parts of well-managed inpatient care (WHO, 1953). The Department of Health (2002) outlines the need for the provision of social, recreational and occupational therapies and activities based on assessment of need. There are no minimum standards for this provision set by the government. The Healthcare Commission (2005) stipulated the need for a 'fair', 'good' or 'excellent' range of therapies and activities. The Royal College of Psychiatrists' Centre for Quality Improvement produces a voluntary accreditation scheme, now in its third edition (2009), the Accreditation for Acute Inpatient Mental Health Service (AIMS). A number of the standards refer to activities and psychological interventions, for example each patient should be invited to therapeutic group contact with both staff and fellow patients for at least one half-hour each day and be involved in negotiating an activity and therapy programme. The AIMS accreditation scheme is an impressive attempt to improve the standard of provision. It is however voluntary and the focus is on access and provision rather than overall attendance levels. The need for such a scheme reflects the historic fact that activities are generally of lower priority on wards than practical ward management such as dealing with requests, administrative tasks and maintaining safety. Our study of a number of hospitals described below shows that activity programmes are still variable and poorly attended. Medication is seen as the most significant aspect of treatment by nurses, OTs and psychiatrists (Bowers et al, 2005) and psychological therapy is provided to a minority of patients.

An absence of engagement in meaningful activities means that there is little reason for patients to get out of bed and the normal rhythms of life are not maintained or established. Organised activities are a vehicle for social engagement. A brief period of withdrawal from social activity may be helpful for some patients in the most acute phase of their breakdown but continued withdrawal is associated with isolation, frustration, low morale, and is a wasted opportunity for meaningful activities and contact with others. The National Survey of Violence (Chaplin, 2006) found that patients named boredom as a factor that could make violent incidents more likely to occur and meaningful activities reduced their likelihood.

The problem of patient inactivity is not new and it is an international problem. In this chapter we give a historical perspective and describe more recent developments. We report on previously published research on the impact of disengagement and describe the findings from our study of 16 wards in a large London mental health trust in 2004. We conclude by discussing what types of activities are helpful and some of the practicalities of running activity programmes.

A historical perspective

The history of the treatment of patients in mental health institutions in England and other parts of the developed world has progressed through a number of stages. The first stage beginning roughly in the fourteenth century consisted of incarceration, physical restraint, and physical treatment. The second stage beginning in the second half of the eighteenth century consisted of the gradual introduction of more humane treatment and psychological explanations of mental health problems. The third stage beginning in the nineteenth century was the growth of large asylums with a variety of social, recreational and occupational activities. The fourth stage from the nineteen sixties to the present consisted of the gradual closing down of most of the large asylums and a move to care in the community and wards in local hospitals.

Early hospitals

The Priory of Saint Mary of Bethlem was confiscated by Edward III in 1375 and became a hospital for 'lunatics' in 1377. This made it the earliest hospital in England solely for the treatment of mental health problems. Ward activities were minimal. Patients were generally on locked wards with physical restraints for the uncontrollable patients. Patients who were permitted to leave Bethlem could be identified by their distinctive badges enabling them to be returned to the hospital should they become lost. In 1676 the new Bedlam was opened in Moorfields in a building designed by Robert Hooke and modelled on the Tuileries in Paris. Two statues by Caius Gabriel Cibber, 'Melancholy' and 'Raving Madness', were placed at the entrance to the hospital to excite the sympathy of passers-by. Patients were expected to beg from visitors or passers-by to support the operating costs of the establishment. Physical treatments such as emetics, blood-letting, hot and cold baths were common but of dubious effectiveness (Rutherford, 2008). Some importance was placed on the availability of fresh air and led to the creation of 'airing courts'. Anyone could visit Bethlem to watch or abuse inhabitants of the asylum for a small fee. It was not until 1770 that a written permission from a hospital governor had to be produced to visit. The word 'patient' was not generally applied to people suffering from mental health difficulties until the eighteenth century.

Moral treatment

This influential humanising liberal movement was pioneered towards the end of the eighteenth century firstly by Pinel in France and then by Tuke in England. 'Moral' was used in the sense of emotional or psychological and meant compassionate and understanding treatment (Bockoven, 1972). Pinel used a psychological approach to the care of mental health patients rejecting the routine chaining of patients. Pinel reported improvements in patients of the Bicêtre Hospital when they were provided with work by Paris merchants. Moral treatment usually included meaningful employment of time, outdoor exercise, a 'family environment' and social interaction between patients and staff. William Battie advocated good food, clean fresh air, exercise, employment and distraction from family stresses as a treatment for patients at St Luke's Hospital and the private asylums that he ran in Britain. Structured activity was seen as having a calming influence providing a basis for relating to others, being part of a group, and providing the sense of achievement and purpose, each of which are sources of self-respect (Borthwick et al, 2001). The Retreat was built by the Quaker Tuke family in York in the 1790s and showed some of the development of Battie's ideas about the importance of the regimen (Tuke, 1813) and on the ideas of Pinel (Berrios & Freeman, 1996). Patients were Quakers or were referred by Quakers. Medical interventions such as restraint or purging were minimised. The Tuke family used social activities such as taking tea with the superintendent, walking, talking to staff and other patients, exercise and work in the garden or on the farm. They felt that activities, especially those reflecting the Quaker life of the Tuke family, were beneficial in diverting patients from irrational thoughts (Rutherford, 2008).

Large asylums

John Conolly (cited in Morris, 2008) wrote two books in the nineteenth century which influenced the development of asylums built during the Victorian era. He emphasised the importance of activities and argued against the routine use of physical restraint. The 1845 Lunatics Act gave rise to the development of the Lunacy Commission, which issued instructions for asylum builders. The Commission insisted that land was provided for therapeutic activities such as gardening, agriculture and recreation, with views from both the grounds and wards. Buildings were modelled on grand country houses in order to have a positive effect on patients' mood. Ornaments, lodges, fields, kitchen and flower gardens, shrubberies, walks and flower borders were all considered beneficial. Exercise through the 'airing courts' and exposure to fresh air were considered important. Patients were expected to take part in activities and a system of rewards was instituted, for example they were given tobacco and access to dances for work in the garden. These institutions provided shelter, food, activity and entertainment, in contrast to the workhouses and prisons, which were the alternatives for many mentally ill patients. Activities in the large asylums were more concerned with the life of the institution itself rather than being seen as of direct benefit to patients. Thus activities such as working on the farm, in the laundry, kitchens, kitchen gardens, grounds, and cleaning duties reduced the operating costs of the establishment. The small scale domestic environment of asylums such as the Retreat of the previous century was superseded by the creation of ever larger asylums such as the second Middlesex Asylum at Colney Hatch which opened in 1851 and had a main corridor that was a quarter of a mile in length.

Under-funding and the passing of the early leaders of the moral movement meant that the kindly compassionate care could not take place in the large asylums. Instead, they became large custodial centres or 'bins' where patients frequently became isolated and deprived of nurturing interactions. Around the same time the earlier romantic view of innocent suffering was replaced by a positivist scientific view of mental illness as a biological phenomenon that was amenable to physical treatments. There was diminishing interest in social or psychological aspects of treatment and on reintegrating patients into society. Indeed in the latter part of the nineteenth century mentally ill patients were often seen as being incapable of achieving independent living.

Milieu Therapy

The twentieth century brought a new kind of moral treatment known as milieu therapy. In Germany, Simon (1927, in Rice & Rutan, 1987, p.4) developed 'activere behandlung' or 'more active therapy' whereby patients were given tasks to perform with gradually increasing levels of difficulty, based on their previous work experience. Thomson (1986, p.35-36) described milieu therapy as a non-hierarchical environment, which can act as a supportive family. The advantages that he describes of removing patients from a home environment that may be contributing to their problems are very reminiscent of Battie's suggestions (Morris, 2008). Milieu's emphasis on involvement and the provision of opportunities for interaction influenced nursing in many countries during the nineteen sixties and seventies (Gunderson, 1983). More recent surveys have shown that patients value and want milieu aspects of inpatient care such as closeness with staff especially in the context of therapy (Lelliott & Quirk, 2004). Haigh (2002) makes a strong case for more emphasis on creating a therapeutic atmosphere, and the importance of human relationships as opposed to organisational arrangements.

Therapeutic Communities

The therapeutic communities movement, developed by Main (1946) and Jones (1952) amongst others, has overlapping characteristics with milieu. It emphasises egalitarianism between patients and staff with joint decisions made about many aspects of running the community. All the patient interactions that take place in the community are considered to reflect individuals' difficulties and characteristic ways of relating and these become part of the treatment, with group meetings of various formats taking central importance. The therapeutic community ideas were influenced by work in military hospitals during World War II, where staff shortages showed how effectively these institutions could be run with the help of patients (amongst others: Bion, 1948; Foulkes, 1948). Therapeutic communities have continued to exist in their pure form in the UK in specialised units such as the Cassel Hospital and Richmond Fellowship hostels. The movement also influenced acute care in local hospitals, for example seen in the weekly 'community' meetings and in ideas of democratisation seen in service-user involvement and empowerment. Haigh (op cit.) outlines some of the principles of therapeutic communities. He points out that the 'principles used successfully to understand the work in modern therapeutic communities are translatable into practice that may help thinking about solutions to the crisis in acute care'.

Anti-psychiatry

The anti-psychiatry movement of the nineteen sixties rejected hospitals and the medical approaches to mental illness. Proponents led by R.D. Laing and others believed that what patients essentially need is support, space and an absence of pressure, or medical / professional interventions. Natural healing would occur with emotional and practical support and without any form of coercion.

De-institutionalisation

The closure of the large asylums in the last decades of the twentieth century represented a major change in psychiatric care in the UK and in many other parts of the world. Patients who were formerly living in the large hospitals moved into hostels, supported accommodation and their own flats. In the last two decades in the UK there has been a huge increase in the number of mental health professionals working with patients living in the community. The local wards replacing the asylum care provide briefer admissions, and are intended to be less institutionalised. Current approaches to ward activities reflect in part a reaction against the institutionalised activities of the asylums. Many occupational therapy departments which traditionally ran activity programmes now focus more on work with individuals aimed at improving independent living skills. Occupational therapies in the large asylums such as basket-weaving became associated with 'institutional mind-numbing', although in fact, art activities can be valuable means of expression as well as vehicles for social interaction. Acute admissions are now far shorter than in the past, averaging two months in wards in the trust we studied (reported below). The population of patients present on the ward is constantly changing with four new patients joining a typical 18-bed ward each week. Quirk et al. (2006) have written about the permeability of acute wards compared with the previous closed institutions, with patients keeping in closer contact with friends and family who visit and by using mobile phones. When they are well enough patients are encouraged to leave the ward for periods each day to acclimatise them to life outside and build up independence. Other patients are prevented from going out. Nurses spend a great deal of time in tasks such as processing and assessing new patients, and note-keeping. The emphasis is on safe containment. There is pressure to free up beds for new admissions.

Following deinstitutionalisation, a major influence on government mental health policy has been public safety concerns. High profile media coverage of murders by patients led to fears of insufficient monitoring and control of potentially violent patients. The UK government response has been to propose more powers to detain and treat patients. Against this has emerged a large and effective coalition (Mental Health Alliance) opposing such coercive powers (Pilgrim, 2007), and the service-user movement has become an active and influential force. At the same time consumer choice has become a key organising principle of healthcare policy, imported from America (Pilgrim, op. cit.) based on the principle that allowing patients to choose hospitals and treatments will drive up quality. This has yet to have a major impact on psychiatric care in the UK. However there are increasing expectations for professionals to discuss options with patients and involve them in decisions. This occurs against a backdrop of a tightening of control over health-care professionals and the treatments they deliver, linked to the increasing primacy of evidence-based treatment. Treatment is increasingly determined by National Institute for Health and Clinical Excellence (NICE) guidelines based on medical diagnoses with evidence derived from randomised controlled trials. These have promoted cognitive behavioural therapy, although anecdotal evidence suggests that the NICE recommendations for psychological therapy are not being implemented on wards to the same extent as in the community. Not providing psychological therapies for inpatients denies the most severely ill patients therapies of proven effectiveness that are recommended by NICE. Having said this, the NICE recommendations can undermine other approaches which lack the evidence of efficacy provided by randomised controlled studies.

Competing influences on inpatient care

As has been seen, there are numerous ideologies and political influences affecting inpatient care. The biological view is that medication is the essence of treatment and other activities should be subordinate to it. Moral treatment with its kindly, humane care in a family atmosphere emphasises the benefits of purposeful activity. Milieu varies according to different writers, with some emphasising the importance of therapeutic programmes whilst others de-emphasise them in favour of relations with individual staff. The influence of the large asylums is largely in the reaction against them; anti-institutionalisation sees less demanding occupational groupwork as being irrelevant to the knowledge and skills needed for independent living. One consequence of government moves to detain and control potentially dangerous patients combined with the service user movement is that coercion in detaining patients may be accompanied by staff being reluctant to impose attendance at activities even when this may be in patients' interests. Anti-psychiatry, the user-involvement movement and the patient-as-customer approach all emphasise choice and lack of strictures and prescription, but this can lead to a laissez-faire approach. Inpatient group therapy has waned in recent years and psychologists and group therapy practitioners have tended to put their efforts into working with outpatients where the ability to select committed patients and work with them longer leads to more satisfying results. Finally, positivist approaches to psychological therapy emphasise the need for research evidence for treatment, which can lead to a devaluing of approaches that do not have sufficient empirical evidence of efficacy.

Activity and social interaction

The beneficial relationship between activity and mood has been long known. Seneca, writing in about 44 AD, advocated activity as an antidote to despair and grief (Seneca, 44/1996). Much of modern cognitive behavioural therapy (CBT) can be traced back to tenets of Stoic philosophy, of which Seneca was a proponent. Activity (sometimes called behavioural activation or activity scheduling) has an important role in the treatment of mood disorders such as depression (Fennell, 1989; Fennell et al, 2004) in combination with the cognitive aspects of CBT. There is evidence that inactivity is a risk factor for depression (Farmer et al., 1988) and that physical exercise can improve mood (Dimeo et al., 2001).

Although surveys show that many patients are dissatisfied with the sparseness of activity programmes, health managers often want more than evidence of improved patient satisfaction in order to justify spending money on activity programmes. Unfortunately demonstrating that high quality organised activity programmes lead to better mental health outcomes is not straightforward. The fact that active patients recover more quickly than less active patients does not prove causality, as the healthier patients are likely to be the ones who are more active and energetic. Comparing outcome between wards with and without activity programmes is problematic as wards vary on numerous dimensions and patient populations also vary between wards.

Conclusions can be drawn from large-scale comparisons although due to the pace of change care must be taken when making comparisons with today's wards. A large-scale study was carried out by Collins et al (1985) on 79 wards in America, where 4589 patients were assessed on admission and three months after discharge. Pre and post-measures were carried out using four patient questionnaires plus questionnaires completed by relatives. 191 ward characteristics were compared with patient outcome, 11 of which were significantly correlated to positive outcomes on both sources of outcome measure. The overall picture was that wards with more interactions of a positive nature were associated with better outcome and wards with more social passivity had poorer outcome. Eight of the 11 factors related to ward attributes including orderliness and good organisation, nurses sticking to regular shift patterns and informal relations between patients and staff. Social passivity was measured by periodic observer ratings of the percentages of patients deemed socially passive, e.g. watching TV, watching other people or engaged in self-care e.g. doing the laundry. Wards with higher percentages of socially passive patients were found to have poorer outcomes. Three other characteristics indicated that positively engaged relationships were associated with better outcome; wards where patients called staff by their first names, wards where there were fewer negative feelings expressed by patients and staff in response to a questionnaire, e.g. 'patients often gripe', and wards where chairs were arranged so that patients interacted rather than watching TV. It is possible that some of these characteristics were markers for well-run wards rather than being significant themselves. However, the overall picture was clear; ward regime clearly makes a difference to recovery.

The findings of a recent study on the perceived effectiveness of scheduled activity were that scheduled activities had a beneficial effect on the mood of depressed inpatients (Iqbal & Bassett, 2008). Most patients also reported increased satisfaction and pleasure in taking part in the activities. Staff attitudes were a mixture of feeling that they did not have time to undertake such activities or uncertainty about the benefits. This may partly explain the lack of activities or staff enthusiasm in delivering them as reported elsewhere in this discussion.

STUDY: Patient activity and social engagement

Our study was carried out on 16 adult acute locality wards in six hospitals in a large inner city mental health trust in 2005 (Radcliffe & Smith, 2007). Firstly, we observed what each patient was doing during the day, focussing on activity and social interaction. Secondly, we audited attendance at organised activities.

Ward context

The number of beds on each ward was between 13 and 25 with a median of 18. Mean bed occupancy rates were 118% including patients sleeping at home on leave (range 96%-150%) and 95% excluding patients on leave (range 80% - 120%). The average length of stay was 60 days. There were on average four new patients admitted or transferred to each ward each week (range 8-26) with the concomitant load placed on staff to assess and process these patients.

Social engagement

Each ward was observed three times a day over the course of a 9 a.m. to 5 p.m. week excluding lunchtimes and weekends. Timings were randomly determined and the observer followed a set route around the ward, categorising each patient's behaviour in one of ten categories (Table 1). Reliability was found to be good, with intra-class coefficients of between 0.60 and 0.93 during piloting for two observers carrying out observations simultaneously. Across 16 wards, 4103 individual patient observations were made, equating to an average of 17 patients per ward visit. An identical patient

Table 1
Percentages of patients observed in different activities

% Socially engaged (n=656)		% socially disengaged (n=3447)	
Interacting with staff	4	Standing/ walking	12
Interacting with other patients	7	Alone in bedroom	46
Negative interaction	1	Self-care	4
Receiving care	1	Sitting socially disengaged	22
Interacting in bedroom	1		
Organised activity	2		
	16		84

Table 2
Categories of activity

Type 1: Talking groups
Ward community meeting, psychodynamic, depression-management, anxiety-management, coping with psychosis, hearing voices, substance misuse, pre-discharge.

Type 2: Non-verbal therapies
Music therapy, art therapy, drama therapy.

Type 3: Creative/expressive
Arts and craft, woodwork, pottery, creative writing, drumming.

Type 4: Skills and information
Cooking, careers advice, local college education advice, outings to local resources e.g. mental health community resource centres.

Type 5: Physical/Relaxation
Aerobics, gym, yoga, walking group, relaxation, meditation.

Type 6: Recreational
Videos, table tennis, pool competitions, table football, music appreciation, leisure outings.

group was not necessarily seen on each ward observation due to patient turnover and because some patients would have been off the ward on leave when we visited.

We found that across 16 wards on average 84% of patients were socially disengaged at any one time. The other 16% were mostly interacting informally and a small number were engaged in an organised activity. 'Socially disengaged' consisted of being alone in the bedroom (46%), walking around or sitting in a communal area, predominantly passively (34%) or engaged in self-care such as washing or making tea (4%; see Table 1). The percentage of socially disengaged patients was consistent across the six hospitals with a variation of three percentage points between the highest and lowest, which

Table 3
Number and types of organised activities provided on each ward

Ward*	1	2	3	4	5	6	7	8	9	10	11	12	13	14	15	16	average
Talking	2	1	2	1	5	3	5	1	1	2	1	1	1	0	1	2	1.8
Non-verbal therapy	1	1	1	3	3	2	0	0	0	0	0	1	1	1	0	0	0.9
Creative- Expressive	0	1	3	0	0	1	4	4	2	7	1	5	5	5	4	4	2.9
Skills or Information	0	0	1	0	3	3	0	2	2	2	3	3	1	3	2	2	1.5
Physical or relaxation	2	1	2	2	3	4	2	3	0	2	2	3	2	1	4	4	2.3
Recreational	0	0	0	0	0	2	1	2	2	1	4	0	0	0	3	2	1.1
Totals	5	4	9	6	11	15	12	12	7	14	11	13	10	10	14	14	10.4

*Wards in same hospitals grouped with bold lines

is not statistically significant (χ^2=1.42, d.f. =5, p>.05). A logistic regression analysis showed that there were significant differences between wards within hospitals for three out of the five hospitals with more than one ward (χ^2= 5.46, p<0.05 d.f.=2; χ^2=6.13, p<.05, d.f.=1; χ^2=40.6, p<.0001). The highest and lowest levels of social disengagement across the trust were found in two wards in the same hospital (91% and 75%).

Organised activities

We audited attendance registers over three-week periods, again focussing on the Monday to Friday working week. We looked at how many activities were offered, their take-up, type, who ran them and how the programme was organised. We placed each activity into one of six categories (Table 2).

The number of weekly activities on each ward varied from four to 15 with an average of ten (Table 3). Between one and three activities were timetabled each day although sometimes these were cancelled. Attendance registers are the most reliable method of showing whether groups take place and for how long. These showed that take-up was low; the average patient spent 90 minutes each week in organised activities, equating to 4% of the 9-5 working week. On one ward the proportion was 2% whilst the highest was 7.5%.

Table 4 shows variation between hospitals. These averages hide wide differences in attendance by patients on the same wards. A minority of patients on each ward attended several activities each week. Detailed audits of three wards showed that 28% of patients attended no activity each week, 25% attended one activity (generally the community meeting), 20% attended two, and 27% attended three or more groups per week.

Table 4
Patients' time spent in organised activities each working week

hospital	no. of wards	%
A	3	6
B	2	7
C	2	3
D	3	2.5
E	5	4
F	1	3
Average		4

There was wide variation in provision of the different types of activity on different wards (Table 3). Talking groups were poorly provided. These mainly consisted of the ward community meeting held weekly and in one case daily. Eleven out of the 16 wards had no other talking group. Two wards had groups run by clinical psychologists. There were no other psychological therapy groups and no groups run by psychiatrists at that time. The other types of talking group were women's groups run on two wards and discharge planning meetings also run on two wards, and a problem-solving group. Seven wards had art, music or drama therapy run by peripatetic professionals. Creative-expressive activities such as art or creative writing were better provided. These were run by nurses or occupational technicians (OT techs) working on the wards. Although all the wards had access to gyms, typically only two or three patients used them once or twice a week.

A range of workers including OTs and psychologists, qualified and unqualified, and peripatetic staff members such as a relaxation therapist and a music therapist delivered activities (Table 5). The largest group delivering activities unsurprisingly were OTs. However, four wards had no OT groups. A key factor was the time-allocation of professionals from local occupational therapy and psychology departments and this varied. Some OT departments concentrated more on patients living in the community whilst others provided a traditional ward OT programme. One hospital had a centrally provided OT service, but not all wards accessed this, and patients were referred individually to the service rather than it being offered to all patients on the wards. Eight wards had no psychologist, one ward had a full-time psychologist and the remainder had one and a half days of psychologist's time. Ward OTs or psychologists decided departmentally or individually how to spend their allocated ward time; some ran groups whilst others concentrated on individual work. Most wards had some peripatetic run activities such as music therapy or relaxation therapy. This was determined by the budget and the priorities of the budget holder, for example the ward manager. In one hospital a decision had been made some years previously to have no art therapy.

Eight wards employed a full-time staff member employed to organise and deliver activities. These wards had a better range and take-up of activities. These were OT technicians (see Table 4, Hospitals A and B and two wards from E), or nursing assistants (Hospital D). Hospital D had previously been audited and improved since nursing assistants were appointed to run activities a few months earlier. This had led to a marked increase in patient activities, albeit largely recreational activities such as karaoke, as well as some arts and crafts and escorting patients to the gym. The OT technicians had art backgrounds and provided art activities as well as organising guest speakers and outings. They individually assessed and reviewed each patient's engagement with the programme, an important aspect of good practice. Psychology assistants ran talking groups under supervision of qualified psychologists as well as seeing individual patients (Hospital C). Eight wards had no worker dedicated to organising and delivering activities. These wards had fewer activities and lower attendance rates. Although regular shift nurses helped run groups, on most wards they did not run other groups other than the community meeting.

Summary of findings

Consistent with findings from patient surveys, our study showed that most patients were socially disengaged and inactive most of the time and took part in few organised activities. Levels of social disengagement were strikingly similar between hospitals although there were differences between wards. There was a marked variation in organised activity provision between wards including those in the same hospital, with some programmes having twice the patient engagement rates as others, as well as considerable variation as to the types of group activities provided. Over half of a sub-sample of patients attended one or no activity each week. The results are consistent with the findings from patient surveys in the UK and elsewhere. The range and quality of activity programmes reflects the priority placed on this as well as resourcing and local OT and psychology department provision. The patchiness of provision suggests that a wider organisational response is needed at trust and national level.

Engaging patients in activity programmes

Who should provide activities?

In terms of costs and benefits, unqualified staff can provide a significant proportion of what is needed if the structure and support is in place. Our study revealed that the fullest programmes were led by an OT technician who delivered activities and over-saw the programme, supervised by a qualified OT. Art, music and drama therapists have much to contribute. There were no psychotherapists running patients groups that we were aware of at that time, and we believe that they would have much to offer especially those with group training. The core inpatient professions of nursing, social work, OT, psychology, psychiatry each potentially have valuable knowledge and skills that can be delivered to patients in groups. The last three professions often combine ward work with community work and have limited time for ward work. Psychiatric registrars routinely ran groups in the same trust ten years earlier (Robertson & Davison, 1997) but we found that consultant psychiatrists and specialist registrars were not running groups. If representative nationally, this situation will lead to a

Table 5
Numbers of timetabled ward-based groups run by profession

Ward*	1	2	3	4	5	6	7	8	9	10	11	12	13	14	15	16	Totals
Nurses	1	1	1	0	0	5	1	6	5	2	1	2	5	1	1	1	33
OT / OT tech	0	0	3	12	11	0	0	0	2	2	3	3	2	7	5	4	54
Psychology	1	0	1	0	0	0	0	0	0	0	0	0	0	0	0	0	2
Peripatetics	2	2	3	2	2	3	5	5	1	0	0	0	0	2	2	2	31
Totals	4	3	8	14	13	8	6	11	8	4	4	5	7	10	8	7	120

*Wards in same hospitals grouped with bold lines

generational gap in psychiatrists' experience of running groups. OTs may get some experience of inpatient groupwork during their training but this is not guaranteed nor necessarily taught on the OT training. Psychologists and psychiatrists are unlikely to have specific training in running inpatient groups.

Nurses are by far the largest group of staff. There are many demands on nurses' time that take them away from direct patient care, including practical tasks, note-keeping and dealing with enquiries. In general nurses tended not to run groups apart from the community meeting. The authors' clinical experience is that nurses can play a key part in supporting patients attending groups run with other professionals, forming a communication bridge between the group and the ward. There is clearly a tension between the demands of containing and managing patients and taking time out to run groups. Sustained contact with disturbed patients also creates anxiety and institutions and individuals develop defences to reduce the intensity of the emotional contact (Menzies Lyth, 1959). Workers who are not based on the ward full-time may find it easier to deal with the feelings stirred up by running difficult groups as they can escape afterwards. This makes the specific role of running groups more manageable although they are less integrated into the ward system and do not know the patients as well. For nurses to run therapeutic groups both training and support would be needed as well as supervision and sufficient time for debriefing after the group. A specialist psychological group intervention role with specific training in different types of groups may be one way forward.

The group programme

As Parahoo et al. (1995) point out, it is not just the number of activities and attendance levels but also their nature and quality. Staffing levels, training and skills, group protocols, support and supervision all affect the quantity and quality of what is offered. Without proper funding, programmes will not meet the needs of most patients. The ideal is for patients to attend an activity after breakfast to give them a reason to get up and another in the afternoon. A lesson from institutionalisation is that activity should not be for activity's sake or a substitute for thought and reflection.

The purposes of activities can be categorised in various ways, for example: meaningful occupation to prevent demoralisation and institutionalisation; exercise which is mentally and physically health giving; the acquisition of new skills to help the person manage socially and with employment outside hospital; rehabilitation to reacquire lost skills; and psychological therapy to address psychological difficulties. Both normalising and rehabilitating activities are needed as well as psychotherapeutic groups and expressive activities (art, music, and drama); broad-based talking groups as well as theory-based therapy groups. Activity programmes need to cater for patients who are functioning at a higher and lower levels. Having a range of groups provides a variety of contexts for interacting and learning as well as meeting the needs of patients with different types of problem. Schwartzberg et al (1980) compared three formats of groups facilitating social interaction and found that the quantity and type of interaction varied according to format. They concluded that patients learn skills in one format and then practice them elsewhere. Innovative practice such as parallel groups in hospital and in the community can provide continuity across the boundary. As a minimum, physical exercise should be available for physically active patients and exercise classes for all should be considered. As a rule, recreational activities should be provided at evenings and weekends and not during the working day.

The paucity of talking therapy groups found in our study is a concern. The commonest talking group was the ward community meeting. Anecdotal evidence suggests that these vary in quality, and that they have become nurse and patient only business-type meetings where practical information is communicated such as information and complaints. Potentially these meetings can form a valuable integrating function, spanning both the practical aspects of ward life as well as social and emotional issues (see Klein, 1981; Russakoff & Oldham, 1982). Community meetings are an area for staff development and could be extended to daily or twice weekly, as was the case on two of the wards.

A key issue is many inpatients' reluctance to engage in organised activities. A minority are too unwell to attend, whilst others are anxious and demoralised. Many are resentful about being in hospital and may be less likely to cooperate with non-essential aspects of treatment. Psychiatric breakdowns are by their nature traumatic and leave patients feeling vulnerable. Withdrawal can be seen as a defence against excessive stimulation when personal resources are needed to deal with an internal crisis. Staff cannot force patients to take part against their will, but they need to work together to create a group culture where attendance is the norm. Patients need support and care but also to re-engage socially and engage with their problems in order to help them to regain their independent functioning. We believe that respecting patients' wishes to remain withdrawn for too long may be unhelpful. Whilst it is widely believed that engaging in meaningful activities and with others is empowering, the culture of many or most patients opting-out makes it very difficult for staff to establish ambitious programmes of activity. An active approach of organising leave around an individual timetable of activity is one way of dealing with poor attendance.

Sundram (1987) writes:

The type of assertive clinical judgement that has led psychiatrists to challenge a patient's refusal to take psychotropic medication should carry over to dealing with other aspects of treatment including a patient's refusal to participating in therapeutic activities … If the programs and activities offered challenge the human spirit, harness human potential and restore human dignity, there would not be any sizable problem of refusal to participate.. the reality is that some patients will refuse participation in all forms of treatment.. (Our) job is to raise expectations, to open new horizons to which we should collectively aspire.. existing standards or expectations should be viewed as evolving standards of decency that mark the progress of a maturing society ... a concerted array of options in therapeutic programs and skill building activities ... (are needed, which) will require a critical re-examination of staffing levels and types of staff available.

Conclusions

Admissions are a chance for patients to learn knowledge, skills and behaviour and they are an opportunity for professionals to deliver therapy to patients who would not normally attend groups. Groups allow learning to take place alongside others in the same situation. Our study showed that this opportunity was not being taken up for most patients. The reasons include the view that medication is the primary treatment, the lack of consensus about what constitutes therapeutic activities and the view that patients essentially need time and space to recover. Professionals may take a user-empowerment view that patients know what is best and should not be pressured into attending activities. This leads to patchy attendance, lack of continuity and lowered expectations and sets up a negative cycle. Resourcing, ward culture and lack of staff skills also contribute. Managers are often more concerned with other issues such as safety and the ward environment. Assertive strategies with support at all levels of the service are needed to create a culture of participation. Becoming ill affords a necessary respite from demands. In the case of mental health problems after a suitable pause for dealing with the trauma of the breakdown, the work of recovery needs to begin. This should be an active process of re-engaging with the world. Inpatient care needs to extend beyond looking after patients, keeping them safe and giving them medication, to the psychological work of recovery, of which passivity and isolation are enemies. If the task of engaging with the problems that caused the breakdown is started, with good follow-up care, change and growth is possible.

References

Berrios, G.E. and Freeman, H. (Eds.) (1996) *150 years of British Psychiatry 1841-1991. Volume II: the Aftermath.* London: Athene.

Bion, W.R. (1948) Psychiatry at a time of crisis. *British Journal of Medical Psychology*, 21, 81-90.

Bockoven, J.S. (1972) *Moral Treatment in Community Mental Health.* New York: Springer.

Borthwick, A., Holman, C., Kennard, D., McFetridge, M., Messruther, K. and Wilkes, J.

(2001) The relevance of moral treatment to contemporary mental health care. *Journal of Mental Health*, 10, 4, 427-439

Bowers, L., Simpson, A., Alexander, J., Hackney, D., Nijman, H., Grange, A. and Warren, J. (2005) The nature and purpose of acute psychiatric wards: the Tomkins Acute Ward Study. *Journal of Mental Health*, 14, 6, 625-635.

Chaplin, R. (2006) The National Audit of Violence: in-patient care for adults of working age *Psychiatric Bulletin*, 30, 444-446.

Collins, J.F., Ellsworth, R.B., Casey, N.A., Hyer, L., Hickey, R. H., Schoonover, R.A., Twemlow, S. W. and Nesselroade, J. R. (1985) Treatment characteristics of psychiatric programs that correlate with patient community adjustment. *Journal of Clinical Psychology*, 41, 299-308

Department of Health (2002) *Mental health policy implementation guide: Adult acute inpatient care provision.* London: HMSO

Dimeo, F., Bauer, M., Varahram, I., Proest,G. and Halter,U. (2001) Benefits from aerobic exercise in patients with major depression: a pilot study. *British Journal of Sports Medicine*, 35,2,114-7

Farmer M.E., Locke, B.Z., Moscicki, E.K., Dannenberg, A.L., Larsen, D.B. and Radloff, L.S. (1988).Physical activity and depressive symptoms: the NHANES I Epidemiological Study. *American Journal of Epidemiology, 128*,1340-51

Fennell, M. (1989) Depression. In: Hawton, K., Salkovskis, P., Kirk, J. and Clark, D. (Eds.) *Cognitive Behaviour Therapy for the Treatment of Psychiatric Problems: A Practical Guide.* Oxford: OUP

Fennell, M., Bennett-Levy, J. and Westbrook, D. (2004) Depression. In: Bennett-Levy, J., Butler, G., Fennell, M., Hackmann, A., Mueller, M. and Westbrook, D. (Eds). *Oxford Guide to Behavioural Experiments in Cognitive Therapy.* Oxford: Oxford University Press.

Foulkes, S.H. (1948) *Introduction to Groupanalytic Psychotherapy: Studies in Social Integration of Individuals and Groups.* London: Heinemann.

Gunderson, J. (1983) *Principles and Practices of Milieu Therapy.* Hillsborough, NJ: Jason Aronson.

Haigh, R, (2002) Acute wards: problems and solutions: modern milieu: therapeutic community solutions to acute ward problems. *Psychiatric Bulletin*, 26: 380-382

Healthcare Commission (2005) *Acute Inpatient Mental Health Service Review: Final Assessment Framework* London: Healthcare Commission. http://www.cqc.org.uk/_db/_documents/Final_assessment_framework.pdf (accessed April 2009)

Iqbal, I. and Bassett, M. (2008) Evaluation of perceived usefulness of activity scheduling in an inpatient depression group [Electronic Version]. *Journal of Psychiatric and Mental Health Nursing*, 15,5, 393-398.

Jones, M. (1952) *Social Psychiatry: A Study of Therapeutic Communities.* London: Tavistock.

Klein, R. (1981) The patient-staff community meeting: a tea party with the mad hatter. *The International Journal of Group Psychotherapy* 31,2, 205-222.

Lelliott, P. and Quirk, A. (2004) What is life like on acute psychiatric wards? *Current Opinion in Psychiatry*, 17: 297-301

Main, T. F. (1946) The hospital as a therapeutic institution. *Bulletin of the Menninger Clinic*, 10-66.

Menzies Lyth, I. (1959) The functioning of social systems as a defence against anxiety. In *Containing Anxiety in Institutions, Selected Essays* (1988) London: Free Association Press.

Morris, A. (2008) William Battie's *Treatise on Madness* (1758) and John Monro's Remarks on Dr Battie's Treatise (1758) - 250 years ago. *British Journal of Psychiatry*, 192, 4: 257.

Parahoo, K., McGurn, A. and McDonnell, R. (1995) Using research to implement change: the introduction of group activities on a psychiatric unit. *Journal of Clinical Nursing*, 4, 195-202.

Pilgrim, D. (2007) New 'Mental Health' Legislation for England and Wales: Some Aspects of Consensus and Conflict. *Journal of Social Policy*, 36, 1, 79-95.

Quirk, A., Lelliott P. and Seale, C. (2006) The permeable institution: an ethnographic study of three acute wards in London. *Social Science and Medicine*, 63, 2105 - 2117

Radcliffe, J. and Smith, R. (2007) How do patients spend their time on acute psychiatric wards? An observational study of social interaction and audit of attendance at organised group activities, *Psychiatric Bulletin*, 31, 167-170.

Rice, C. and Rutan, J. (1987) *Inpatient Group Psychotherapy: A Psychodynamic Perspective*, New York: McMillan.

Robertson, S. and Davison, S. (1997) A survey of groups within a psychiatric hospital, *Psychoanalytic Psychotherapy*, 11, 2, 119-134.

Royal College of Psychiatrists' Centre for Quality Improvement (2009) *Accreditation for Acute Inpatient Mental Health Services (AIMS)*. London: Royal College of Psychiatry. http://www.rcpsych.ac.uk/clinicalservicestandards/centreforqualityimprovement/aims.aspx (accessed April 2009)

Russakoff, L. and Oldham, J. (1982) The structure and technique of community meetings: the short-term unit. *Psychiatry* 45,1, 38-44.

Rutherford, S. (2008) *The Victorian Asylum*. Oxford: Shire.

Sainsbury Centre For Mental Health (1998) *Acute problems: a survey of the quality of care in acute psychiatric wards*. London: The Sainsbury Centre for Mental Health.

Sainsbury Centre For Mental Health (2002) *An executive briefing on adult acute inpatient care for people with mental health problems*. London: The Sainsbury Centre for Mental Health.

Schwartzberg, S.L., Howe, M.C. and McDermott, A. (1980) A comparison of three treatment group formats for facilitating social interaction. *Occupational Therapy in Mental Health*, 2, 4, 1-16

Seneca, L.A. (44/1996) *Moral Essays Book VI: To Marcia on Consolation*. Cambridge, Mass: Harvard University Press.

Sundram, C.J., (1987) Patient idleness in public hospitals. *Psychiatric Quarterly*, 58, 243-254

Thomson, I.G. (1986) Milieu Therapy. *Bulletin of the Royal College of Psychiatrists*, 10, February.

Tuke, S. [1813] (1996) *Description of the Retreat*. London: Process Press

World Health Organization (1953) *Expert Committee on Mental Health. 3rd Report*. Geneva: WHO.

2

Is it possible to make acute wards into therapeutic communities?[1]

Leonard Fagin

Tuesday morning, and my first day on return from leave. I have 10 patients under my care on the unit at the moment, but only two are around at the time when the group is about to start. Even though we remind everybody regularly that our groups happen twice a week, starting at 9.30 for an hour, a number of patients still regularly fail to turn up, and others amble in, between 10 and 40 minutes late, which is definitely a statement of sorts. Phil McManus, a recovering patient with a paranoid religious preoccupation, is in a voluble but more friendly state of mind than when I left for my holidays. He uses the silence requesting leave and for me to rescind his section. The other patient, Yuen Cheng, a seriously ill patient with schizophrenia, is in a world of her own, laughing at times incongruously, and then making eye contact with me, asks me whether I am alright and also makes a request to leave the ward to spend time with her parents. I take that as a welcome back! I wonder, however, how we are going to proceed with only two patients in the group, when Alan James and Shaheeda Hussain come in escorted by a nurse, telling me that they had mistakenly gone into another group. They are followed by Obi Oganseye, an African woman, also recovering from a serious schizophrenic illness. Throughout these arrivals, Phil continues to talk as if he is the only member of the group, addressing all his comments to me and making me feel forced to answer. Yuen occasionally interrupts laughing at her own jokes which she does not share. I ask myself how we are going to use the group in a reflective manner. Somehow, however, the theme of conversation starts to revolve around the reasons that led people to come into hospital, and what can be done to prevent another crisis when the time comes to leave. Phil is beginning to recognize that it is not necessarily a homosexual anti-Biblical conspiracy out there, and that his continuous preaching sometimes provokes others to distraction. Much to my surprise, he admits that since he's been taking his olanzapine regularly and has been refraining from cannabis, which he used to import on the ward, he is feeling a lot better, and that he has made up his mind to continue taking his medication when he leaves. I wonder whether this is a real change, or whether he is playing the game to ensure an early discharge, but he seems genuine enough. Alan, who was admitted in a suicidal frame of mind after another alcohol binge following which he started to experience auditory hallucinations, then butts in. He describes how shortly after his divorce 6 years ago he was involved in an accident at work, when a tunnel he was surveying caved in, and his world also completely crumbled. 'I feel a total failure'. We start talking about how when people are in a negative frame of mind they can make decisions they could later regret, which could have a crucial effect on one's life and self-confidence. I also have in mind Shaheeda, who was attending the group for the first time and was looking quite intimidated, as I knew she had recently impulsively given up her job in a big Government Department on the advice of friends, and now rued her decision. I was aware she was listening intently to what was being said, but didn't have the confidence to speak. The group is starting to work on more thoughtful lines now. I introduce the idea that it is very easy to get into a negative frame of mind, and ignore all the resourceful aspects of ourselves, which in that mood begin to lose importance. Phil speaks about his need to get a driving licence back, because it reminds him of when he used to feel competent as a lorry driver. Alan says that he has to start building up his confidence somehow, because up to now he has been afraid of taking risks again in case he meets up with failure, and resolves to start by redecorating his flat. At that point Shaheeda walks out. It leaves me wandering whether she is ready to think more positively about her problems at this stage. Up to that point, Obi has not said anything at all during the group. I invite her to comment. She looks at me pensively and says 'We see the world in our own eyes'.

It never ceases to amaze me how effective inpatient groups can be with patients who are in acute stages of their illnesses. Despite this, it is fair to say that inpatient groups are not widely available in our acute inpatient wards, and even when they are, they are rarely attended by senior medical or nursing staff. Are we ignoring the potential benefit of a unique therapeutic tool, which can have a considerable impact on patient's welfare and the therapeutic atmosphere on our increasingly disturbed units? In the group session I have described, consisting of patients with mixed diagnoses, some of them still experiencing florid psychotic symptoms, it was possible, even in the short period of an hour, to establish some sort of connection, a dialogue, an opportunity to reflect on the reasons that led to their admission and even with those that remained silent, or those that avoided the group altogether, it was possible to respond to their silent or resistive communication. In the time that I was there I could ascertain how patients were progressing, how they were relating to others and thinking about themselves and their situation, if they were showing side effects from their medication, if they were potentially violent, depressed or suicidal, and so forth. In perhaps more analytical terminology, I was able to see how they were projecting, and often reliving their problems in the context of the group, transferring and identifying their problems through others, using the group as 'a cathartic garbage bin,' or simply using it as a way of containing their anxiety or relating to others in their isolation.

Brief historical background

The history of therapeutic communities goes back some time, right at the start of the creation of units such as that of pioneering psychiatrists Pinel in France and Tuke at the York Retreat, but in the UK they gathered increasing momentum during the 60s when a number of hospitals (Henderson, Cassel, Dingleton and Claybury) started to introduce measures to create therapeutic environments and change the style of care in traditional asylums, so that patients had more opportunities to express themselves and staff became more aware of the importance of dynamic thinking in the interaction with patients. In patient groups were a natural extension of this development.

I had the opportunity of joining Claybury Hospital as a training psychiatrist in the mid 70s, and although by then the major impetus of the therapeutic community approach had faded, groups were still a major part of the acute ward activities. I especially gained experience in joining in with these groups, ably led by Dr John Pippard to whom I am indebted and whom I eventually replaced as consultant psychiatrist when he retired. It seemed so obvious to me at the time that groups were essential in the management of acute care that I have continued to participate in them, even after the closure of Claybury and its replacement by community inpatient services. I eventually left the NHS in 2006, but still miss my work in group settings with acutely disturbed patients.

Unfortunately in the UK the influence of these therapeutic inpatient experiments has waned with the advent of community approaches, and with it the tradition of psychodynamic group work. If they do happen, in most acute facilities they are led by occupational therapists and tend to be for a very specific objective, such as relaxation, anxiety management, leisure activities, and so forth. Exceptions to this are the occasional inroads made by creative therapists, art or movement, who explore non-verbal avenues to self-expression.

With the advent of functional teams and emphasis on short admissions, wards have become places for care for the most disturbed patients, more often than not admitted under compulsion, their conditions frequently affected by the use of street drugs, inevitably imported into the ward setting. In large conurbations, wards also have a very varied cultural and ethnic mix, with different and sometimes perplexing approaches to mental health issues and attitudes to reflecting on the reasons for a crisis or an admission to hospital. These circumstances can create serious, but not insurmountable obstacles to the creation of a therapeutic environment.

The title of a Royal College of Psychiatrists report, 'Not Just Bricks and Mortar' (1998), quite rightly indicated that there was much more to planning or refurbishing an acute psychiatric unit than design considerations. In surveys carried out by different organizations there have been serious concerns expressed about what goes on and what does not go on in these units, and in particular the quality of interaction between patients, carers and staff (MIND, 2000).

The therapeutic environment

The atmosphere in an inpatient environment is in constant change, often determined by the emotional and mental state of the patients. The ward can be quiet and tranquil one minute, and become a frightening, persecutory, noisy bedlam the next. Patients come and go often within days, and new arrivals or departures affect those patients who have longer inpatient stays, particularly if they have established trust or have bonded with others. A crucial therapeutic task is welcoming newly admitted patients, providing them with orientation to the unit, an explanation of its aims and its routines, in a way that is sensitive to their mental state.

The obvious aim in planning is to create an environment which is safe, containing and therapeutic enough for people who are in various states of distress, as well as a setting in which staff can be enabled to meaningfully carry out their responsibilities. In a previous paper, I have outlined factors that contribute and conspire against the creation of a therapeutic milieu and I refer the reader to it (Fagin, 2001)

Staff-patient interactions and staff groups

Experience suggests that the emotional nature of work in inpatient units tends to make staff become complacent or inured to the distress experienced by their patients. This is often reflected in the nature of interaction between them. To some extent it is understandable, but not justifiable, to see staff retreating from patient interaction, or developing officious, unresponsive, rigid and sometimes overtly aggressive attitudes towards very demanding, crisis-prone, attention-seeking patients. Much can be done at the time of planning ward environments, and subsequently in supporting them, to address these emotional staff developments, in order to prevent escalations of risky behaviour which often follow when patients feel misunderstood or ignored. Staff support groups give an opportunity to discuss these difficult issues, especially if they feel free to raise uncomfortable feelings without prejudice, giving time for 'dynamic reflection' on incidents and reactions to events on the ward. As in other fields of psychiatry, inpatient work is fundamentally an interdisciplinary activity, and this can sometimes lead to difficulties when inter-professional rivalries create obstacles to effective therapeutic practice, particularly as patients are very able to pick up tensions when they exist. Support groups can also help to ventilate unspoken problems and prevent them from becoming entrenched. My own experience is that these staff groups are often resisted and extraordinarily problematic to maintain, but when they do become a regular feature of the ward they reap very observable benefits in terms of staff morale.

Patients usually are admitted in a state of extreme vulnerability and helplessness, and this often creates barriers between those in receipt and those offering care, particularly in the sense of power and control. However, successful therapeutic outcomes usually follow an agreement to enter into a collaborative partnership with patients. Somehow what needs to be overcome is the notion that all the solutions lie in the hands of the professionals. Whilst it is important to convey clear jargon-free information about the nature of mental disorder, and involve patients and their carers actively in the Care Programme Approach, it is especially incumbent on them to take responsibility over their treatment and encourage them to think about ways in which they can restore a sense of self-control and direction. A useful recent development in this area is the introduction of Advanced Directives, allowing patients and carers to decide on the form of care they can receive or object to should they become unwell again. A realistic and hopeful attitude to treatment and recovery should be strongly conveyed. This emphasis on recovery, rather than a cure which is professionally led, can transform the therapeutic aims of the inpatient unit.

Thoughts on therapeutic groups

Specific characteristics of inpatient groups

We must ask ourselves, why have these talking groups disappeared from the inpatient scene? Perhaps a great deal has to do with the paucity of psychotherapeutic experience available to psychiatrists and senior nurses, who are then likely to feel out of their depth when participating in a group. Training in psychotherapy, and particularly in group psychotherapy, is not available as a matter of course to psychiatric or nursing trainees. Even those psychiatrists who are fortunate enough to have a psychotherapeutic placement as part of their pre-membership rotations are unlikely to have the opportunity to participate in inpatient groups, as they are expected to prioritise assessments, duty calls and ward rounds as their responsibilities. Nurses, whether fully qualified or in training, are also not encouraged to join in these groups, often handing them over to other staff, especially occupational therapists. But this is not the whole picture.

As a form of psychotherapy, it is fair to say that inpatient groups are very different from similar, stable and structured groups available to patients in community or private settings, who are probably there because they want to and because they have a psychological attitude towards their difficulties and prepared to reflect and learn from them. By contrast, inpatient groups are likely to be very disturbed and disturbing at times, as behaviours can be unpredictable, patients may be unable to express themselves coherently, and may in fact find groups challenging or frightening in an altered frame of mind, without any desire to stay the full hour. One has to be prepared for the fact that these groups may have different patients every time, that patients will have a panoply of diagnoses, may be heavily sedated or responding to side effects of their medication, have varied levels of psychological sophistication and be at dissimilar stages of recovery, and that their commitment to therapy is ambivalent to say the least! To cap it all, staff shifts pre-empt stable input from nurse therapists. Each session therefore has to practically stand on its own, without a great deal of continuity from one group to another. Inpatient groups can be scary experiences, and not surprisingly one finds some staff avoiding them. This invites the question about what can be done to help staff overcome this fear. Perhaps some of the following comments can be helpful.

Inpatient group processes

I would like to comment now on the main group processes revealed in these very unique circumstances, and some lessons that I have learnt over the years. The following points are by no means exhaustive.

Starting the group

Groups of this nature can be very intimidating and frightening to the inexperienced, both patients and staff, and some induction and explanation is always necessary. For example, I start off by welcoming new patients and staff, explaining that this is a regular group that we hold on the unit twice a week for an hour, that we are here to help one another, and that people are invited, if they wish, to share what is on their minds and what may be worrying them. I request that patients try and stay for the whole hour, even though in my experience the group never starts with the same number of people as when it ends. I sometimes suggest that it might be useful to speak about the reasons that led to admission, and their understanding of events. I then ask for people to introduce themselves if there are new arrivals.

We tend not to disclose information revealed to us outside the group and only use the material that is offered and that is shared by all group members. I make a point of saying that the issues discussed in the group are confidential to the group and staff on the ward, and ask other patients to bear this in mind when discussing matters with other patients on the ward.

One of the difficult hurdles we are often faced with are language difficulties, especially for those patients who have recently arrived in the UK, and this can sometimes be insurmountable if there is no one on the ward who can speak the language and can join the group. Despite this, I have been in many groups with patients who do not speak a word of English and yet seem to be comforted by their participation in a group experience: the group has become for them a virtual, non-verbal container for difficult feelings.

Basic requirements

In order to preserve some intimacy, groups need to be between 8-10 patients at the most. I am joined by an SHO, occasionally a nurse and a Specialist Registrar. I have had psychotherapy trainees in from time to time, and they have always been stimulating participants and have found these experiences invaluable in their training. I sometimes worry if the number of staff exceed the number of patients, but only occasionally I have had to ask some staff to leave when patients obviously feel intimidated.

I always make sure that the group starts on time. Groups are only cancelled in exceptional circumstances, and need to be a regular and predictable feature of ward therapeutic activities. We have identified two rooms for therapy and we all sit in a circle. It is interesting to note where people choose to sit. Very often patients will be lined up on one side of the room, leaving the 'therapists ' to sit on the other side, underlining a 'them and us' feeling. At other times, patients who are very dependent or those who wish to focus attention on themselves will choose to sit somewhere where they will keep a close eye on the person they feel is the main therapist, in many cases myself. When possible I will draw attention to the sitting arrangement and what this can possibly indicate. Staff who feel apprehensive will sometimes try and sit outside the circle, or hold a clipboard and study it, making their discomfort obvious and reminding me to discuss their anxieties about the group in the staff feedback meeting. New staff will often feel very confused about what is going on, and feel uncomfortable about participating actively in the group for fear of 'saying the wrong thing'. It is comforting to tell new staff that there is hardly anything that will be considered 'wrong' as long as it does not show indifference or cause offence. Patients are as alert as ourselves to the inner feelings of all those who are participating in the group. The basic dictum is applicable to both patients and staff: the more you participate and become engaged, the more you are likely to gain.

There is an understanding that this is a group to share and discuss feelings and preoccupations. Intimidating, violent or offensive behaviour is not condoned. When the meeting gets heated, as it can very occasionally do, it is important to have discussed with staff how violent behaviour can be contained, and be prepared to seek outside help when necessary. To put this in some context, I can remember only having to resort to this on three occasions in 25 years of practice.

Another 'rule' worth re-enforcing is that participants should respect the right for people to speak and not to interrupt or divert attention when someone is holding the floor.

Group dynamics

As I already mentioned above, one has to be prepared for the fact that group composition is always different, as patients come in and others are discharged. Each group stands alone, to an extent, and the nature, atmosphere and attitudes may change radically from one group to the next. One day, the group may be feeling suspicious, showing lack of trust in the staff and the treatments provided, acrimonious and combative, and the following group patients appear to be prepared to do some emotional work on themselves and offer support to each other. Invariably the group is a reflection of what is going on in the rest of the ward. If the ward is disturbed and fractious, it is likely that the groups will be expressing this in some way. At the time when staff are leaving, when patients feel unsure of who will be there for them, the group will often deal with the need to seek reassurance and containment. It is also not unusual for these groups to reflect unspoken difficulties or disagreements among staff, or general uncertainties about the service as a whole. This will highlight the need to explore these issues in separate staff groups.

Groups at times become predominantly 'psychotic' in character, consistent with the participants' state of mind. The psychotic communication is sometimes a form of defence that blocks understanding and any form of personal awareness of emotional pain, which often includes a range of psychotic symptoms, such as command hallucinations, persecutory delusions, ideas of reference or passivity experiences. Very often the conversation will initially strike one as confusing and irrational but although the content appears at times to be unintelligible, it is worthwhile paying attention to the verbal and non-verbal aspects of communication, because sometimes meanings are disguised and only 'make sense' at a later stage. Even in the midst of a psychotic flow of conversation, patients are often trying to communicate to others what their experiences are like, so that if the therapists feel scared, confused, angry, despondent, bored or repelled, it is highly likely that these are projected feelings which offer invaluable clues as to what patients are going through. At another level, when the group is feeling safe and containing, patients will often share their psychotic experiences and visibly feel relieved to find out that they are not alone in listening to voices, in thinking that the world is against them, in feeling totally powerless or isolated.

The groups become a stage for re-enactment, and it is up to the therapists to pick up what is being offered. These forms of distorted communication deposit on the therapist the responsibility for 'understanding'. It leaves the group therapist with the difficult dilemma of deciding whether to link in with the psychotic or non-psychotic part of his patient. In my experience the invitation to enter or to stay away at a distance is often communicated in veiled and non-verbal cues. Meaning may then be shared and mutually explored, or at times require to be put in 'safekeeping' until patients are ready, even though in many cases the event may never come to pass. It may well mean that even before this, a state of meaninglessness has to exist between patient and therapist, a situation where the patient does not feel 'imploded' on with external understanding, leaving the therapist to have to join the patient in a discomfiting, drifting and apparently aimless voyage (Fagin 2005).

Participation in the group will also vary depending on the stage patients are going through in their mental state. There is an expectation for all patients to participate in groups during their hospital stay, but patients are not forced to attend. Patients with high levels of suspiciousness, in the throes of personal disintegration, or in a state of heightened anxiety or confusion may exclude themselves from the group for good reason, and I tend to encourage them to join when they feel they are ready to do so. We place no restrictions on people leaving the group mid-course, although we will ask them why they are leaving to explore if something that we are discussing is particularly troublesome for them. I am always amused by the alleged weakness of bladders when the group is going through a difficult patch and patients excuse themselves to go the toilet. Only in exceptional circumstances I have had to ask patients to leave the group. Occasionally a patient in a frank manic state becomes so disruptive that it becomes impossible to hold the group, and we have to explain why we are suggesting for a time that they should not attend. In rare situations patients may become so intimidating that the group becomes unsafe, particularly if they are unresponsive to being challenged about their behaviour.

As was apparent in the example given above, and perhaps not uncommon to all group processes, there are some regular patterns to the progress of each group which are important to bear in mind. The initial stage of the group is often characterized by resistance behaviour and communication, manifested for example in prolonged silences, delays in coming to the group, or attempts to draw the therapist into a dialogue to get specific answers about leave, medication or diagnosis. It is during this time that group therapists will feel uncomfortable and/or irritated and begin to wonder whether the group can get into 'emotional business'. Minutes seem to drag on and one wishes the group to end at this stage. Bringing the group into the notion of speaking about feelings does require some skill and tolerance of this resistive behaviour, as well as alertness to the possible inner turmoil of some of the participants, and the timing of a comment or an invitation to speak. More often than not, however, it is the participants themselves that eventually bring these concerns into the group, often reserving the most poignant insights to the last few minutes of the group, and then the time runs out, and one wishes the group could go on!

The therapeutic task

The main job of the therapist is to ensure that the group feels safe enough to do some work and discuss feelings in the 'here and now', particularly in terms of interpersonal group relations. If the group feels unsafe, the feeling can be discussed and verbalised. An unsafe group is a non-working group. The specific considerations of the inpatient group requires that the main therapist adopts a directive approach, often inviting members to comment and being openly supportive. The therapist has also to be attentive to those who are not able to feel comfortable about talking to others in a group, and ensure that there is some equity in distribution of time for all those that attend. The therapist also has to be attentive to the not unusual tendency for patients to enter into frank denial of their difficulties, or attempts at excessive rationalization, moving the discussion to more profitable areas.

Obviously groups are working at their best when patients are interacting with each other. The tendency however, is for patients to direct their conversation to the therapists. Therapists can respond to these attempts by asking other patients if they identify with what is being said. A view expressed by another patient carries very strong weight, particularly if they have had similar experiences. As mentioned above, it is extremely reassuring to hear from someone else that they have heard voices too, that they have ambivalences about taking medication or trusting psychiatrists, that they have come through a period of hopeless, black depression, and that they can get some support from others when they leave hospital by keeping in touch. On the other hand, it helps patients to have a realistic assessment of what is in store by discussing employment prospects, stigmatisation, misunderstanding from friends or families, or simply the notion that those suffering from mental illness may relapse.

Silences are difficult to manage. I do not believe that long silences are helpful with our client group, and although I do not rush in to fill the gaps, I do not let them extend too far without commenting on them. Very often one can pick up barely hidden feelings of resentment, suspicion, plain stubborn mindedness or avoidance in these silences. As I mentioned above, the style I adopt does not follow traditional psychodynamic lines, and at different times I adopt an interventionist approach, inviting people to talk about themselves. I hardly ever use analytical jargon or interpretations, and feel comfortable moving between cognitive and psychodynamic standpoints, dependent on circumstances.

Some patients are very effective group participants, I call them 'catalysts', because they have the knack of reading in between the lines of what people are saying and are prepared to challenge others. One has to be careful, however, that they do not transform themselves into co-therapists, as this may be a way in which they may be avoiding personal disclosures, or placing themselves in a different status to others.

As mentioned above, the group will tend to focus on here and now issues, mostly related to the experience of admission and what led to it. In this process, different cognitions and assumptions about what led to the crisis of admission can be confirmed or challenged, both by therapists and patients alike. It is less common for patients to bring in material from their early development and distant past, although occasionally issues to do with faulty parenting, early sexual and physical abuse, feelings of rejection, abandonment and loneliness, disastrous relationships, or even sexual feelings may emerge if the group is feeling safe and reasonably settled. In my experience, it is not helpful to identify and share transference processes, but close attention to one's own counter-transference is helpful and productive in trying to make sense of what is being projected.

Psychodynamic understanding

Although I do not necessarily use traditional psychoanalytic techniques in everyday group involvement, such as transference interpretation, I do find it useful to recognize psychodynamic processes during the course of a session. Most common of these are *splitting* (separating opposite or contradictory feelings into different, 'all good and all bad' camps), *projective identification* (a complicated three step process where 1. unwanted or unbearable feelings are projected onto others, usually but not necessarily the therapist, who is felt by the patient able to contain them, 2. these emotions are then processed and reacted to by the person on whom this is projected, who begins to 'feel' or 'behave' in a way determined by this projection, and 3. feelings are re-introjected by the patient once it has been modified by the person on whom it was projected in the first place), *introjection* (where aspects of others are internalised and experienced as part of oneself) and *denial* (complete disavowal of reality considerations).

In this context and as in all therapeutic groups, it is interesting to observe how different patients are likely to take different roles in groups, often reflecting their own internal conflicts and previous history of important relationships. Some will become spearheads for voicing their anger and frustration, often directed at staff as substitutes for other important figures in their lives, others will adopt nurturing roles to members who may be considered passive, vulnerable or weak and take them under their wing, others in turn will act as saboteurs to try and destroy the group's therapeutic atmosphere and not allow time to reflect or think, and yet others will take on the role of catalysts and challenge those that convey a denial of feelings or difficulty in coming to terms with their situation. I am of the opinion that groups are an excellent vehicle for the deposition of unwanted and unbearable feelings, and that they have a major impact in reducing acting-out behaviour on the unit, or the need to use other measures, such as the reliance on p.r.n. ('as needed') medication or increased levels of observation.

Post group reflection

We ensure that after each group the staff had an opportunity of a few minutes to reflect on what has been going on in a short, interactive, post group session. On our ward , two groups met simultaneously, so this gave us a chance of feeding back to the other therapists (in the same and different groups) what has happened during the session, and getting their responses, as well as sharing feelings, often unexpected, uncomfortable, embarrassing or anxiety-provoking. This is a time to reflect on group processes and group dynamics. It also enabled us to notice running parallels between both groups, an indication of what was going on in the ward as a whole, and often an early warning sign of impending difficulties ahead.

Intervening in a group is a courageous act, for both patients and staff. But this is an act that carries with it distinct rewards. Groups can be the most effective ways of containing unbearable feelings and emotions at particularly distressing times which can have lasting effects on patients and on-going therapeutic relationships. It is also important to recognize that there is no 'single correct' intervention, but a range of possibilities according to circumstances and one's own distinct style, and that it therefore introduces an opportunity to be creative in our work and engage in very personal ways.

Ward assemblies and crisis meetings

Apart from small group psychotherapy, we also held a ward assembly every week, attended by all patients and chaired by one of them, agreeing on an agenda, and someone to take the minutes. Senior staff were in attendance. The regular themes were about life on the ward, and the resolution of practical problems, such as the state of kitchen or bathrooms, the absence of cups, the quality of the food. They are extremely useful when patients who intimidate by their behaviour are challenged, as well as confronting those who bring drugs or alcohol into the unit. However, they are sometimes used as opportunities to scapegoat vulnerable patients, who are then seen by others as responsible for everything that is bad on the ward. This makes the large group occasionally veer into more traditional therapeutic lines, and senior staff need to be aware of when to intervene and suggest that some issues are addressed in the more intimate sessions of small groups. Conversely, when subjects of a practical nature are brought up in the psychotherapy group we invite people to raise them in the ward assembly.

On occasions, when there was a crisis on the ward, such as a massive importation of drugs, escalation of violent behaviour, a suicide or major moves for refurbishment we have held crisis meetings to inform the whole ward about what was going on, to give staff and patients a chance to discuss their immediate worries and concerns, and to suggest possible solutions. These very occasional meetings have the obvious function of containing anxieties at times when there is a danger of feelings getting out of control.

Other therapeutic hurdles and opportunities

It is useful to be aware that not all therapeutic interactions occur at planned or structured times. Many patients refer to helpful comments made by other patients when they need to talk well into the night, or during a spontaneous chat with a member of staff over a cup of coffee, or in the smoking room. Staff need to ensure that they are supported to give time to patients when this happens, and that there are suitable quiet places on the ward where it can take place. Such opportunities may also have to be extended to anxious carers when they visit their relatives on the ward requesting support or explanation, reminding us that carers are not nuisances and that therapy is not confined to the person that has been admitted.

Boredom is often mentioned as one of the greatest negative factors of inpatient experience. The provision of meaningful activity, not necessarily always with a therapeutic aim, well planned and structured throughout the day and night, weekdays and weekends, not forgetting plain and simple entertainment, can do much to foster interaction and a return to everyday normal social intercourse. This is not solely in the province of occupational therapists, and there is much to be said for jointly planned programmes between doctors, nurses and OTs, incorporating other professions when appropriate, for example, providing educational opportunities in different aspects of mental health care, inviting welfare advisors to discuss financial problems or voluntary services who offer befriending and other activities in the community.

Everyday ward routines, based on ritual, tradition or professional habit can be experienced by patients as impersonal and at times personally humiliating or intrusive. Examples of this are medication or food queues, waking up procedures, excessive preoccupation on paper-work, shift and rotational schedules with unavailability of staff and intimidating ward rounds. Careful consideration of these practices from a therapeutic standpoint can often come up with alternatives which are more respectful and humane. Some rules have obviously to be enforced in order to ensure patient involvement or safety (for example, patients not staying in bed all day, providing escorted leave for patients still at some level of risk, introducing close observation, the proper and judicial use of minimum restraint, etc) but it never goes amiss to explain the reasons to patients who might not be able to understand their logic. Sometimes there may not be practical alternatives, and it is helpful at least to ensure that when appropriate these aspects are sufficiently explained if patients find them disturbing or perplexing.

In the comments I have made so far I have emphasized aspects which I think can change the therapeutic atmosphere on the ward. I have not, however, ignored the real problems our over-burdened acute inpatient wards have to face. In the UK acute admission wards are filled with patients who are homeless, unemployed and penniless. An admission is not only an episode to help them with their psychotic symptoms and emotional difficulties, it is also a request, often verbalized, to secure accommodation and regular income. The symptom becomes the entry ticket into a 'mothering welfare system,' and guidelines provided by government support this by ensuring that the admission episode is only concluded when these provisions have been met, under the Care Programme Approach. At the same time there are economic pressures demanding short admissions. Primary Care Trusts, who now hold the purse strings for mental health services, present benchmarked indices to staff creating expectations of swift episodes of inpatient stay, with quick discharges to Home Treatment or Crisis Resolution Teams. Treatment unsurprisingly relies heavily on psychotropic medication. Failure to comply with these expectations could end up with financial penalties for Mental Health Trusts. The culture of litigation in Great Britain, whilst not as extended as in the USA, invites users and carers to make complaints and for these to be investigated and dealt with within set time limits. Good staff are difficult to keep in our acute settings, with many excellent nurses experiencing burnout and seeking other opportunities in community settings, creating an exodus with undue reliance on agency staff. In this maelstrom of forces there is little space or time to delve into the inner life of the person who is admitted, let alone to discuss feelings in response to the demands placed on staff. To maintain a therapeutic stance in our modern inpatient services is becoming a real uphill struggle (Fagin 2001) and recent surveys have confirmed that patients find admissions to be scary and unpleasant experiences, with high levels of staff sickness and turnover.

Conclusion

Is it possible, therefore to make modern acute ward settings into therapeutic communities? In a strict sense of the word, I believe that changing conditions in society and in the NHS make it unrealistic and unlikely that traditional therapeutic community principles, with its culture of open wards, flattened hierarchy, and lengthy admissions can be re-created in inpatient units. But I do believe that the ward 'community' can become much more therapeutic than it presently is. The initiative from the Royal College of Psychiatrists in raising standards of care in inpatient settings can be seen as an opportunity to travel in this direction (AIMS, 2008). In this context, an admission to hospital may be seen as an opportunity to change rather than a traumatic experience. For this to happen, the professionals involved in inpatient care need to have their status as practitioners acknowledged as one of the most demanding and skilled areas of psychiatric expertise. Much will also depend on enabling talking opportunities between all parties. As Elizabeth Shoenberg mentioned in the introduction to a pivotal book on hospital therapeutic communities, written in 1972, but still applicable to this day:

> All this breaks down (traditional patient/staff barriers) if staff and staff, staff and patients, patients and patients begin to communicate meaningfully to each other. We find that patients can do an enormous amount to help themselves and each other, can teach the staff a lot, and work with them as active partners. We find that staff have more personal and interpersonal problems than they previously dared to acknowledge. But they also have deep, unsuspected resources within themselves of love and insight and initiative, once they cease to be gagged by the hierarchical structure of the traditional hospital setup. Frank recognition of these difficulties, and the use of all the skills and talents of all the staff and all the patients is fundamental to the therapeutic community. It implies mutual respect, mutual responsibility- a kind of loving which springs from the fullest possible opening of communications. (Shoenberg, 1972, p.10)

Note

This chapter is based on a paper given to Suffolk Mental Health Services in 2005.

References

Accreditation for Acute Inpatient Mental Health Service AIMS (2008) http://www.rcpsych.ac.uk.

Fagin, L. (2001) Therapeutic and counter-therapeutic factors in acute ward settings. *Psychoanalytic Psychotherapy*, 15, 2, 99-120.

Fagin L., (2005) Suffering insanity: Psychoanalytic essays on psychosis (Review of Hinshelwood, B (2004) *Suffering Insanity*. Brunner-Routledge, Hove). *Intenational Journal of Psychoanalysis*, 86, 4, 1223-8.

MIND (2000) Environmentally friendly? Patients' views on conditions in psychiatric wards. London: MIND.

Royal College of Psychiatrists (1998) *Not Just Bricks and Mortar* Council Report CR62 . London: Royal College of Psychiatrists.

Shoenberg, E. (Ed.) (1972) *A Hospital Looks at Itself. Essays from Claybury.* London: Cassirer.

3
Inpatient groups: Working with staff, patients and the whole community. Reflections of a group analyst

Bob Harris

Introduction

This chapter is not only about groups in inpatient settings, but it is also about groups generally to some extent. Inpatient groups are a very special and intense sort of experience; for that reason they are both extremely useful and valuable and also attract a good deal of fear and apprehension. There are many reasons for this ambivalence, and I will discuss some of these later. But it is worth mentioning at the start that a group that is run on the basis of free-group discussion, in other words, where the content is not decided in advance by someone, may well generate material that is difficult and complex and not amenable to simple solutions. Many inpatient groups fail, or have very rocky and precarious existences; I want to discuss and highlight some of the reasons why groups fail, and suggest ways of thinking about and managing difficulties in forming and maintaining groups.

I am going to say something about the usefulness and desire for inpatient groups, as well as about some of the problems that these groups encounter, some of the 'anti group' processes, as Morris Nitsun imaginatively calls them (Nitsun, 1996). The thoughts in this chapter are mine, however, drawn largely from my own experience. Over time I have, of course, used the work and thought of many others to help inform my views.

Case study 1: Groupwork in the traditional asylum.

Many years ago, at the beginning of the eighties when I was beginning my group analytic training, I was required to run a group in a psychiatric setting. So not knowing any better, I talked my way into a local psychiatric hospital; one of the large institutions that used to circle London and that have now been sold off for housing developments. One of the friendly and helpful psychiatrists suggested that they could do with a group for inpatients on the acute admissions ward, and that I could work with a doctor who was also interested in running groups. How lucky was I! And I mean that without a trace of irony.

It was my first incursion into the 'wacky world' of a psychiatric institution and I had no idea what to expect. I'd seen some of Hogarth's pictures of the Harlot's and the Rake's Progress, of course, but nothing more recent, so, like the paying visitors to Bedlam, I possessed a freshly tuned curiosity with just a hint of voyeurism. The Ward Sister was very keen, and asked if she could join in. She enthusiastically recruited patients for the group and commanded that her nurses do likewise. There was little or no history of group therapy in the hospital, so far as I knew, although there was a well-established Occupational Therapy department. The staff nurse knew that it was just as important for patients to be in a group as it was for them to be well fed, clean and take their medicines: and so we arranged a time for the group that seemed to best suit the ward business, and my availability, and began.

As it happened, the patients turned out to be relatively everyday members of the local community, not in the main shaven headed, and none that I can recall with visible black spot signs of syphilis like Hogarth's characters. They were just local people who because of unbearable stresses of various kinds were given sanctuary, temporary or long term, in the hospital. The hospital was near quite a wealthy town; the catchment area, and consequently most of the patients, could not be thought of as economically impoverished in any way, although psychologically and emotionally impoverished they most certainly were.

We ran the group for well over a year, and it became very well established, and very well liked by the patients and staff. The patients, in the main, were surprised to find that there was a place where people were actually interested in who they were and what had brought them there, rather than in curing or stopping some odd symptom that they had developed.

We had what felt like the exclusive use of a large, quiet, warm room with comfortable armchairs and big windows that let in the daylight. I'm sure the room was shared with other users, but it was always much the same for us, clean and well kept. It felt like we were being thought about and taken care of. We had a sense of consistency and reliability of the setting that helped our fragile and often frightened group members to feel safe and protected.

Although the group was intended for the 'Acute Admissions Ward', after a while, because this was a large hospital with a well-developed internal structure and interpersonal communications network, one or two patients from the back wards started turning up, perhaps out of curiosity to see what was going on. The doctor, whose attendance was intermittent, also told people whom she saw for 'front-line' assessments at the day hospital that they could go to the group. These patients would just turn up and I didn't have the heart to turn them away. In the group, we discussed these visitors, and the issue of whether or not to accept them into the group. The consensus was to be welcoming to our 'passers-by', but to point out that commitment and confidentiality were also important, so after a while we had quite a stable sort of intergenerational community group consisting of newcomers to the mental health services who weren't yet inpatients, people who were probably short term inpatients in crisis and a couple of people who had been on a back ward for some time.

One of my favourite memories is of a thirtyish chap from the back wards who for several weeks would stand at the door, often for the duration of the group, slowly opening and closing it, uncertain about whether or not to come in. Somebody suggested that we make a place and set out a chair for him. Eventually, he came fully through the door and took his place amongst us. He spoke in a strange, strangulated voice. Someone said, 'You've swallowed your voice, Richard. Come on, cough it up.' He told us a story about living in a shed at the bottom of his parent's garden. He couldn't be with them. And he couldn't leave them either. The tension in the house was unbearable, and yet he didn't have the confidence to leave. When our group ended, at the final session, he said, 'I've liked being here. Thank you for the atmosphere. I've been able to breathe.' And, in fact, although no one had paid much attention, his voice had become much more ordinary. He had come in from his back ward shed.

Another person was a woman whose husband was a City banker. She had come into hospital because she was spending 24 hours a day scrubbing and cleaning the house and preparing food that wasn't necessary. The house was spotless and the fridge and freezer were full to overflow. She was exhausted and her hands were red raw. In a well-meaning attempt to help, her husband had taken her on a holiday trip to Africa. She told us about this in the group. They had visited an African village, and it had made a deep impression on her; the way in which the women all did their washing together, chattering and gossiping, the children ran about freely, playing with the animals, and the men sat around talking, playing dice, drinking beer and apparently doing very little. People seemed to be cheerful although they had none of the material things that she and her husband worked so hard for. She wondered if it would be better to be like the villagers. The group listened to her attentively. I thought about our funny little group-village where we could get to know each other, where we had several generations, and where we could do our washing in public, but I didn't say anything.

Reflections on the group experience

Understanding, or rather the *attempt* to understand is far more important than demonstrating that you understand, or trying to give words too soon to very complex matters. Bion talks about this in his concept of minus K (Gordon, 1994). Incidentally, the patient mentioned above may have been an undiagnosed early victim of the Affluenza virus (James, 2007).

In the group, the questions that arose most frequently were 'How did you get to be here? Who are you? How did this happen?' It is strangely easy to ignore the fact that to be in a psychiatric inpatient unit of any kind something must have gone badly wrong. This happens because people in inpatient units are *all* there because something has gone badly wrong. If we lose that sense of surprise, of shock even, then we are in danger of accepting the breakdown of ordinary life as ordinary; of entering a meaningless universe. In the group, 'I'm here because I've got depression, or OCD, or because the drugs aren't working' or whatever, more usefully becomes a question: 'How did you get it? What does it mean?' Even the most thoughtless person would have to consider that if you are suffering from something unpleasant, it might have been caused by something that needs to change. Experience teaches us that change is very difficult, and usually painful.

When you become an inpatient you are a person who has become estranged from your group. For some reason or another, your usual groups can no longer hold you.

You may have become intolerable to them, or they may have become unbearable to you. This is very often a humiliating or shameful experience. You become part of a community of people who have lost their group, or their group has lost them. So most inpatient settings are full of people who find it difficult to be in groups, and who generally speaking, don't much want to be there at all. These groups are full of people who cannot be in groups. However, we were able to run a very useful group, usually containing eight or nine people, with a slow-open membership for well over a year, only ending when my placement finished. (*Editorial note*: slow open group: a group where the membership changes in a thoughtful and managed way. The group is open to changes in membership, but the process of joining and leaving the group is done 'slowly').

If the only value of medium to long term groups were to help people improve and integrate over time the essential competence of being an integral member of human groups, they would serve a vitally useful purpose on this criterion alone. This group enabled some very distressed people to feel part of relevant human interactions again, to feel that they could learn from talking with others about their problems and to feel less isolated as a result, to feel that they could understand and help others as well as receiving help (a vital aspect of building self-esteem), to explore, understand, give words to and communicate strong, difficult, confusing and problematic emotions, and to feel worthy enough to be valued, looked after and taken care of. Group members naturally *repeated and enacted* some of their basic problems in relating to others in their interpersonal relations in the 'here and now' of the group sessions. Problematic relationships, like Richard's, were able to be explored and thought about, and to a small extent, perhaps, re-solved through the re-enactment. The group helped patients to explore and understand the realities, difficulties and potentials of their position as persons and patients in a psychiatric setting and to think about their situations and problems in a benign, respectful and helpful environment. The group itself being the primary medium of treatment, meant that each participant shared responsibility for the success or otherwise of the group, thus providing a genuine opportunity for the development of personal empowerment.

So why did this work?

'*Treatment is about how you treat people*'. RD Laing

You can see that this group was set up in a very benign environment. I was very lucky. I was 'bright eyed, enthusiastic and bushy tailed,' delighted to be given this opportunity to be a proper group therapist, although I'd had several years experience in social group work and group relations training and experience as a participant in quite a few short term therapy groups by then. I had weekly supervision from a helpful and tolerant newly appointed Consultant Psychotherapist, and I was also in the early stages of training at the Institute of Group Analysis. Both of the Consultant Psychiatrists who shared duties on the acute admissions ward were wonderfully kind and helpful gentlemen, and 'prescribed' the group to suitable new patients. I had a surprise friend and enthusiastic ally in the Ward Sister, who wasn't afraid to boss her underlings and the patients around to some extent, and who gave the group a good press on the ward! I later found that this sort of group-positive ward 'insider' relationship was extremely useful, if not invaluable, in other inpatient settings. The patients already knew someone, hopefully whom they trusted and liked. (This is all the more important when working with more disturbed and psychotic patients.)

I had a co-therapist who was a doctor, which gave our group additional status in the wider medical matrix. The Occupational Therapy Department which offered groups and experiences of various kinds to patients, were happy to synchronise their offerings so that the patients did not have to deal with 'timetable clashes'. The Admin. Secretary who administered the room bookings and also had a sort of receptionist role was very helpful and well liked by patients and staff alike. She allotted us a room near the Day Centre so that patients got away from the ward for their group (something which I came to feel was very important) and the room was always clean, tidy, light and airy with comfortable chairs. The heavy red-bricked hospital that contained the group had been there for about 100 years and felt as if its foundations had well and truly sunk into the earth. There was no hint yet of the hospital closures and the huge changes in the levels of general social insecurity that was to come in the eighties and beyond; the individualistic and 'dog-eat-dog' competitiveness that is in some sort of meltdown at the time of writing in Autumn 2008. We were also lucky to have very few group members or staff, who were actively destructive or aggressive towards the basic aims, structures and process of the group. The prevailing attitude of most of the group members was positive and well motivated, and this was also true of the supporting staff in the institution in which we existed; again, we were fortunate in this respect. I shall say more about inevitable negative influences on groupwork later on.

It is an African saying that 'it takes a village to raise a child', and much the same can be said about nurturing and growing a healthy group. This hospital village did a very good job of getting our group going, feeding it and looking after it. To operate a group where the aim is to provide a safe place where people can talk freely with one another about what is happening to them and explore their thoughts and feelings about their lives, we needed the support of the hospital village.

This group, interestingly, grew its own extension into the outside world of the hospital via the small number of day patient members, and also extended itself further into the body of the institution with visits from the long-term inpatients. I think the group would have worked well anyway, but these additions gave the group an additional sense of reality and context, and also brought more overt psychosis into play, which was worked with in a surprisingly understanding and thoughtful way.

Because of the very fortunate nurturing factors outlined above, the group survived and flourished. The group needed the benign involvement of aspects of virtually the whole hospital community in order to evolve into a therapeutic medium where personal, relational, social and institutional realities could be explored and thought about. The helpful institutional context of the group enabled the group itself to become the medium of treatment, which is the main aim of good groupwork. When the group itself becomes the medium of treatment, this process facilitates genuine patient empowerment and maximises the opportunity to enhance the maturational development of individuals.

Case study 2: Groupwork in an inpatient secure unit.

Quite a few years later, post qualification, after 8 years as a Principal Psychotherapist in the NHS, I became a group analyst in a secure inpatient setting. One of my jobs was to run a group for very disturbed patients on a long-stay ward. I was fortunate again in being able to work with an enthusiastic and highly competent co-therapist who worked on the ward and who had done some intensive groupwork training. We managed to get a pleasant room down the corridor, not far from the ward, and started to recruit for our group. Of course, we began by working the network.

The Ward Manager treated us with a certain amount of polite suspicion, and seemed to like the idea of a group. But we couldn't be quite sure. The ward nurses smiled and nodded and said, 'What a good idea, but you'll never get them to come'. We thought it best to interview patients ourselves to see what they made of the idea of a group, so we set up a series of appointments with likely candidates. We let the Consultant Psychiatrists who were responsible for the patients know what we were up to; that I was a group analyst and we were going to run a group under the auspices of the psychotherapy department. About half a dozen patients said they would like to attend. We set a start date.

Just the one man turned up, very smartly dressed in suit and tie. Despite the pre-group interview, he appeared to think that we were a review body of some kind, which was one of the types of hospital groups he had previously experienced. We spent a very uncomfortable hour, the three of us. The following week, nobody turned up. We checked with the ward. Our group members had gone off to do other things; playing football with the nurses being one of them. The week after that, two people came. Then three. We stuck at three non-footballing members for a while. Not much of a group, but a start. Nothing much happened for some time; our 'referral stream' appeared to have dried up.

Following some enquiries, we discovered that one of the psychiatrists was actively discouraging patients from attending because he didn't want them distressed by 'having to talk about their childhoods'. My 'analyst' tag had worried him. I went along to see him to explain that the group was just a place where patients could talk with each other and perhaps learn to communicate their feelings a bit better. Nothing much, really. This produced a marked effect, the psychiatrist's anxiety was alleviated and more patients started to attend.

We also discovered that the nurses were not exactly being encouraging. It seemed that they were concerned about patients being taken off the ward, stirred up and then dumped back with them again. Apparently a previous therapist of some sort had done this at some time in the past. Football was a much safer option, and the nurses could play too.

We thought about all this in supervision, in a weekly group composed of two or three pairs of co-workers, and group numbers gradually crept up. Supervision was a vitally important part of the work and provided an essential thinking-space with a very experienced and expert senior colleague.

Something else really seemed to make a difference. In response to a suggestion from my supervisor, I began a group for the nurses on the ward where they could reflect upon and think about their own experiences. Now they had their own group!

Our numbers in the patients' group continued to increase and held at between six and eight with a fairly consistent 'slow-open' membership for almost two years. Attendance at the staff 'reflective practice' group was also very high and consistent. Patients began to feel safe enough to start thinking about some extremely problematic and difficult material, including their 'index offences'; the term given to the often bizarre and violent illegal behaviours that had brought them to the institution. Psychotic processes became more visible and able to be tolerated, or confronted and to be thought about. Communication developed and became deeper. From a professional and theoretical standpoint, it was sometimes stunning to see psychotic splitting, dissociation and projection happening in the group in front of our eyes.

We had to be very fast on our psychological feet to keep up, frequently didn't, or got lost, and often we were completely exhausted at the end of a session. We had to work hard to maintain our own sense of reality and ordinary social behaviour in a setting infused with psychosis and grossly distorted and disordered personal, interpersonal and social values.

We co-therapists had to do considerable work protecting and maintaining the boundaries and space of the group. It helped a great deal that there were two of us to spread the workload, and the fact that one of us worked on the ward was a huge benefit. We would always spend at least 15 minutes together after the group to get our breath back and review the session before going to formal supervision.

As an aside here, it unfortunately needs saying that the worst possible reason for co-working is so that the co-working pair can 'cover' for each other in case of absence. This naïve attitude drives a truck through the essential attempts to maintain consistency and reliability in group leadership. If the group is co-lead, the co-leading pair should always be there to help and support each other, and be related to as a pair by the group as a whole.

The role of supervision

Supervision from an experienced clinician is essential when running groups, especially the more difficult kinds like inpatient groups. A good supervisor will help you keep your feet on the ground and help you not be too swayed by the powerful unconscious processes that are at work in groups, especially those containing very disturbed patients with psychotically fractured reality testing.

In the second group described above, we were very fortunate in having our weekly supervision session almost immediately after each group. This model, of supervision immediately after the therapy group, which was adopted initially for logistical reasons, proved very effective in processing the psychotic material that the group produced.

When you are doing very intensive work, especially if developing your professional interests in an unfamiliar area, you become a 'beginner' again and should have more or less the same time in supervision as in the clinical work: an hour doing therapy; an hour of supervision. Expert supervision is essential for the mental hygiene of therapists working in emotionally toxic environments; it is not an 'optional extra'.

Many organisations and institutions quite simply do not take this fact seriously enough, and on the grounds of cost or lack of time (which amounts to the same thing) will allow only the minimum amount of supervision time that is recommended by professional bodies. Beginning, or neophyte therapists, and those new to working with severe pathologies need *much the same time in supervision with an experienced and expert supervisor as the time spent with patients.* Anything less is putting patients and therapists at risk.

If there is anything at all in the theory of projective identification, which is a situation in which disturbing and often damaging feelings are forced into or induced in therapists as a primitive means of communication by patients, then this is a genuine risk factor that must be taken very seriously by managers and clinicians alike. Expert clinical supervision is the means by which potentially damaging aspects of projective identification and the re-enactment of trauma and abuse dynamics can be thought about and understood, thereby assisting a movement towards understanding and creative thinking in both patients and therapists alike.

Formal training and personal group experience is also of great importance; to be able to work with strong emotions and psychotic processes you need to be properly trained and supervised, and to have had as much personal group experience as possible.

Envy, attachment and nurturance

Therapy groups seem to be responded to within institutions in fairly predictable ways. Groups are often welcomed, and even idealised, and then treated in ways that can undermine them and even attack their existence. In institutions which deal with psychosis (which is most mental health units) the psychotic processes of idealisation and denigration can run unchecked. Therapists and groups may be treated as messianic saviours by patients and the institution at one moment, and then rapidly feel undervalued, undermined and 'up against it', enjoyment of their work and enthusiasm sapped and drained.

It may be that this effect is the result of unconscious envy in the interpersonal matrix that surrounds the group. Envy is a very strange emotion; often unconscious. We attack in others that which they have and we don't.

What exactly is it about groups that may be envied?

A group can be a generator and container of experience; a place, or an organ that can help us to think about and process emotions. Envy of this marvellous ability may well prove detrimental to the group process to the point of the destruction of creative potential. Open and covert issues of control and power may predominate, usually not to any good effect. Institutionalised responses, that is, behaviour and activities that serve the interests of the institution rather than the human beings within it, may well denigrate creativity and free communication in groups of both staff and patients, and may work against the need to provide space and time where people can communicate openly with one another and perhaps find new thoughts. Simple reflective spaces where we can meet regularly and reliably to talk openly with each other may be highly desirable, but also fragile within an institutional or relational context that demands predetermined outcomes. This is already difficult and heady stuff! Sometimes you have to go back in order to go forward, so that is what we shall do.

Human beings have a very basic need for attachment. The work of Bowlby and others, (Bowlby, 1979) and the current burst of research in neuroscience, especially that of Allan Schore (Schore, 2003; Gerhardt, 2004), seems to indicate strongly that attachment to a figure (or possibly a group) *felt to be protective and attuned to our emotional states* (or at least trying to understand us) may be a pre-requisite to the desirable ability to think about feelings (let alone the joy of simply feeling loved and protected). And unless we can experience and think about our feelings we cannot function cognitively as effectively as we might otherwise be able to. As the poet E.E. Cummings put it, 'feelings come first.'

Schore calls this process of experiencing and thinking about our feelings 'emotional regulation', a difficulty especially prevalent in borderline, narcissistic and personality disordered states. In *psychotic* states, the defensive process of *dissociation* of distressing feelings that are too painful to bear, means that the patient is *actually unable to experience feelings*, and thus can only communicate feelings and emotions by evoking them in others, via the process of projective indentification, much as a baby's cry evokes feelings of distress in an empathic parent.

Unless we are able to identify our own feelings, empathise with those of others and regulate our emotions, we cannot engage in free-flowing social interaction, have relationships with other people, and function in groups.

Groups, which offer the potential for group members to enjoy attached, attuned, empathic experiences are highly valuable objects, and may be subject to unconscious envious attacks from what may be an emotionally impoverished surrounding environment. Groups also may well be an Object of Desire (Nitsun, 2006), and as such subject to the usual idealisations and denigrations of loved objects.

If you are felt to possess such an object of desire, you may well be envied and you or your object or both of you destroyed. If you are unlucky enough to possess a malevolently envious internal object you may well attack yourself!

In the institutional context, if all staff enjoy the opportunity to be in a well run group, this goes some way to alleviating the problem of unconscious envy and negativity. Groups not only offer the *potential* for a reflective and emotionally attuned experience, but also provide a creative space, where ideas and thoughts and words can be put out into the group, taken back in, and where group members can safely play with ideas. This can help build a gradual internalisation or 'store' of 'good' emotional experiences, creating good internal objects in the context of a reliable relationship (Celani, 1994, also Fairbairn, 1952) which is part of the psychotherapeutic aim of our work. Following Fairbairn, the interpersonal and intrapsychic realms create, interpenetrate and transform each other in a subtle and complex manner. This is a desirable process and a major aim within the overall objectives of good clinical practice. An effective institutional environment will include the provision for all staff to be involved in groups run with the same skill, care and attention to detail as those provided for the patients, or the entire clinical work is at great risk of being undermined by a build up of negativity which, within very emotionally toxic environments can rapidly reach a destructive critical mass.

Many things can adversely affect the nurturing function of a group, even one that has had the best and most assiduous attention paid to its setting, context and dynamic administration. (*Editorial note*: dynamic administration is a term which is used to describe the sum total of all the things you have to pay attention to when setting up and maintaining your group, from room bookings and timetable clashes, to managing referral pathways). When working with very emotionally deprived and damaged patients, the potentially destructive processes of splitting, and especially projective identification, can infect a group and easily spill out into the surrounding staff teams and institutional dynamics, leading to defensive staff behaviours or enactments as bits of the patients' mental processes are pushed into staff teams and unconsciously played out.

Abuse dynamics are especially pernicious in this respect. Dealing in depth with pathological processes in groups and institutions is beyond the scope of this chapter, and would be something of a digression; but it should be said that our current social and institutional climates are far from the ones prevailing 25 years ago; our global culture is in a state of flux, with deep uncertainty about the viability of established economic, social, relational and political structures. The social, as SH Foulkes (1948) concluded, does indeed permeate the individual to the core.

Conclusions

This chapter describes two successful and useful group experiences with very disturbed patients in inpatient environments. They show how the context and setting of the group is profoundly important, how the surrounding professional matrix must be supportive, understanding and benign, and the therapists enthusiastic, reliable, well trained and properly supervised. Processes which work both for and against successful groupwork are discussed, and emphasis placed on the need for work with staff teams in order to preserve a constructive and positive emotional and administrative climate.

The Institute of Public Policy Research report published in 2006 and other research (Palmer, 2007) indicate that, apart from a few impoverished ex Soviet States, Britain is the worst place to grow up in the western world. British children also face more tests and achievement targets than anywhere else in the world. We are surrounded by a relentless culture of winning and competiveness. We are confronted by 'achievement' targets, tick-boxes, pre-determined outcomes and mass-consumed media fixated on the inanities of 'reality shows' with their manufactured exclusions and close-up humiliations. Our wider consumer-driven and affluent society faces economic insecurities, family and community breakdown, deeply problematic gender relationships and gross social and economic inequality where fear of failure or exclusion dressed up as 'performance appraisal' is used to generate and motivate compliance.

Groupwork approaches which emphasise thoughtfulness, reflection, consistency, inclusion, tolerance, reliability, free-speech, free group discussion, open-ended exploration and which take fully into account the inter-connectedness and complex contexts of the 'virtual villages' of modern human life can go some way towards understanding and alleviating distress. This means that we may have to work harder than ever to form and maintain our groups, and also that properly constructed, thoughtful and well maintained groupwork approaches are needed like never before.

References

Bowlby, J. (1979) *The Making and Breaking of Affectional Bonds.* London: Routledge.
Celani, M. (1994) *The Illusion of Love.* New York: Columbia University Press.
Fairbairn, W. (1952) *Psychological studies of the personality.* London: Routledge Kegan Paul.
Foulkes, SH. (1948) *Introduction to group analytic psychotherapy.* London: Karnac.
Gerhardt, S. (2004) *Why Love Matters.* London: Routledge.

Gordon, J. (1994) Bion's post-Experiences in groups thinking on groups : a clinical example of minus K. In Schermer, V.L and Pines, M (eds) *Ring of Fire*. London: Routledge.

James, O. (2007) *Affluenza*. London: Vermillion.

Nitsun, M. (1996) *The Anti-Group*. London: Routledge.

Nitsun, M. (2006) *The Group as an Object of Desire*. London: Routledge.

Palmer, S. (2007) *Toxic Childhood*. London: Orion.

Schore, A. (2003) *Affect Regulation and the Repair of the Self*. New York: Norton.

4
Acute wards: Context, pressures and satisfactions

Frank Holloway

Introduction

In this scene-setting chapter I look at the current inpatient acute ward and in particular the challenges and opportunities that have over the years faced staff and patients alike. In seeking an understanding of complex phenomena, context is all. I therefore begin with a subjective personal account of my engagement with inpatient psychiatry, which dates back some 35 years. I go on to present some data on inpatient psychiatry. I discuss the state of the contemporary acute inpatient ward, about which there has been a fair amount of moral panic. I will end with some speculations about the future. Throughout I allude to the various ideologies and policies that have underpinned changes in practice over this lengthy period.

I write as a General Adult and Rehabilitation Psychiatrist. Although I am not a group-work practitioner I am acutely aware of the dynamics of acute inpatient settings, the significance of group processes and institutional culture in the work that we do. These issues are ably summarised in a brief paper by Davenport (2002).

What is an acute ward for?

It is perhaps worth pausing here to consider what is the acute psychiatric ward for?

This is not a trivial question. One answer comes from mental health legislation, which in England and Wales allows for compulsory admission to hospital for treatment of mental disorder provided the disorder is of sufficient severity to warrant compulsion, appropriate treatment is available and admission will be in the interests of the health or safety of the patient or the safety of others. Appropriate treatment here is broadly defined and, as the Mental Health Act Code of Practice states, includes 'nursing, psychological intervention and specialist mental health, habilitation, rehabilitation and care' (Department of Health, 2008: 23.32) as well as medication. Psychological interventions, habilitation and rehabilitation may, of course, all be delivered in group settings as well as individually.

Bowers (2005) has identified seven reasons for admission to the acute ward: dangerousness, assessment, medical treatment, severe mental disorder, self-care deficits, respite for carers, and respite for the patient. He concludes that therefore the role of the staff (his interest is in nurses) is in

> providing safety for the patient and others; collecting and communicating information about patients; giving and monitoring treatment; tolerating and managing disturbed behaviour; providing personal care; and managing an environment where patients can comfortably stay.

Others might well identify different roles and functions for acute psychiatry and a simpler definition might be (1) to provide care and treatment to people presenting in severe emotional distress whose community supports have broken down, (2) to provide treatment for people who are demonstrably ill and cannot be cared for in less restrictive settings and (3) to protect the individual and the public from risks of harm. The primary aim of the acute ward, as for all mental health services, will be to become unnecessary as far as the patient is concerned, since they will have successfully rejoined their lives.

Looking back

I first stepped onto an acute psychiatric ward in 1973 when, as an undergraduate studying psychology, a friend who was a student nurse invited me to spend the day on the ward she was working on. My main memory is of a very large room with chairs arranged around the walls where the patients, staff and I spent a challenging hour in a large group meeting that was dominated by a middle-aged woman, who in retrospect was manic. I wasn't to know that this novel experience for me was a quite unusual first exposure to psychiatry as practised at that time (and indeed subsequently). The hospital was Fulbourn, in Cambridge. As I write I have in front of me a battered second hand copy of David Clark's Pelican Original *Social Therapy in Psychiatry*, published in 1974, recommended retail price 45p. This set out a vision that was embodied in the practices at Fulbourn. The book is infused by deep learning in the history of psychiatry, psychodynamic ideas, social psychology and sociology and it is a volume contemporary proponents of the Recovery paradigm would do well to read. Clark was, of course, a firm believer in the possibility of the therapeutic community, in its widest sense.

That initial, perhaps disorienting, experience of acute inpatient psychiatry could not have been too off-putting since as a Medical Student I arranged an elective in psychiatry in 1976, working in Charleston, South Carolina (chosen because they would pay me to come rather than asking me to pay them!). There I saw a spectrum of inpatient services from the well appointed University Medical Centre, through the Veterans Administration Hospital to the local County Hospital and the State Mental Hospital located 200 miles from Charleston. I suspect I saw the best and the worst of care available at the time. At the University Hospital the attending consultant undertook a daily review of all patients and there was a richly resourced multidisciplinary team; security staff at the VA hospital had guns and were clear they needed them; in the County Hospital 'restraint' meant shackling a person to a bed and I was gleefully shown how it was possible to kill oneself even in this position because of a design fault; the State Hospital took anyone who no-one else would take responsibility for.

By 1979 I was a neophyte psychiatric trainee working within an inner London service that was undergoing very rapid demographic change. There were two acute psychiatric wards within the service located on the second and third floors of St Giles Hospital. This was a small former Workhouse Infirmary that had become an NHS General Hospital (the lower two wards were devoted to Orthopaedic patients). St. Giles is known as the patron saint of cripples, lepers and nursing mothers. Proponents of normalisation noted that once the hospital closed for acute care all that was left were outpatients services for drug addicts, people with a mental illness and developmental disorder. In 2008, only those with developmental disorder remain. On one of the wards (the 'Professorial' one – not that the Professor actually went there) once a week a Consultant Psychotherapist held a large group meeting which was replicated in somewhat shadow form later in the week under the slightly dubious leadership of the most experienced psychiatric trainee working on the ward. This was a different geographical setting to Fulbourn, but boasting similarly uncomfortable chairs and similar interjections by manic patients.

Accommodation for people living in each ward was almost entirely in two large single sex dormitories (a side room was available for people who were particularly unwell or a mother and her baby). Twice a week one of the dormitories was off-limits to most patients as it became the venue for ECT, a popular and effective therapeutic option. Risk assessment as we currently understand it was rudimentary (though trainees were thoroughly versed in assessing deliberate self-harm as it presented to the local General Hospitals). Discharge planning was somewhat ad-hoc, though many people went on to spend time in the Day Hospital, a brand new building that had recently been opened by Barbara Castle, the then Secretary of State for Health, who had published a landmark policy document *Better Services for the Mentally Ill* (DHSS, 1975). The other patients would generally be offered follow-up in the outpatient clinic, where a uniformed nurse could also administer depot antipsychotic injections. A population of 80,000 in what became known as 'East Lambeth' was served by one Community Psychiatric Nurse. *Better Services* envisaged a pattern of mental health care based around the District General Hospital Psychiatric Unit, with its associated Day Hospital and Outpatients Clinic and linked Social Services provision.

The wards were completely open and the stairs provided only rudimentary protection against people throwing themselves off the stairwell. No-one was so impolite to do this (the only person who attempted to commit suicide by jumping off a high place kindly did so whilst at home on leave – he survived and we were surprised and perhaps pleased to meet at a CPA meeting almost 30 years after the event when he moved into my catchment area).

In general the atmosphere on the wards was benign. There was a mixture of patients who were well on the way to recovery and those who were acutely ill, of social backgrounds that reflected the very mixed catchment area and of ages: at times middle-aged people in recovery acted as mentors to their younger fellow-patients. The predominant diagnosis on the unit was of affective disorder. Outcomes, at least as far as the staff were concerned, were excellent and certainly better than those of the orthopaedic wards located below the psychiatric wards. Very occasionally the wards would find that they could not safely manage a patient. These people would be sent to the mental hospital that historically had served the catchment area (Cane Hill Hospital in Coulsdon) to be treated in the 'Intensive Care Unit'. As I remember it they didn't tend to return to us – 'out of sight out of mind'.

This inpatient unit at St Giles Hospital, which I remember with some fondness, closed in the mid-1980s in the context of cuts to health services, leaving only the now not-so-new Day Hospital as a base for local community mental health services. The site was over time redeveloped into rather nice housing. The inpatient wards were relocated to a former workhouse, St Francis' Hospital (later renamed North Dulwich Hospital), which had historically provided one of the two London Receiving Wards for people identified as mentally ill prior to subsequent transfer to the large mental hospitals that surrounded the Metropolis. Following this move conditions for both staff and patients deteriorated significantly, the unit correctly being defined by an observer as 'Dickensian'. At the same time access to the mental hospital that had traditionally served the catchment area ceased for all but Old Age and Forensic Psychiatry. Looking back the St Giles closure and relocation to worse conditions was a tipping point in the quality of inpatient care that we provided locally, which deteriorated quite sharply. This partly reflected an organisational change within which the individual wards became the 'inpatient unit' where consultants shared beds across the unit, multiple ward rounds were held that moved location to follow the patients and previously established ward multidisciplinary teams broke down.

Moving forward to 1987 I became a Consultant Psychiatrist within the same South London service that I had joined as a trainee almost a decade previously. My responsibilities included developing the local community services for people with severe mental illness and working to close Cane Hill Hospital, a task that was achieved in 1991: by 2000 some 116 of the 130 mental hospitals in England and Wales had closed. The dominant ideology of the time was Normalization or Social Role Valorization (Wolfensberger, 1983): this located the problems of people experiencing disability largely within societal reactions to disability and described the desired outcomes for services in terms of providing service users with valued social roles. In that ideological context acute inpatient psychiatry was at best an irrelevance that might soon go the way of the disappearing mental hospital.

I worked as a consultant in the local day hospital, which became the focus for developing community mental health teams to serve the catchment area, and had access to a small number of beds at North Dulwich Hospital: working there was always the low-point of my week. A stark portrait of the quality of inpatient care across London during the late 1980s and early 1990s is provided by the *Ritchie Report* (Ritchie et al, 1994) which documented the care provided to Christopher Clunis in the years leading up to his murder of Jonathan Zito in December 1992, another tipping point for psychiatry in the UK. The Ritchie Report is usually seen as a critique of community mental health services but it might better be read as a catalogue of missed opportunities to arrange effective long term treatment for a man with a severe mental illness. The pressures on beds in London during this period have been vividly documented (Powell et al, 1995).

A takeover of the small local service by the then Bethlem and Maudsley Special Health Authority resulted in an improvement in our resource base. I took on responsibility for a Psychiatric Intensive Care Unit (PICU) at the Maudsley and later worked as a catchment-area psychiatrist for East Lambeth with access to acute beds within the Maudsley and the Bethlem. Multidisciplinary teamwork on the wards was again a possibility, and I had the unheard of luxury of working with ward-based psychologists.

During the late 1980s and 1990s with colleagues I was able to document some of the experiences we had in both closing the mental hospital and developing what were then innovative community mental health services. The focus of interest for me and my contemporaries was on our work within community-based services, where it was felt the action was, though we did do our best to document what was happening within our acute services over these turbulent times (Holloway et al, 1988; 1992;

Patrick et al, 1989).

Funds released by the Cane Hill closure were largely spent on improving the range and quality of community-based services. However it was apparent to anyone working in inner-urban psychiatry during the latter part of the 1990s that, despite the undoubted advances occurring in community mental health services, there was a crisis in inpatient care. This was reflected at the most obvious level in extreme bed pressures that saw patients being denied admission as the thresholds for admission were increased, very high levels of bed occupancy and a reluctant, and expensive, reliance on private psychiatric hospitals that expanded and opened to meet the demand for 'overspill'. Less obvious but apparent in the tales our patients returning from a spell of private sector care had about the quality of the physical environment (and the food) that they experienced was a message about the impoverished care environments that we had grown used to within NHS psychiatry. Slowly issues about the atmosphere on the wards, relationships between staff and patients and in particular violence and sexual assault came to the fore. (In the pre-Clunis era many 'difficult' patients had simply been precipitately discharged, often with a diagnostic relabeling as suffering from a personality disorder – an option that was increasingly less feasible to take.)

In 1999 I moved from the Lambeth service to work in Croydon, an outer London Borough with a different demography to Lambeth and historically much lower levels of mental health service funding. Inpatient services had been scaled down as the local mental hospital, Warlingham Park, was shut. Acute beds were relocated to the Bethlem in refurbished accommodation. Locally and nationally the past decade has seen significant investment in community services along the lines set out in the *Mental Health National Service Framework* (Department of Health, 1999), the *NHS Plan* (Department of Health, 2000) and the subsequent original *Policy Implementation Guide* (Department of Health, 2001). For some years the inpatient service retained a somewhat second-class status locally with, for example, all the acute ward consultants having the bulk of their responsibilities within their community teams. That second-class status adhered to the nursing staff, always by far the most important staff group within inpatient services: ambitious nurses, it was believed, would and should move as rapidly as possible after qualification to posts within community services that offered both higher grading but substantially more professional autonomy. It never proved possible to obtain investment in a full ward multidisciplinary team, although we were able to maintain and even expand Occupational Therapy support to the wards (at a time when it was being withdrawn in other services).

It is only in the past few years that the centrality of the acute inpatient ward to an effective community mental health service has been thoroughly reaffirmed. *Policy Implementation Guides* were published both for acute wards and PICUs (Department of Health 2002 a,b). These provided a critique of current practice and set standards for service improvement. Locally this has been marked by a service redesign that has brought us single-sex wards, dedicated inpatient consultants and enhanced status for the staff working within what remains an extremely pressured, demanding environment. It has been possible to invest in Occupational Therapy for the wards, focusing on enriching the daily activity programme on the wards, as well as encouraging nursing staff to spend protected time in one-to-one interactions with their patients. Perhaps paradoxically a major reason for this shift was the development of the gate-keeping function of the Crisis Resolution/Home Treatment Team. In the latest service change locally there have been clear winners and losers. No longer is the inpatient unit bottom of the prestige pile: that dubious honour now lies in the era of 'functionalised' mental health services with our generic Community Mental Health Teams.

Data

How many beds?

The outstanding and obvious feature of psychiatric practice over the past 50 years has been a move away from an institutional base in the large mental hospitals to a much more complex and pluralistic system of care. Table 1 documents the decline in NHS psychiatric beds in England and Wales from a peak in 1954 of well over 150,000 to some 24,000 recorded in 2007 (including 2,000 in Wales). Most of this decline has come about by a reduction in long-stay and elderly care beds but the past 20 years have undoubtedly seen marked reductions in the numbers of acute beds in England whilst in recent years intensive care, low security and medium security bed numbers have expanded significantly. The National Service Mapping exercise for 2008 identified some 16,000 NHS adult mental health beds serving England (excluding the High Secure Hospitals, which this exercise did not capture accurately) – see Table 2. Only 9000 of these were acute beds – the rest were intensive care beds, low and medium secure beds and rehabilitation and continuing care provision.

To this contemporary picture must be added beds in the Independent Sector purchased by Mental Health Trusts as acute overspill and Primary Care Trusts (PCTs) for longer-term Out of Area Treatments. There is no readily accessible data on the size of this market, but a reasonable estimate would be some 3000 additional beds, almost all of which provide longer-term care for people with complex needs that cannot be met locally. Many of these individuals are the responsibility of the Forensic Mental Health Services. However some people who cannot adequately be cared for in local acute wards end up in the Independent Sector. Typically they move on to this provision after extended periods within general adult acute wards after

Table 1

Decline in psychiatric bed numbers in England and Wales 1954-2007

1954	155400	
1959	142500	
1964	131000	
1969	117000	
1974	85000	
1979	75000	
1984	65000	
1989	50000	
1994	40000	
1999	36000	
2002	30000	
2007	22000	(excludes beds in Wales - approx. 2000)

Table 2

NHS Inpatient Provision in England for Adults in 2008

	Number
Acute Inpatient Beds	8796
Psychiatric Intensive Care Units	931
Low Secure Beds	1309
Medium Secure Beds	1671
Rehabilitation Beds	3078*
Total	15785

* combines Residential Rehabilitation and 24 hour nurse staffed care

Note; High Secure provision excluded

Source: Mental Health Strategies National Service Mapping 2008

http://www.mhcombinedmap.org/ReportsProvisionUnweighted.aspx (accessed 8/12/08)

fraught negotiations with service managers and local PCTs. Anecdotally these people often present very challenging problems associated with co-morbid autistic spectrum disorder, severe personality disorder or acquired brain damage.

Where does the money go?

We work in the era of community care. Epidemiological studies tell us that 27% of the adult population experience diagnosable mental disorder in a year (Wittchen and Jacobi, 2005): this is of the order of 10 million people in England. Although a much smaller percentage of the population receive some care within specialist mental health services including substance misuse services, perhaps 4% of the adult population a year, this still represents over a million people. Of these million people 20,000, give or take, will be inpatients at any one time – about 5% of those in contact with mental health services and far less than 1% of all adults experiencing an episode of diagnosable mental disorder in a year. Analysis of the spending on adult mental health, including social care, identifies inpatient services as three of the top four budget lines that together account for well over 40% of the total spending (taking into account indirect costs such as capital charges on the NHS estate, Mental Health Strategies, 2006). Any business where 40% of its costs were associated with a particular activity would pay great attention to understanding how to optimise the efficiency and effectiveness of this aspect of the business.

What happens as acute beds reduce?

Twenty years ago my colleagues and I observed from a local study that as acute bed numbers reduced and as an inevitable consequence the morbidity (or 'acuity' as it is often now termed) of inpatients increased the environment on acute inpatient wards might become more difficult for patients and staff, amplifying levels of disturbance on the wards and making them progressively less therapeutic (Patrick et al, 1989). There is no dataset available to confirm or disconfirm this hypothesis but most mental health professionals, patients and carers would agree that over time inpatient wards became, despite everyone's best efforts, more difficult places in which to live and work. Our somewhat surprised observation coming from enthusiastic proponents of community care has become a truism.

One study of an inner urban service found that in the decade from 1988 there were significant demographic changes in the inpatient population, who in 1998 were younger, more likely to be unemployed and less residentially stable than inpatients in 1988 (Fitzpatrick et al, 2003): in contemporary parlance they had less social capital. Median length of stay halved over this period (from 30 days to 15 days). The authors' finding that admission thresholds had not changed over time (using retrospective expert ratings) does not reflect the experience of clinicians during that decade but their observation that the local demography is a powerful determinant of demand for inpatient care is very pertinent.

Very high bed occupancy levels, which became typical in London in the 1990s (Powell et al, 1995), require inpatient staff to take responsibility for larger numbers of patients than their establishment was nominally set up for. In addition to patients resident on the ward staff have to be aware of the needs of people sleeping out in a variety of settings (for example at home, with friends or carers, in local bed-and-breakfasts or in elderly care wards: all expedients I have had to have recourse to in the past). In this

Table 3:

Where does the money go? Mental health expenditure for England, 2005-06

	Expenditure (£'000s)	% total costs
Direct Costs		
Secure and High Dependency Provision	660,634.99	14.1
Acute Inpatient Unit/Ward	574,860.74	12.2
Community Mental Health Teams	549,206.91	11.7
Continuing Care	384,263.64	8.2
Housing and Residential Care	361,770.27	7.7
Day Services (including NHS)	210,287.09	4.5
Crisis Resolution/Home Treatment Teams	155,225.32	3.3
Psychological Therapy Services	142,047.13	3.0
Assertive Outreach Teams	101,423.87	2.2
Psychiatric Outpatient Clinics	97,451.98	2.1
Home Support Services	91,440.73	2.0
Specialist mental health services	56,739.94	1.2
Early Intervention in Psychosis Services	41,893.40	0.8
Community Services for Mentally Disordered Offenders	37,906.34	0.8
Carer's Services	18,697.79	0.4
A&E Mental Health Liaison Service	17,902.26	0.4
Personality disorder services	10,401.07	0.2
Mental health promotion	3,146.40	0.1
Direct Payments	2,484.49	0.1
Other direct costs	233,951.90	5.0
Indirect Costs	395,047.23	8.4

situation decision-making can become entirely reactive to the overwhelming demand to find a bed for someone presenting to the service in enormous need.

Keown et al (2008) have carried out an interesting analysis using official statistics for England to explore the relationship between changes in bed numbers, patient characteristics and rates of detention in patients admitted between 1996 and 2006. Bed numbers reduced by 29% over this time. The total number of admissions fell from 1998 but compulsory admissions increased both absolutely and more markedly as a proportion of total admissions. They concluded that:

> The case mix has shifted further towards psychotic and substance misuse disorders, which has changed the milieu of inpatient wards. Increasing proportions of involuntary patients were admitted to private facilities.

The proportion of admissions involving compulsion continues to increase: Department of Health data shows that in 2006-7 there were some 162,000 admissions to NHS mental illness and learning disability beds of which approximately 25% involved detention under the Mental Health Act at some time during the inpatient episode.

There has been a general trend throughout Europe for inpatient beds to decrease whilst compulsory admissions, Forensic beds and supported housing places have increased. The process has been termed 'reinstitutionalisation' (Priebe et al, 2005). The European-wide increase in compulsory admission deserves particular note since inevitably the fact of compulsion casts a shadow on the nature of the relationship between the patient and the service however benign the intentions of that service.

Although the picture is not entirely clear a pattern emerges from the available data. Better initial treatment of mental illness, improvements in community care that can support people experiencing an exacerbation of their mental illness out of hospital and reductions in available acute inpatient beds will together result in a change in the characteristics of people coming into hospital. Changes in local demography will also have an effect as will Governmental and societal attitudes towards mental illness that, for example, favour coercive interventions. (It will be intriguing to follow changes in case-mix and compulsory admission following implementation of the Mental Health Act 2007, which has been interpreted as representing a strong governmental steer towards risk avoidance and coercion). Bed pressures will raise admission thresholds and demand staff increase throughput, with the metric of success being to make length of stay on the ward as short as possible.

Ward atmosphere and environment

Numerous reports have documented the patient/service user perspective on life on an acute ward. Patients report being bored, frightened, looking for therapeutic inputs that are absent and not infrequently becoming the victim of violence or sexual harassment (Sainsbury Centre for Mental Health, 1998; Baker, 2000; Quirk and Lelliott, 2004). Physical conditions on wards have often been described as poor, with people reporting a cramped, poorly maintained rather dismal environment. One early study noted, perhaps depressingly, that the thing people most valued about inpatient care was being allowed a pass or leave from the ward (McIntyre et al, 1989). However patients do consistently report valuing the quality of the nursing care that they receive, particularly the empathy, warmth and respect that they experience. These positives are balanced by negatives when patients experience apparently arbitrary behaviour by nurses, coercion and punishment and a tendency for staff to congregate in the office to the exclusion of the patients they are there to support (Quirk and Lelliott, 2004).

Staff have also reported their concerns, which have striking parallels with the patient perspective. The first *National Audit of Violence* (Royal College of Psychiatrists Research Unit, 2005) identified the main concerns from staff as poorly designed and unsafe environments; inadequate levels of staffing with unacceptably high vacancy factors and a reliance on bank and agency staff; overcrowding and inappropriate client mix; high prevalence of substance misuse on many wards; lack of access to relevant training for staff; and high levels of boredom for patients. A picture comes through from this and other reports that inpatient psychiatry, particularly for the nursing profession, is a low-status occupation.

Radcliffe and Smith (Chapter 1) discuss in detail the issue of occupation and activity on inpatient units. Throughout this book a theme will be the centrality of effective personal engagement between 'staff' and 'patients', albeit mediated by the particular concept of group work. Group work may be an effective medium for delivering specific evidence-based psychological treatments to inpatients (Kinderman, 2004), although the short average duration of stay presents a formidable practical barrier to this. Ward groups and community meetings that adopt a modified psychodynamic approach may be of value in improving ward atmosphere and, in particular, addressing serious untoward events (Holmes, 2004). High quality wards often, as a matter of routine, bring all patients and staff together when an adverse event occurs that involves a patient or member of staff.

Environmental issues are of great importance in effective inpatient psychiatric practice: people respond to and respect high quality physical environments (as our patients who spent time in private sector facilities intended for a fee-paying clientele attested). To these positives need to be added the fear of and actual violence perpetrated, witnessed and experienced by inpatients.

Violence and self-harm

There is a substantial literature on violence in psychiatric inpatient settings. Guidelines have been developed surrounding the prevention and management of violence in inpatient settings (Wing et al, 1998; National Institute for Clinical Excellence, 2005). Violence has been associated with factors related to patient characteristics, staff behaviours, environmental factors and interactions between these variables (Johnson 2004). The two National Audits (Royal College of Psychiatrists Research Unit, 2005; Royal College of Psychiatrists Centre for Quality Improvement, 2007) document the sheer scale of the problem, with 80% of nursing staff and 36% of patients reporting having been attacked, threatened or intimidated during their time on the inpatient units surveyed in 2003-5. In the 2006-7 audit 46% of nursing staff and 18% of patients reported having been physically assaulted. The 2006-7 audit concluded that '*recent national policy and practice drivers that have emphasised the use of prevention and de-escalation, rather than physical interventions, were firmly embedded in ward-based practices in many services. Staff, patients and visitors were clearly aware of this changing culture, and were responding positively to it*'. The standards developed for the 2006-7 National Audit sets out standards of good practice surrounding being treated with respect and dignity, and given privacy and choice; being offered meaningful occupation; being given adequate information; staff training and supervision; supports from other colleagues; environmental safety; both staff and patients being supported in relation to actual incidents. One major shift in thinking has been the realization that sensitive post-incident discussion with the perpetrator of violence can be very valuable.

Environmental safety has been a major emphasis in another policy programme, that to reduce suicides by psychiatric patients, particularly current and recent inpatients. A major programme has been undertaken to ensure the removal of ligature points on wards following the publication of reports from the National Confidential Inquiry into Homicides and Suicides which noted the significant numbers of people dying by hanging whilst on an inpatient ward (Appleby et al, 2001).

Substance misuse

A further aspect of life on inpatient wards is the extent of substance misuse (Abou-Saleh 2004). Some people are admitted to acute wards with primary substance misuse problems but co-morbidity is a much more common problem. Co-morbid substance abuse is associated with increased rates of impulsivity, violence and deliberate self-harm. People with schizophrenia who are admitted having abused cannabis or stimulants spend longer in hospital than those whose illness is not characterized by co-morbidity and those who continue to abuse drugs whilst in hospital have even longer stays (Isaac et al, 2005). Despite its evident importance we know that historically adult mental health staff have felt deskilled at managing people presenting with co-morbid substance misuse and mental illness. To plug that gap the Department of Health (2002c; 2006) has issued good practice guides and encouraged more substance misuse training for adult mental health staff.

Long-stay patients

Although lengths of stay within acute wards have continued to decline there is a small but important sub-group of patients who have extended inpatient stays. They are a heterogeneous group, including some with treatment-resistant psychosis, a small number of individuals with severe behavioural problems that occur in the context of severe personality disorder and others with very complex co-morbidities and/ or forensic histories. Such individuals often do very badly on acute wards and may require specialist rehabilitation services (Holloway, 2005).

Ethnic minorities

An issue of particular concern, which is rarely clearly articulated, is the experience of people from black and minority ethnic groups who become inpatients. There is good evidence that people from some minority groups, particularly African-Caribbeans and Black Africans, are over-represented amongst people admitted to psychiatric hospitals, detained in hospital, experiencing seclusion and restraint and moving through the system to secure hospital settings (Sainsbury Centre for Mental Health, 2002). One point that does need to be made is that whatever the factors are for the often additionally difficult engagement between people from ethnic minority groups and inpatient services (and these will be very complex) inappropriate racial stereotyping by inpatient staff is not a root cause of the problem (Feinstein and Holloway, 2002; Gudjonsson et al, 2004)

The acute inpatient ward now

Casual readers of this chapter might be forgiven for thinking that I believe acute inpatient psychiatric services to be irredeemably broken, barely more than warehouses which briefly hold people who are extremely disturbed before dispatching them unchanged, or possibly further traumatised, back into an uncaring community. This is far from the case: people have always come into hospital in extreme distress and admission has always resulted (on average) in a marked decrease in distress, albeit thresholds for admission have changed over the years as have the social and clinical characteristics of inpatients.

Indeed recent initiatives, some of which have already been outlined, do appear to be driving up standards in acute wards. Of particular note is the Star Wards programme (http://starwards.org.uk/). The website describes Star Wards as

> a project which works with mental health trusts to enhance mental health inpatients'
> daily experiences and treatment outcomes. We discover, celebrate, share, publicise and
> inspire excellence in inpatient care, and there is plenty of that all round the country.
> Our members use and adapt our resources to stimulate and structure therapeutic and

enjoyable daily programmes for inpatients in the full range of wards including elderly, rehab, learning disability and secure.

Technology is here being used to join people of good will, with good practical ideas together. *Star Wards* is clearly imbued with Recovery principles (Care Services Improvement Partnership, 2007).

Another important development has been the Accreditation for Acute Mental Health Services (*AIMS*) project. This has seen the elaboration of standards for acute inpatient services and an associated accreditation system (Lelliott et al, 2006). The standards cover four interlinked domains: General Standards that relate to aspects of staffing, policies and procedures; Timely and Purposeful Admission (relating to admission, assessment, care planning discharge planning, management, skill-mix); Safety; and the Therapeutic Environment (Cresswell et al, 2007). Wards achieving accreditation through AIMS will be providing a safe environment but beyond this will be offering effective treatments (not just medication) to their patients.

Both *AIMS* and *Star Wards* emphasise the importance of engaging patients in structured activities (often provided in group settings) and the life of the ward, through regular meetings of the ward community. Therapeutic community principles, evident in my early experience at Fulbourn, are being rediscovered and reinterpreted in the light of contemporary concerns (Firth, 2004). It is now, for example, routine to draw the ward community together when a serious untoward incident has occurred within the unit.

The complex role of the inpatient Consultant Psychiatrist (soon to be joined by Approved Clinician colleagues from other disciplines in the statutory responsibility for people detained under the Mental Health Act) offers a great deal of satisfaction. Most obviously, as I have already noted, people arrive on the ward in great distress and, generally, leave much less distressed. Even in this era of community care the inpatient unit lies at the heart of any mental health service. The Consultant role demands a very wide range of clinical and managerial skills. Every day on an acute inpatient unit will offer new challenges.

The future inpatient ward

It is always dangerous to predict the future but it is possible to extrapolate from clear current trends. Inpatient psychiatry will continue to be a challenging area within which to work. There will be continuing pressures on a relatively small stock of inpatient beds. However staff will be able to take pride in working in a field that attracts high prestige with ready access to information about good models of practice.

Multidisciplinary working will strengthen and the inpatient workforce will become more diverse in terms of professional (and indeed non-professional) background. Specific time-limited psychosocial therapies may be more frequently offered either individually or in group settings on units, although this requires staff to have received appropriate training and have adequate supervision arrangements in place.

After early successful experience (Dratcu, 2002; Ingram and Tacchi, 2004) it is becoming the norm for wards to have dedicated inpatient consultants. As I have already noted this has been implemented in my own service. The change has brought perhaps predictable positives and negatives – our wards function better but the interface issues between ward and community teams have become more problematical. One unresolved issue is whether inpatient psychiatry will become a speciality in its own right (Holloway, 2006): readers of this book may develop a view of the competencies that the psychiatrist will require to offer leadership to an inpatient unit.

We are working in an era of increasing specialisation. Some very highly specialist psychiatric services offer treatment packages to patients with very particular problems: wards dedicated to perinatal psychiatry and eating disorders are common whilst other units are emerging that provide inpatient care for first onset psychosis, severe anxiety disorders and obsessive-compulsive disorder, personality disorder, neuropsychiatry and autistic spectrum disorder. Further specialisation reflecting specific care pathways (for example for schizophrenia and bipolar disorder) may well emerge. In all these specialist areas there is a potential for the development of further evidence-based group work interventions. Another form of specialisation has been the 'triage' ward, which takes and assesses all acute admissions, discharging those who do not require longer inpatient stays to community-based alternatives (Inglis and Baggaley, 2005).

One necessary change that remains difficult to implement is better engagement between the inpatient unit and carers. This links in with another area where service improvement is required: the quality and timeliness of discharge planning. A 'good practice toolkit' has recently been developed to encourage improvement in care planning and discharge planning (Care Services Improvement Partnership, 2007). A further area for improvement is the way that inpatient services address the issue of capacity. A high percentage of inpatients lack decision-making capacity at some stage during their admission (Owen et al 2008). The *Mental Capacity Act 2005* sets standards for staff in making decisions where people lack capacity: recording of decisions has to be adequate and decisions need to be taken in the 'best interests' of the person. In addition staff need to be aware of the existence of advance decisions/directives that people have made about their care and act appropriately where advance decisions are in place (although broadly speaking the Mental Health Act, only relevant to the treatment of mental disorder, 'trumps' the Mental Capacity Act).

Although much has been learned over the past 25 years about how best to run a psychiatric inpatient unit and standards have undoubtedly improved in recent years the past has a lot to teach us. A quarter of a century ago Martin (1984) summarised what had been learned from a series of scandals that had occurred in learning disability, old age and psychiatric hospitals over the preceding two decades. Inpatient units that went to the bad tended to have similar characteristics: physical isolation of the unit, lack of openness of the unit to external scrutiny, poor nursing and medical management and lack of vision from senior leaders within the local service (in both senses – not seeing what was going on and not having any view about what should be going on). Hopefully these conditions will not recur in the future and the quality of care will continue to improve despite the pressures that will always be there.

References

Abou-Saleh M.T. (2004) Dual diagnosis: management within a psychosocial context. *Advances in Psychiatric Treatment* 10, 352–360.

Appleby J., Shaw J., Sherratt J., Amos T. and Robinson J. (2001) *Safety First: Five Year Report of the National Confidential Inquiry into Homicides and Suicides by People with a Mental Illness*. London: Department of Health.

Baker, S. (2000) *Environmentally friendly? Patients' views of conditions on psychiatric wards*. London: MIND.

Bowers, L. (2005) Reasons for admission and their implications for the nature of acute inpatient psychiatric nursing. *Journal of Psychiatric and Mental Health Nursing*, 12, 231-236.

Care Services Improvement Partnership (2007) A common purpose: Recovery in future mental health services. Joint Position Paper 08. Leeds: CSIP.

Clark, D.H. (1974) *Social Therapy in Psychiatry*. Harmonsdworth: Penguin.

Cresswell, J., Beavon, M. and Hood, C. (2007) *Standards for Acute Inpatient Wards 2nd edition*. London: Royal College of Psychiatrists' Research and Training Unit.

Davenport, S. (2002) Acute wards: problems and solutions. A rehabilitation approach to inpatient care. *Psychiatric Bulletin*, 26, 385-388.

Department of Health and Social Security (1975) *Better Services for the Mentally Ill*. London: DHSS.

Department of Health (1999) *National Service Framework for Mental Health. Modern standards and service models*. London: Department of Health.

Department of Health (2000) *The NHS Plan: A Plan for Investment, a Plan for Reform*. London: Department of Health.

Department of Health (2001) *Mental Health Policy Implementation Guide*. London: Department of Health.

Department of Health (2002a) *Acute Inpatient Provision Care Provision: Mental Health Policy Implementation Guide*. London: Department of Health.

Department of Health (2002b) National Standards for PICU and Low Secure Environments.

London: Department of Health.

Department of Health (2002c) *Mental Health Policy Implementation Guide: Dual Diagnosis Good Practice Guide.* London: Department of Health.

Department of Health (2006) *Dual Diagnosis in Mental Health Inpatient and Day Hospital Settings.* London: Department of Health.

Deapartment of Health (2008) *Code of Practice Mental Health Act 1983.* London: Department of Health.

Dratcu, L. (2002) Acute hospital care: The beauty and the beast of psychiatry. *Psychiatric Bulletin,* 26, 81-82.

Feinstein, A. and Holloway, F. (2002) Evaluating the use of a psychiatric intensive care unit – is ethnicity a risk factor for admission? *International Journal of Social Psychiatry,* 48, 38-46.

Firth, W. (2004) Acute psychiatric wards: an overview. In *From Toxic Institutions to Therapeutic Environments: Residential Settings in Mental Health Services.* P. Campling, S. Davies and G. Farquharson (Eds.). London: Gaskell pp 174-187.

Fitzpatrick, N.K., Thompson, C.J., Hemingway, H., Molloy, C., Higgit, A. and Hargreaves, S. (2003) Acute mental health admissions in inner London: changes in patient characteristics and clinical admission thresholds between 1988 and 1998. *Psychiatric Bulletin,* 27, 7-11.

Gudjonsson, G.H., Rabe-Hesketh, S. and Szmukler, G. (2004) Management of psychiatric in-patient violence: patient ethnicity and use of medication, restraint and seclusion. *British Journal of Psychiatry,* 184, 258-62.

Holloway, F. (2005) The Forgotten Need for Rehabilitation in Contemporary Mental Health Services. http://www.rcpsych.ac.uk/college/faculty/rehab/frankholloway_oct05.pdf.

Holloway, F. (2006) Acute inpatient psychiatry: dedicated consultants if we must but not a specialty. *Psychiatric Bulletin,* 30, 402-403.

Holloway, F., Davies, G., Silverman, A.M. and Wainwrigh,t A.W. (1988) How many beds? *Bulletin of the Royal College of Psychiatrists,* 12, 91-94.

Holloway, F., Silverman, A.M. and Wainwright, A.W. (1992) 'Not waving but drowning', The East Lambeth Inpatient Survey. *International Journal of Social Psychiatry,* 38, 131-137.

Holmes, J. (2004) What can psychotherapy contribute to improving the culture on acute psychiatric wards. In *From Toxic Institutions to Therapeutic Environments: Residential Settings in Mental Health Services.* P. Campling, S. Davies and G. Farquharson (Eds.). London: Gaskell pp 208-217.

Inglis, G. and Baggaley, M. (2005) Triage in mental health – a new model for acute inpatient psychiatry. *Psychiatric Bulletin,* 29, 255-258.

Ingram, G. and Tacchi, M.J. (2004) Service innovation in a heated environment: CATS on a hot tin roof. *Psychiatric Bulletin,* 28, 398-400.

Isaac, M.B., Isaac, M.T. and Holloway, F. (2005) Is cannabis an anti-antipsychotic? *Human Psychopharmacology,* 20, 207-210.

Keown, P., Mercer, G. and Scott, J. (2008) Retrospective analysis of hospital episode statistics, involuntary admissions under the Mental Health Act 1983, and number of psychiatric beds in England 1996-2006. *British Medical Journal,* 337, 1837.

Kinderman, P. (2004) Delivering psychological therapies in acute in-patient settings. In *From Toxic Institutions to Therapeutic Environments: Residential Settings in Mental Health Services*. P. Campling, S. Davies and G. Farquharson (Eds.). London: Gaskell pp 197-207.

Johnson, M.E. (2004) Violence on Inpatient Psychiatric Units: state of the science. *Journal of the American Psychiatric Nurses Association*, 10, 113-121 DOI: 10.1177/1078390304264959.

Lelliott, P., Bennett, H., McGeorge, M. and Turner, T. (2006) Accreditation of acute inpatient mental health services. *Psychiatric Bulletin*, 206, 361-363.

McIntyre, K., Farrell, M., and David, A.S. (1989) What do psychiatric in-patients really want? *British Medical Journal*, 298, 159-60.

Martin, J.P. (1984) *Hospitals in Trouble*. Oxford: Blackwell.

Mental Health Strategies (2006) *The 2005/6 National Survey of Investment in Mental Health Services*. London: Department of Health.

National Institute for Clinical Excellence (2005) *Violence: The short-term management of disturbed/violent behaviour in psychiatric in-patient settings and emergency departments*. Clinical Guideline 25, NICE.

Owen, G.S., Richardson, G., David, A., Szmukler, G. and Hotopf, M. (2008) Mental capacity to make decisions on treatment in people admitted to psychiatric hospitals: cross-sectional study. *British Medical Journal*, 337, a448.

Patrick, M., Higgitt, A., Holloway, F. and Silverman, M., (1989) Changes in an Inner City Psychiatric Inpatient Service Following Bed Losses: a follow-up of the East Lambeth 1986 Survey, *Health Trends*, 21, 121-123.

Powell, R.B., Hollander, D. and Tobiansky, R.I. (1995) Crisis in admission beds. A four-year survey of the bed state of Greater London's acute psychiatric units. *British Journal of Psychiatry*, 167, 765-769.

Priebe, S., Badesconyi, A., Fioritti, A., Hansonn, L., Kilian, R., Torres-Gonzales, F., Turner, T. and Wiersma, D. et al (2005) Reinstitutionalisation in mental health care: comparison of data on service provision from six European countries. *British Medical Journal*, 330,123–6.

Quirk, A. and Lelliott, P. (2004) Users' experience of in-patient services. In *From Toxic Institutions to Therapeutic Environments: Residential Settings in Mental Health Services*. P. Campling, S. Davies and G. Farquharson (Eds.). London: Gaskell pp 45-54.

Radcliffe, J. and Smith, R. (2010) What actually happens on acute wards? An observational study. In *Psychological Groupwork with Acute Psychiatric Inpatients*. Radcliffe J, Hajek K, Carson J and Manor O (Eds.). London: Whiting & Birch pp. 1-20

Ritchie, J. H., Dick, D. and Lingham, R. (1994) *The Report of the Inquiry into the Care and Treatment of Christopher Clunis*. London: HMSO.

Royal College of Psychiatrists Research Unit (2005) *The Healthcare Commission National Audit of Violence (2003-2005)*. London: Royal College of Psychiatrists Research Unit.

Royal College of Psychiatrists Centre for Quality Improvement (2007) *The Healthcare Commission National Audit of Violence 2006-7 Final Report – Working Age Adult Services*. London: Royal College of Psychiatrists Centre for Quality Improvement.

Sainsbury Centre for Mental Health (1998) *Acute Problems: A Survey of the Quality of Care in Acute Psychiatric Wards (ACIS)*. London: Sainsbury Centre for Mental Health.

Sainsbury Centre for Mental Health (2002) *Breaking the Circles of Fear: A review of the relationship between mental health services and African and Caribbean communities*. London: Sainsbury Centre for Mental Health.

Wing, J.K., Marriott, S., Palmer, C. and Thomas, V. (1998) *The Management of Imminent Violence: Clinical Practice Guidelines to Support Mental Health Services. Occasional Paper OP41*. London: Royal College of Psychiatrists.

Wittchen, H-U. and Jacobi, F. (2005) Size and burden of mental disorders in Europe – a critical review and appraisal of 27 studies. *European.*

Neuropsychopharmacology, 15, 357–76.

Wolfensberger, W. (1983) Social role valorization: a proposed new term for the principle of normalization. *Mental Retardation*, 21, 234-239.

5
Bearing the unbearable

Understanding and working with individual and organisational resistances to groupwork on acute psychiatric wards

Richard Duggins

'A' Ward in the asylum is
a place full of wanderers with deluded minds,
slashed wrists and singed arms;
a place not for the faint of heart
('The Revolving Door' In *Poems From The Madhouse*, 1993, by Sandy Jeffs.)

Introduction

My aim in this chapter is to describe, and attempt to understand, the challenging human interactions that tend to repeatedly occur on acute psychiatric wards, and to consider the implications of these interactions for groupwork.

My fascination with this subject grew from my wish to understand my own painful experiences as a junior doctor working on an acute inpatient ward, and I start this chapter with a description of those formative experiences. I then consider my experiences in the context of some qualitative research I undertook and a review of the wider research literature on inpatient wards. My personal experience and the research lead me to put forward the opinion that there are fundamental difficulties with forming therapeutic relationships on many acute wards. I present an understanding based on a psychodynamic approach to psychosis that helps me make some sense of these difficulties.

I suggest that psychosis is a defence that protects a person against unbearable emotions, and as a result, unless there is a safe and robust ward environment, both patients and staff tend to avoid any therapeutic activity that may risk engaging with these unbearable emotions and the intolerable states of mind they induce. I argue that patients and staff do wish to engage in therapeutic relationships, but fear their mental survival is threatened by such engagement. The powerful anxieties of staff and patients are reduced by behaviours in the institution, known as institutional defences, which unfortunately act against real human contact, and therefore threaten any therapeutic intervention, including groupwork. I argue that groupwork has an essential role in managing these destructive institutional defences on acute psychiatric wards, and it is only through effective groupwork, with both patients and staff, that human therapeutic activity can be helped to hold sway over defensive isolation.

First impressions

I was a relatively junior doctor when I commenced my six-month placement on Ward A, a mixed-sex acute psychiatric ward. I was enthusiastic and motivated, and I had found working in community mental health teams rewarding.

I will describe two of the behaviours of staff that were repeated again and again on the ward; these behaviours were sedating and the ward review. I wish to make it clear that I am not presenting a full picture of the complex and varied interactions of the staff and patients on Ward A, and that, despite the pressures I describe, I encountered some inspiring human contact on that ward.

I was introduced to the 'sedation behaviour' within ten minutes of entering the ward. I saw a nurse face-up to an agitated middle-aged gentleman and shout, 'back-down' at him, first once, and then twice. The patient seemed to step-back a little, and the nurse grabbed his medicine chart and asked me to prescribe an injection for sedation. I was told that he normally had sedation when he 'gets manic' like this.

Sedating was a daily occurrence on the ward. It was usually initiated if a patient threatened to invade a staff member's personal space. The patient then had two choices, either to calm him or herself down and withdraw, or to be injected with a sedative.

The other repeated behaviour I wish to describe is the weekly ward review. During the ward review each patient was invited to enter a room containing four or more multidisciplinary professionals. Before the patient entered the room, there was a quick discussion amongst the professions to formulate a care-plan involving concrete issues like medication, risk and leave. The patient then had five to ten minutes in the spotlight. A 'good' patient, to the ward review's relief, quickly accepted our care plan and left. 'Difficult' patients raised the anxiety of the ward review by wanting to discuss their feelings, especially their distress. Such patients were told that this was not the forum for such discussions, and that ward reviews were about reviewing care plans, which meant making decisions.

Initially, on the ward, I tried to keep my involvement in these repeated behaviours to the minimum, and instead spend my time talking to the patients, and finding out about their distress. My patients on the ward invited me into worlds that were often horrific and tortuous. Their lives in the outside world were mostly chaotic, poverty-stricken and lonely, but it was their internal worlds that had the most significant impact on me. For example, one patient I got to know told me that he had the constant feeling of animal semen being ejaculated into his mouth. I was shocked, and unable to make sense of this communication, and the feelings it stirred-up in me. (I return to this example later in this chapter.)

Getting to know my patients did not appear to be a role the staff expected of me. In fact, some staff seemed to feel such behaviour by a doctor was a sign that I was unfocussed, or had too little to do. Some staff even suggested that my frequent talking with patients might be dangerous, because it did not demonstrate clear boundaries between staff and patients.

It was understandable that the staff were concerned about danger; the ward felt like a threatening place. On a daily basis, I witnessed patients making threats and behaving in an intimidating manner, and at times this would explode into physical violence directed towards other patients or staff.

A few months into my placement on the ward, I started to struggle. My contact with my patients seemed to be making me feel overwhelmed. Horrific worlds invaded my waking mind, and my dreams. I was struggling to think. I needed something to change, and I started to find relief by retreating into a less threatening world, in which I became increasingly willing to sedate patients and dropped much of my contact with them outside of ward reviews. I felt shame as I retreated to the 'sedation' and 'ward review' behaviours, but the horror in my mind calmed.

Soon my only interactions with patients were in ward reviews, and in prescribing medications. I lacked curiosity about my new patients, and knew little about them. I noticed I was not alone; I started to recognise that many of the nurses, like me, were struggling, and despite their best intentions, had also retreated to these safer interactions. Looking through the multidisciplinary case notes of many of the patients seemed to confirm this; mostly the notes were full of practical plans such as medication, risk and leave, and lacking in personal details and descriptions of how the patient was feeling. There was hardly any psychological activity of any kind on the ward, and nurses would often cancel their 'one-to-one' sessions with patients because of other demands; there was no groupwork. Although patients were told that the ward-review was not the forum for them to discuss their distress, I soon realised there was no other place on the ward for them to discuss their feelings either.

My increasing emotional distance from my patients and my colleagues seemed to help me survive for a few more months, but soon I felt unbearably isolated and also deeply unsettled by the knowledge that I was not helping anyone. Even more concerning was my growing fear that I was in danger of breaking the 'golden rule' of healthcare; 'first, do not harm.' I applied for another job, and although leaving was intermingled with a heavy heart and a sense of failure, I mostly felt great relief when I walked out of Ward A.

A qualitative study of the experiences of patients on inpatient wards

After leaving Ward A, I found out it was widely recognised by my colleagues as a ward that was struggling. I have since gone on to work in other acute psychiatric wards that have maintained a more therapeutic culture for patients, and a more supportive environment for staff. I have worked with staff members on acute wards that are able to retain a human touch and not retreat too much into repetitive interactions, like sedation and the ward review. However, although I now appreciate my experiences on Ward A represent an extreme, I have recognised the pressure and tendency to retreat towards repetitive anti-therapeutic reactions as a feature of all the wards I have worked on, and especially at times when the staff team is under increased stress.

It was my interest in this tendency to retreat towards anti-therapeutic relationships on acute wards that motivated me to conduct some research exploring the experiences of patients on acute psychiatric wards. This qualitative research published in a peer-reviewed journal (Duggins and Shaw, 2006) used grounded theory to examine the experiences of ten patients with a diagnosis of schizophrenia on six different inpatient wards. The opportunity to listen to patients describe in great detail their inpatient stay was an incredible privilege, and I was struck by how their experiences resonated so clearly with mine. A key theme that repeatedly came across in the interviews was the lack of human contact and communication on the wards. One participant summed-up powerfully his inpatient experience as:

> *It's like being a sausage in a sausage machine, put in one end, processed and put out the other.*

All the participants complained about the lack of therapeutic contact with staff, and believed staff prioritised other activities. For example:

I was just put in a room. They seemed preoccupied with their job, their office job, getting all the work done.

The saddest finding for me was that the majority of the participants did not expect anything therapeutic to happen on a ward. A participant, who had just left hospital following his first admission that had lasted six months, told me stoically:

I would have liked someone to talk to, but that's psychology, you don't expect it on the ward. The ward is psychiatry; you know - medicines.

Wider research findings

A review of the wider research literature confirms my personal experience and the experience of the participants in my research. Recent reports describe inpatient care as demoralised, unsafe, and sometimes untherapeutic (Sainsbury Centre for Mental Health 1998; Department of Health 2002). Quantitative and qualitative studies suggest a lack of communication between staff and patients on wards (Weinstein 1981; Goodwin et al. 1999), and the Mental Health Act Commission (1997), in a visit to 309 acute wards, recorded that on 38% of wards there was no staff contact with patients except observation of high-risk patients. Numerous reports have highlighted the absence of therapeutic activities on inpatient wards (Department of Health 2002; Sainsbury Centre for Mental Health 2002), and one report found that psychosocial interventions were routinely available in only 35% of wards (Garcia et al., 2005). Radcliffe and Smith (2007), in a survey of 16 acute inpatient units in six hospitals in South London, found that on average only 4% of a patient's time was spent in group activities.

Several studies have highlighted patients' frustration with the lack of opportunity for discussion at ward reviews (Sainsbury Centre for Mental Health 1998; Goodwin et al. 1999), and the frequent use of sedation has been identified in several studies (Weinstein 1981; Rose 2001). It is a common finding that patients and staff perceive inpatient units to be dangerous and frightening (Shepherd et al. 1997; Sainsbury Centre for Mental Health 1998; Barker 2000).

Using a psychodynamic model of psychosis to understand experiences on wards

Everyone on a ward, including patients and staff, can be considered to be constantly participating in an inter-group event (Farquharson 2004). A number of classic studies have highlighted the fact that specific patients elicit specific responses from specific staff (Stanton and Schwartz 1954; Main 1957). However, it is interesting to note that despite the fact that approximately 75% of patients on an acute ward have a psychotic illness (Shepherd 1997), and it is recognised that people with psychosis have a profound effect on those around them (Hinshelwood 1987; Martindale 2001), there has been only limited interest in considering the influence of the dynamics of psychosis on the ward environment.

I will examine the potential influence the dynamics of psychosis can have on the therapeutic ward environment by exploring separately how they affect patients and staff.

Influence of the dynamics of psychosis on patients

In his later work, Freud (1924: p.151) described psychosis as a turning away of the mind from reality, and that the 'nature for this dissociation from the external world is some very serious frustration by reality of a wish – a frustration which seems intolerable'. In the same paper, Freud described this turning away of the mind from reality as a 'rent' (tear or laceration) appearing in the mind's relation to the external world, and psychotic experiences as a 'patch' over this rent. Freud appears to view psychosis as a way of escaping an intolerable experience (because innate instinctual forces are too strong, or reality is too traumatic). A related view of psychosis is held within the 'Need-adapted' treatment of psychosis in Scandinavia. This treatment uses the stress-vulnerability model (Zubin and Spring 1977) as a paradigm for understanding psychosis, and states that certain individuals require a high degree of triggering stress before they reach psychosis, whereas others, who are more vulnerable, require less. Such a model makes it possible to understand psychotic symptoms as an adaptive strategy used by a mind that is trying to cope with overwhelming stresses. Cullberg (2001: p.118) explains that:

> One must understand for a patient in this situation, the feeling of meaning is more important than a feeling of reality – this is not a question of intelligence, but merely one of mental survival.

Both these models contend that the patient has encountered a personally overwhelming stress that has led to an unbearable state of mind. It is to avoid this unbearable state of mind that the patient has found it necessary to prefer psychotic explanations to rational ones (Jackson 2001).

Example: Brenda

For example, Brenda suffered a psychotic breakdown following the birth of her first child, and developed the delusional belief that she was a prophet of God. Clearly having a baby is a time of great stress, but the triggering stress was probably finding out her husband was having an affair and planning to leave her. This stress led her to feel she was worthless and alone, and cruelly resonated with her experience as a baby of being left alone in an orphanage by her mother following her birth. The feelings of worthlessness and isolation she had to bear were absolutely overwhelming for her, and her psychosis stepped in as an adaptive strategy used by her mind to survive.

Wilfred Bion (1967) can be considered to add a further dimension to this view of psychosis. He extended Melanie Klein's work (Klein 1946), and described the aim of psychosis as attacking or preventing links. These links are not just between the mind and the representations of the unbearable experience in the external world, but are also links within the mind (Bion 1967). By attacking links within his or her mind, a person with psychosis stops the links between his or her thoughts, and thus makes thinking about the unbearable experience impossible. Bion believed a person with psychosis needs to try to break links with anything that might allow him, or her, to think about the unbearable experience, and this includes trying to break links with any member of staff behaving in a therapeutic way.

Example: John

For example, John had recurrent admissions for a chronic psychotic illness in which he believed the security forces were monitoring his every move and plotting against him. He found it immensely frightening to engage with staff, and refused offers of medication and therapeutic work. Engagement with John was made even more challenging because of his persistent thought disorder, which made it hard for him to think straight, and hard for staff to understand what he was saying. Eventually, a gentle and long-term therapy was established, and through this therapy it slowly became clear that John's psychotic experiences, although immensely distressing, protected him from the unbearable pain of getting in touch with his sense of terrible isolation and loneliness. In his psychotic state, John was the centre of the security forces' attention, and his thought disorder stopped him thinking about his deeper difficulties. However, when his psychosis receded, and his thoughts cleared, he became painfully aware of the reality of his current social isolation, and he suffered extremely distressing feelings that emanated from a childhood in which he felt lonely, insignificant and unwanted.

I believe much of my experience on Ward A, and the wider research findings, start to make sense if psychosis is viewed as a defence from an experience felt to be unbearable. For a patient with psychosis, like John above, making potential therapeutic links with a member of staff can feel like a threat to his mental survival, because such therapeutic links allow the patient to start to become aware of, and make links with, his own underlying unbearable distress. Under the threat of such primitive anxieties patients are likely to project aspects of their experience, and the staff will pick-up these projections. For example, on several occasions, when I was talking to a distressed patient with psychosis on Ward A, I found myself unable to think, and this may be understood as my action of taking inside myself the patient's own struggle to think about his, or her, unbearable feelings (in psychodynamic terms this taking inside of the patient's experience is known as projective identification). The lack of curiosity I developed about my patients may too have reflected a projective identification with their fear of being curious about themselves.

I believe that some of the violence encountered on acute wards could also be linked to the patients' fear for their mental survival. Here I find Glasser's (1998) views on self-preservative violence helpful. Such violence focuses on a danger that threatens the survival of the individual. Glasser explains:

> This kind of violence has a single-minded, narrow-visioned quality like a laser beam, which focuses on the dangerousness of the object rather than the object itself. If it is the victim's look that is experienced as threatening through accusation, it is the eyes that are attacked; if what is been said is intolerable, the mouth is punched; on so on. (Glasser 1998: p.888)

I propose that on the ward, it is potential therapeutic contact with a member of staff that is seen as dangerous, because such contact makes links that threaten to provoke intolerable psychic pain. Thus, there can be a strong self-preservative desire to 'attack' this potential therapeutic contact through threats and physical violence. Also, we may use the concept of self-preservative violence to explain some of the violence between patients, because such violence may represent a self-preservative attempt to attack meaningful contact with other patients in order to protect against seeing oneself in them. There are, of course, other reasons for violence on acute wards; for example, we should not be blind to the importance of frustration, sadomasochism and substance misuse.

Influence of the dynamics of psychosis on staff

Menzies Lyth's (1960) study of nursing on a medical ward clearly demonstrated that, within an organisation, systems are created that appear to offer staff the promise of protection from the emotional pain of their work. She called such systems 'institutional defences'. Emotional pain is intrinsic to the work on psychiatric wards, and staff are required to engage with unbearably painful states of mind. As Hinshelwood (2001: pp.42-43) clearly states:

> *We must do first what the patient, his intimate relatives, or his friends and neighbours, and other professional helpers cannot do – that is to bear his experiences. This is a tall order, and it faces the service with the problem that staff must face unbearable suffering.*

Such extreme psychic pain can feel impossible for staff to bear, not only for what it represents internally for each patient, but also because of the way it resonates with each staff member's own defended psychotic aspects. It is likely, in such situations, that staff will also start to feel concerns for their own mental survival. For example, when I made contact with my patient who described animal semen in his mouth, I not only felt overwhelmed with more familiar emotions, such as sadness, fear and anger, I also found myself dealing with more primitive anxieties such as a nauseating disgust, and the fear I might sexually or physically assault this man. At the time I had no way of understanding my frightening emotions (in psychodynamic terms, my countertransference), but I have since wondered if my feelings of sexual and physical violence may have said something about this man's perceptions of his earliest experiences. I am struck by how far a mouth full of animal semen is removed from a mouth full of mother's milk. The repeated behaviours on Ward A of sedation and ward reviews could be understood as institutional defences evolved within the organisation to protect me from such frightening feelings, and therefore reduce my fears for my mental survival.

Glasser's views on self-preservative violence, discussed earlier, may also explain some of the attraction of sedating. There may be a strong self-preservative desire in staff to prevent therapeutic contact with patients by 'attacking' the patients' mind with sedation, because such therapeutic contact is sensed as dangerous for staff members' mental survival.

'Task drift'

The concept of the primary task can be defined as the task that a specified human system must perform at any given time if it is to survive (Bion 1961), and it makes a link between the phenomena of development and survival. Campling (2004: p.32) suggests the primary task of a psychiatric ward is 'to process suffering'. This primary task is common to many fields of healthcare, and would still be appropriate even if we were to conceptualise psychotic illnesses in purely biological terms, and consider such illnesses analogous to other chronic relapsing painful illnesses such as rheumatoid arthritis. 'Task drift' (Menzies 1979; Hinshelwood 2004) may occur on psychiatric wards because the dynamics of psychosis encourage both patients and staff to avoid therapeutic contact. Such 'task drift' results in the processing of suffering becoming overshadowed by the task of surviving the unbearable states associated with psychosis. I experienced a personal 'task drift' during my time on the ward; initially I engaged in the primary task of processing suffering, but I soon found myself unable to bear the work, and started to defend myself from the contact with patients inherent in the primary task.

An example of an organisational representation of 'task drift' may be my observation that some of the nurses thought my frequent talking with patients was unfocussed, and perhaps dangerous. 'Task drift' may promote the reduction of the role of the doctor away from therapeutic contact with his, or her, patients towards the more limited interactions of ward reviews, medication and risk assessment.

Staying with the primary task of processing suffering

I find both Wilfred Bion and Donald Winnicott's theories regarding the mother-infant interaction useful in thinking about ways in which staff may be helped to stay with the primary task. For Bion, an infant is able to make links, only once his, or her, mother is able to take-in his, or her, projections of raw emotional states, process them, and transform them. It is this modification of the unbearable projections by the mother, which allows the infant to feel able to receive them back in a now bearable form. This containing function of the mother eventually enables the infant to tolerate (contain) his, or her, own feelings and develop the capacity to think. If a mother is unable to contain her infant's projections, the infant experiences 'nameless dread' and is unable to develop the capacity to think.

Winnicott (1952, 1971) suggests that the basis of the mental health of the personality is laid down in earliest infancy by the natural techniques of a mother who is preoccupied by the care of her own infant. Initially, by active adaptation to the infant's needs the mother allows her infant to be in undisturbed isolation, only aware of his, or her, own subjective reality. The mother must bear the strain of emotions, such as fear and hate, evoked as a consequence of her infant's ruthless use of her in the service of his, or her, development. As the relationship progresses, the infant, in graduated steps, becomes aware of objective reality through the mother's minor failings to adapt immediately to her infant's subjective illusions. The mother's role is therefore to be only a 'good enough mother', and to supply the infant with graduated 'doses' of reality. However, if there is a severe failing of the reactive maternal environment, the infant does not experience this gentle disillusionment, but suffers traumatic impingements that violate of the infant's 'legitimate experience of reality' (Winnicott 1971: p.112), and lead to a threat of annihilation and a retreat from reality. Severe impingements may occur, for example, if the mother is so unwell because of her own mental illness and is unable to react to her infant's needs.

Both Bion and Winnicott propose that a severe disruption in the mother-infant relationship could result in a vulnerability to developing psychotic experiences. Such a severe disruption may have its roots in innate qualities within the infant (for example, an infant with a challenging temperament, perhaps because of genetic influences, or intra-uterine factors), or traumatic external events, or a combination of the two. It is of significance that recent research is once again proposing that early trauma may be important in the aetiology of some patients' psychotic experiences (Read et al. 2004).

Patients have a tendency to unconsciously re-enact their early internal object relations with staff, and it is likely that in inpatient wards, with patients suffering such high levels of anxiety, very early patterns of relationships will be recreated (Thurston 2003). Patients can unconsciously put severe pressure on staff to re-enact with them their early patterns of relating, and if some patients have suffered a severe disruption to the mother-infant relationship, these patients constitute a massive therapeutic challenge for staff. This is because it is very likely that there will be a tendency for such patients to put pressure on staff to recreate the disruption, which can lead to repeated experiences of abandonment, chaos and other emotional abuse. Staff may be required to stand firm against such pressure in order to try to provide a patient with their first ever experience of being effectively contained, or held in a good-enough manner.

Implications for groupwork on acute psychiatric wards

Groupwork inherently promotes therapeutic human contact between patients and staff, and between patient and patient. Therefore, this is a method that can be powerfully resisted by institutional defences because such therapeutic contact can feel as if it threatens the mental survival of patients and staff by engaging with the underlying unbearable mental distress. There is an extremely powerful unconscious pressure to resist the primary task of groupwork, which is to process suffering, because patients and staff fear the unleashing of unbearable states of mind. The challenges we find in initiating and maintaining groupwork on wards directly relate to the unconscious terror that such work holds. The difficulties we find in running inpatient groups, such as competing demands on the ward, unavailable rooms, absent patients, and sedated patients, stem in no small part from these deep unconscious terrors in staff and patients.

A psychodynamic understanding of psychosis also allows an appreciation of some of the specific challenges in working with groups of patients in acute psychotic states. The fear of the confusion and chaos involved in emotional disclosure is universal to any groupwork. However, the groupworker should appreciate that patients with psychotic difficulties can feel an immense terror that they will be forced to bear emotions that are unbearable. For example, Peter was a man in his early twenties admitted to an inpatient ward under the Mental Health Act with his first manic episode, in which he believed he was God and could save the world. Initially, he was very difficult to engage in any therapeutic conversation, and it was only after sensitive and determined input by the Early Intervention Team that he eventually agreed to give therapy a try. During that therapy we gently and gradually understood that Peter's grandiose beliefs protected him from the unbearable painful reality that he felt utterly inadequate in his demanding job and failing marriage, and that this current painful reality also deeply connected with an overwhelming sense of worthlessness stemming from an upbringing by his obsessive-compulsive mother for whom he could never get it right.

The psychodynamic understanding that psychotic experiences protect patients from unbearable emotions that are overwhelming in their intensity and complexity, can help groupworkers on acute psychiatric wards. Such understanding leads to paying particular attention to preparing patients for groupwork, to the structure and framework of each session, and to appropriately pacing the session itself (Manor 2000, and his chapter in this book; Birnbaum and Cicchetti 2005). A ward culture that encourages gentle 'chats' between patients and staff can be a crucial first step in helping patients move towards 'formal' therapeutic groupwork. A structure and framework for groupwork, such as the single session format, can be very containing for patients with psychotic experiences. Particularly so when the framework recognises the necessity of warming-up at the start of sessions, and cooling-down at the end of sessions. The thoughtful and flexible pacing of the emotional depth in sessions is crucial. This stance, when coupled with modest therapeutic aims, allows groupworkers to help minimise their patients' experiences of unbearable mental pain. Consequently, the understandable resistances to further therapeutic work seems to diminish too.

There are considerable emotional challenges for groupworkers in inpatient settings. Groupworkers are placed under immense pressure from the group members' psychotic processes and often groupworkers during a group will loose their ability to think and be curious. The primitive feelings stirred-up in the groupworkers (countertransference) are often bizarre and frightening.

Yet, if the mother-infant relationship is considered as a model for the staff-patient relationship, we can see that the key role for staff is to be able to be appropriately emotionally reactive to their patients, and to be able to survive and process their patients' unbearable suffering without escaping to the excessive use of defensive behaviours. A second role is also necessary; staff must not only have a way of bearing patinets' suffering, they must also have a way of understanding it, and a shared language to communicate it.

Groupwork with patients and staff is essential for both these roles. A well organised and resourced groupwork programme with patients creates a structuring of therapeutic activity that allows both patients and staff to feel safe to work with the frightening states of mind suffered by psychotic patients without fearing for their own mental survival.

A training of the ward staff in a psychological understanding of psychosis and group-processes allows them to better understand, communicate and contain their experiences. Hinshelwood (2004) considers weekly reflective practice with an external consultant to be a crucial intervention, and he believes this can evolve into ward staff developing into their own internal consultants. A weekly reflective practice group allows the staff to feel held and contained, and therefore less likely to retreat permanently into defensive behaviours to protect themselves from their patients' pain. A reflective practice group helps the staff to identify their inevitable defensive behaviours, and feel able to work-through, and learn from, them without feeling blamed.

Ronald Britton (1989), in describing psychotic processes, emphasises the absence of a 'triangular space' that allows observation and thought. He conceptualises a baby as initially aware only of a dyadic relationship with his, or her, mother, but that 'triangular space' becomes opened-up if the baby also can become aware of his, or her, mother having a relationship with father (or another primary care-giver). It is this awareness by the baby of mother also having a relationship with father, which stimulates thought, reflection and knowledge. Groupwork is in a potent position to help patients with psychotic experiences open-up triangular space among themselves because it encourages movement beyond a dyadic relationship by asking group members to listen to one another's experiences, and to observe and reflect on other relationships within the group. An effective group programme for patients, and for staff, can allow staff to maintain this triangular space within themselves, and among the members of the group, despite the influences of the dynamics of psychosis. The triangular space created allows thought in the form of observation, communication, reflection and knowledge. In such an environment, medication and patient reviews can be used in thoughtful ways that become helpful to the recovery of patients, rather than in the unthinking ways described earlier in this paper.

There is a danger in discussing care for patients with psychosis that we get caught up in the dynamic of omnipotence. Staff omnipotence can be an attractive illusion for both patients and staff (including groupworkers!). However, staff do not need to be perfect mothers, and indeed it is important that staff as good-enough mothers do at times gently and gradually disillusion their patients to help them slowly find a way back to reality.

Conclusions

Inpatient wards remain an essential component in the appropriate psychiatric care of our most disturbed and vulnerable patients. However, my experience as working as a junior doctor on Ward A, and recent research findings, indicate that some wards, at least at some times, are struggling to fulfil their primary task of processing suffering. I suggest that institutional defences evolve because both patients and staff feel unable to face and process the unbearable states of mind associated with psychosis. Groupwork inherently promotes human therapeutic contact. Yet, patients and staff, struggling with psychotic states of mind, resist such contact because it feels as if it threatens their mental survival. However, despite this natural resistance, groupwork for both patients and staff is absolutely essential in freeing wards from the dominance of institutional defences, and for nurturing and sustaining a therapeutic environment.

References

Barker, S. (2000) *Environmentally Friendly? Patients' Views of Conditions on Psychiatric Wards.* London: MIND.
Bion, W. (1961) *Experiences in Groups.* London: Routledge.
Bion, W. (1967) *Second Thoughts.* London: Karnac.
Birnbaum, M.L. and Cicchetti, A. (2005) A model for working with the group life cycle in

each group session across the life span of the group. *Groupwork*, 15 (3), 23-43.

Britton, R. (1989) The missing link: Parental sexuality in the Oedipus complex. In: Britton, R., Feldman, M. and O'Shaughnessy, E. (eds.) *The Oedipus Complex Today*. London: Karnac, 83-101.

Campling, P. (2004) A psychoanalytic understanding of what goes wrong: The importance of projection. In: Campling, P., Davies, S. and Farquharson, G. (eds.) *From Toxic Institutions to Therapeutic Environments*. London: Gaskell, 32-44.

Cullberg, J. (2001) 'The parachute project': First episode psychosis – background and treatment. In: Williams, P (ed.) *A Language for Psychosis*. London: Whurr, 115-125.

Department Of Health (2002) *Mental Health Policy Implementation Guide: Adult Inpatient Provision*. London: HMSO.

Duggins, R. and Shaw, I. (2006) Examining the concept of patient satisfaction as an assessment of patient experience in patients with a diagnosis of schizophrenia admitted to psychiatric inpatient units: Qualitative study. *Psychiatric Bulletin*, 30, 142-145.

Farquharson, G. (2004) How good staff become bad. In: Campling, P., Davies, S. and Farquharson, G. (eds.) *From Toxic Institutions to Therapeutic Environments*. London: Gaskel, 12-19.

Freud, S. (1924) Neurosis and Psychosis. In: *The Standard Edition of the Complete Works of Sigmund Freud, Volume 19*. (2001) London: Vintage.

Garcia, I., Kennett, C., Quraishi, M. and Duncan, G. (2005) *Acute Care 2004: A national survey of adult psychiatric wards in England*. London: Sainsbury Centre for Mental Health.

Glasser, M. (1998) On violence: A preliminary communication. *International Journal of Psycho-Analysis*, 79, 887-902.

Goodwin, I., Holmes, G., Newnes, C. and Waltho, D. (1999) A qualitative analysis of the views of inpatient mental health service users. *Journal of Mental Health*, 8, 43-54.

Hinshelwood, R.D. (1987) The psychotherapist's role in a large psychiatric institution. *Psychoanalytic Psychotherapy*, 2, 207-215.

Hinshelwood, R.D. (2001) *Thinking about Institutions: Milieux and madness*. London: Jessica Kingsley.

Hinshelwood, R.D. (2004) *Suffering Insanity*. Hove: Brunner-Routledge.

Jackson, M. (2001) Psychoanalysis and the treatment of psychosis. In: Williams, P. (ed.) *A Language for Psychosis*. London: Whurr, 37-53.

Klein, M. (1946) Notes on some schizoid mechanisms. In: *Envy and Gratitude and Other Works 1946-1963*. (1997) London: Vintage.

Main, T.F. (1957) The ailment. *British Journal of Medical Psychology*, 30, 129-145.

Manor, O. (2000) *Choosing a Groupwork Approach: An inclusive stance*. London: Jessica Kingsley.

Martindale, B. (2001) New Discoveries concerning psychoses and their organisational fate. In: Williams, P. (ed.) *A Language for Psychosis*. London: Whurr, 27-36.

Mental Health Act Commission (1997) *The National Visit*. London: Sainsbury Centre for Mental Health.

Menzies Lyth, I. (1960) *The Functioning of a Social System as a Defense Against Anxiety.* London: Tavistock Institute of Human Relations.

Menzies Lyth, I. (1979) Staff support systems: Task and anti-task in adolescent institutions. In: *Containing Anxiety in Institutions: Selected essays.* (1998, 222-235) London: Free Association Books.

Radcliffe, J. and Smith, R. (2007) Acute inpatient psychiatry: How patients spend their time on acute psychiatric wards. *Psychiatric Bulletin,* 31, 167-170.

Read, J., Goodman, L., Morrison, A.P., Ross, C.A. and Aderhold, V. (2004) Childhood trauma, loss and stress. In: Read, J, Mosher, L.R. and Bentall, R.P. (eds.) *Models of Madness: Psychological, social and biological approaches to schizophrenia.* Hove: Routledge, 223-252.

Rose, D. (2001) *User's Voices: The perspectives of mental health users on community and hospital care.* London: The Sainsbury Centre for Mental Health.

Sainsbury Centre For Mental Health (1998) *Acute Problems: A survey of the quality of care in acute psychiatric wards.* London: The Sainsbury Centre for Mental Health.

Sainsbury Centre for Mental Health (2002) *An Executive Briefing on Acute Inpatient Care for People with Mental Health Problems.* London: The Sainsbury Centre for Mental Health.

Shepherd, G., Beadsmoore, A., Moore, C., Hardy, P. and Muijen, M. (1997) Relationship between bed use, social deprivation, and overall bed availability in acute psychiatric units, alternative residential options: A cross-sectional survey, one day census data, and staff interviews. *British Medical Journal,* 314, 262.

Stanton, A. and Schwartz, M. (1954) *The Mental Hospital.* New York: Basic Books.

Thurston, I. (2003) Developing the therapeutic alliance in acute mental health care. *Psychoanalytic Psychotherapy,* 17, 190-205.

Weinstein, R.M. (1981) Attitudes toward psychiatric treatment among hospitalised patients: A review of quantitative research. *Social Science and Medicine,* 15, 301-314.

Winnicott, D.W. (1952) Psychoses and Childcare. In: *Through Paediatrics to Psychoanalysis: Collected Papers.* (1958, 219-228) London: Karnac.

Winnicott, D.W. (1971) *Playing and Reality.* London: Routledge.

Zubin, J. and Spring, B. (1977) Vulnerability: A new view of schizophrenia. *Journal of Abnormal Psychology,* 86 (2), 103-124.

6

Containing the uncontainable: A role for staff support groups

Ian Simpson

An infallible method of conciliating a tiger is to allow oneself to be devoured. (Konrad Adenauer)

The National Service Framework for mental health services (DoH, 2004) highlights the need for staff who are working within psychiatric services to explore the impact of the work on their general well being and performance. Two recent reports were published reaffirming the importance of this issue. The findings of both reports confirm that working in acute psychiatric wards can be damaging to a staff member's mental and physical health. *Acute Care* (Sainsbury Centre, 2004) and *The National Audit of Violence 2003-2005* (Royal College of Psychiatrists, 2005) both reveal disturbing findings. User surveys also tend to be highly critical of inpatient care. In one survey, 57% of patients said they would have liked more contact with staff, 82% reported less than 15 minutes per day in face-to-face contact with staff, 56% said the ward was an un-therapeutic environment and 45% said ward conditions had a negative effect on their mental health (MIND, 2000). The Audit of Violence report states that, '…staff were fire-fighting as they struggle to work with an increasingly unwell population, some of whom have a dual diagnosis'. This report also found inadequate staffing on wards with high vacancies and inexperienced leadership. In this context, it argues,

> providing a therapeutic environment can become impossible'. The extensive use of agency/bank nurses is highlighted as a problem by both reports. One respondent said: 'I feel unsafe dependent on who I am working with. Most bank staff are unaware of issues in mental health therefore it is often left to you as possibly the only regular staff to try and keep things safe'.

Rufus May, in his paper on the problems of acute wards points out that the National Audit of Violence has shown there are real problems in making psychiatric wards safe and peaceful places for both staff and service users. The report emphasises the need for more meaningful activities for service users. It argues ways have to be found to enable staff to spend more time in one to one contact with service users, 'doing the job they were trained to do'. I would question this assumption that staff are trained to spend time in one-to-one contact with service users. When it comes to helping people who are self harming, hearing voices or having unusual beliefs, I think nursing staff are often poorly trained to engage with these experiences. (May, 2005)

Working in an acute inpatient ward poses several intrinsic problems for staff. There are two basic and daunting issues that must be squarely faced: the rapid turnover of patients and the wide disparity in patient psychopathology. Most wards are characterised by rapid patient turnover. The 'revolving door' model means that patients (although there seem to be many who stay longer) will have an average stay of 4 to 6 weeks on the ward. This means that the therapeutic possibilities will necessarily be limited. Similarly, the wide spectrum of pathology present on a contemporary acute ward must be taken into account when thinking of possible therapeutic aims and objectives and about methods of working in this setting. A typical contemporary inpatient psychiatric ward admits patients with a wide diagnostic spread. Acute schizophrenia, borderline and other personality disorders, severe neurotic conditions, dual diagnosis with substance abuse, bipolar disorders, major affective disorders, eating disorders, PTSD, and situational or adjustment reactions are all likely to be present at any given time. Adding staff turnover, shift patterns, temporary bank staff and changeovers this means that it is always going to be difficult to maintain cohesiveness of treatment and containment. Similarly, in recent years, mental health services have constantly been restructuring their organisational models and processes and this undoubtedly increases uncertainty, leading to fears of lack of containment and raising the levels of anxiety in staff teams.

Thorndycraft and McCabe (2008), in their paper on team development and reflective practice groups, point out that

Constant exposure to psychological disorder can and does disturb mental equilibrium. This not only impacts on the individual's capacity to perform at an optimum level but also seriously impacts on the collective working relationships within the teams.

Dennison, in a paper on organisational burnout states:

Compared to other work groups, such as teachers for example, health professionals in general have higher rates of psychiatric morbidity (see for example, Tillett, 2003), and those working in mental health face additional risks of becoming ill or burnout (Snibbe et al., 1989). These additional risks are related to the often unconscious processes, such as projection or splitting, that can lead to a worker, or indeed the larger organisation, becoming deeply affected (infected) by the client group's pathologies. In extreme cases, the work itself becomes toxic' (Carson and Dennison, 2008).

The National Service Framework guidelines highlight that the quality of therapeutic engagement has a profound impact on the outcome of the treatment in mental health services. Whilst it is accepted that there are patients who are hard to reach, it is also suggested that effective engagement is inevitably a reciprocal process. As such, it is clear that blocks to effective engagement must also be understood as a manifestation of staff struggling to become effective members of the team in order to engage with and reflect upon the demands of their work with patients and within the organisation in which they work.

> Indeed, today's acute wards run the risk of being not so much un-therapeutic as anti-therapeutic (Fagin, 2001), reflecting poor staff morale. Acute wards tend to be seen as unattractive places to work compared with community settings. There is rapid staff turnover and, especially in the inner cities, extensive use of 'bank' staff to make up numbers. The consequent lack of continuity and commitment means that custodial, rather than therapeutic, values prevail. (Holmes, 2002)

In considering these issues it makes more sense to tackle the matter of staff welfare, safety and containment as a primary task. When staff feel contained themselves they are more able to function therapeutically and professionally with their patients, colleagues and also within the wider organisational structure.

The context

> With regard to the NHS mental health system, great care for health and safety is taken where there is a risk of exposure to radiation and/or physical infection. However, little or no account seems to be given to the risks of contamination from working with mental disorder. In fact, it is frequently stated by professionals that the nature of the work is actually not the problem. It is the widespread minimising – or even denial – of the need for appropriate resources for the processing and working through of the potentially damaging emotional residues of engaging in such work, particularly under stressful conditions. (Thorndycraft and McCabe, 2008)

Containment

Containment is a term often used but not always clearly understood. It refers to the process of psychologically 'holding' an individual – or a group of people – who fear that their own feelings are spiralling out of control and could overwhelm not only them but also those close to them. It cannot be achieved by offering bland reassurances. Rather, it requires actively offering an understanding of what is happening and demonstrating that the patient's anxiety or distress is not overwhelming but can be addressed. Setting limits, maintaining boundaries, and not attempting to unnecessarily suppress the patient's distress and/or disturbance are an essential part of the process. It is important to 'stay with' the patient or group and work with and 'through' the issues and the behaviours that arise. It is a dynamic process, which involves feeling, thinking, organising and acting (Bion, 1970). This is helped by staff being available and consistent, not reacting in a punitive or judgemental manner, and not rejecting or avoiding the patient.

In the mental health field, containment is a process that must be constantly attended to by the whole organisation and, accordingly, those staff, working in acute settings, have to be held and supported by robust and formalised structures. Ongoing training, detailed supervision of clinical work and staff support structures are integral to psychologically-informed practice. In the inpatient setting these are more important than any specific programmes or models of work. Regular supervision and staff support are the crucial ingredients in improving the quality of psychological care on acute wards.

The ward setting

A context is a space inside which something can happen. When we think of a therapeutic context we can imagine a comfortable room, secure from interruptions and extraneous noise where patients, individually or in groups, can be seen in a 'safe enough' setting. However, this room needs to be in its own 'safe enough' context (Simpson, 1995) and so on. Staff, working in mental health, need to feel safe and contained by their profession, their organisational support structures and also in their personal lives: in the widest social domain. Nothing happens in isolation. There is a complex relational field at work when we consider the notion of context. A facilitating context is more than just a room it is a complex system encompassing many variables and interlinked structures. An acute ward team must balance their clinical work with the demands of their personal lives, their interaction with their colleagues and their relationship to the wider organisation. They must hold the tension between these, often conflicting, pressures. If they are to achieve some sort of balance in this and maximise therapeutic potential in their work, their welfare and personal and professional health is of paramount concern.

The most pressing need of the psychotic patient at any point in time is to 'contain' the illness so that it does not become overwhelming, causing serious disruption or breakdown in their own or others lives. People experiencing psychotic episodes have periods of stability but may slowly or rapidly move into serious and severe states where they may be either at risk to themselves or to others, they may lose all forms of self-care, be prone to 'accidents' and altercations, and become completely disorientated and incoherent. Medication is the first line of containment for the psychoses because in many cases it quickly and effectively offers some containment and enables easier patient support and management. However, a theoretical understanding of group processes and how to work with these therapeutically can also provide an important basis for support and containment in an inpatient or partial hospital setting. A 'holding environment' (Winnicott, 1976) can be created by attending to institutional and staff needs as well as to the clinical aspects of patient care. In order to better understand this it is necessary to first focus on group theory and then on the 'context' within which work with patients normally takes place.

Group analytic theory and practice

We only know who we are through our intrinsic connectedness to others. As we 'become' we need to 'belong'. Human beings are essentially social. If the individual is the basic biological unit, the basic psychological unit is the small group (family). Our sense of self is formed through interaction with others. Language, communication and particularly dialogue (reciprocally relating – talking to others about ourselves and listening to what they have to say to us about themselves) is key. If a staff team are not talking to one another about the way their daily interactions with patients affects them, in both positive and negative ways, this will limit their ability to empathise with each other and with the patients in their care. For example, if a staff member feels apprehensive and anxious when accompanying certain patients on trips outside of the ward and is prepared to admit that this can often feel embarrassing and anxiety provoking, with an accompanying fear of not handling the situation appropriately, this sharing will inevitably resonate with the feelings of other staff members and relieve some of the individual anxiety evoked by this situation. If staff are not talking or checking out these issues with each other, how can they know what is shared or commonly experienced.

Language use is primarily a creative social phenomenon, an inter-active on-going phenomenon. This dialogic process is outlined by Ryle and Kerr (2002)

In essence, the dialogic approach replaces the ' I think, therefore I am' of Descartes with 'We interact and communicate, therefore I become.

Group analytic theory argues that we can only arrive at a sense of ourselves through our interaction with others. As John Donne said 'No man is an island.' We get meaning and significance from our relationship with others. The notion of someone having a sense of themselves in isolation from others is absurd and theoretically untenable.

The individual is an artificial, though plausible, abstraction: each person is basically and centrally determined by the world in which he or she lives: by the group: by the community of which he or she forms a part. Inside and outside, individual and society, body and mind, fantasy and reality, cannot be opposed: all separation is artificial isolation. The individual is a part of a social network and can only be considered in isolation like a fish out of water. (Pines et al, 1982)

In psychotherapeutic terms this means that individuals must be studied within their own natural/cultural groupings, particularly their family of origin. Patient's problems represent only one aspect of an intricate and complex group phenomenon. We locate patient's disturbance in some aspect of their life situation and interpersonal relationships. We see that psychological disturbances are located with the individual always in relation to others. This, of course, must include the treatment setting. The task of psychotherapy is, as R D Laing (1960) said, to help the individual find 'ontological security' by having a sense of being separate and autonomous while being intrinsically linked and attached to others. The optimum configuration for the individual is to feel a separate, autonomous person with something of value to give and also be able to receive something back in a balanced relationship with the group with which they primarily identify. At any given time this may be their family, friendship or work group. The aim for the individual is to feel a functional sense of security in relation in their group, acknowledging difference and living with a relatively healthy sense of self while not feeling powerfully overwhelmed by or excluded and rejected from the group. This 'ontological security' enables us to function and survive through life's ups and downs in all the interpersonal fields within which we operate.

It is important to say that this is not to elevate the group to the detriment of the individual. The individual, through active participation in the group, always remains the central focus. It is the optimal degree of liberation and integration of the individual, which is the ultimate goal. This is not achieved in a vacuum but in the lived context of daily relationships and in the search for meaning with others, significant and otherwise. Our families, friendship networks and our working relationships constitute this evolving sense of self. This process always happens in the context of others, within the small, medium and large groups in which we live and function. It makes sense to think about ourselves in dynamic, group terms and for us to explore interpersonal relations in that forum when things go wrong. However, while emphasizing the importance of the basic principle of belonging – and the wish to belong – there is another position, which cannot be ignored, which also needs to be considered. That is the wish to be private and separate from others, to have space on our own, to have our own identity and individuality.

Group analysis has always put great emphasis on similarity and difference and managing that relationship. The great fear of involvement in groups lies in the potential loss of self, of individuality and, in the extreme this involves primitive fantasies of either being overwhelmed and losing one's sense of identity in the greater mass of the group or of being found unacceptable and unworthy and being abandoned by the group. In both instances we become 'nothing', we have no sense of 'belonging' or of having any kind of meaningful attachment to others. We have no frame of reference, no sense of self in relation to others. This sense of self in relation to others is essential for our mental and physical health and welfare. We have a basic need to belong, to be accepted and valued, to be 'inside', to be a 'part of' the group as opposed to being 'outside', isolated and 'apart from' the group.

However, there is a tension between wanting to connect and wanting to disconnect, wanting to belong and, at times, wanting to be private and separate; a natural tension between the individual and society, the individual and the group. How we work out that tension, how we reconcile these conflicting needs constitutes the core material of meaningful social integration. In the language of self-regulation and self-organisation the aim is to shift to a more integrated, organised state, a new level of awareness, which optimises the integration of our individual with our social (group) needs. In the working situation, staff team members need to feel that they are respected as valued and valuable individuals within the team and that their individual work contributions are acceptable and effective in the evolving team working context. In this way they can feel an integral part of the team and fully involved in its dynamic developing processes while avoiding a sense that their voice has been silenced by powerful group pressures or being put in positions which result in them feeling excluded or isolated from the group. For instance, if one team member feels that their contributions are under valued or dismissed this may leave them feeling resentful and frustrated. This can often lead them into taking up a pattern of negative or critical responses to the contributions of others. This, in turn, can further ostracise them and result in them becoming the scapegoat for the group. Alternatively, a team member may feel a lack of confidence in voicing their opinions and largely remain silent while passively accepting the decisions made by others. An integrated group member should feel able to challenge others and be challenged without feeling either of the extremes outlined above.

The tension between the often contradictory needs evoked by individual and group pressures, also points to why there can be a powerful ambivalence towards groups, both from potential members and also within organisations. Group analytic theory and practice addresses these issues. When considering teamwork in the mental health field, staff support groups based on a group analytic understanding provide a unique situation that offers patients and staff the opportunity to interact with others and to share and explore the conflicts and anxieties that arise in interpersonal relationships in the working context. An understanding of groups and group dynamics can not only help staff and patients but also help us make sense of what happens in the institutions, which have been set up to work with these patients. It is a fundamental group analytic principle that individual, group, and social contexts are strongly interdependent. If patients are to feel contained, then the institution and staff members working there must be containing and be contained themselves. If the context feels safe and containing then this will optimise the therapeutic potential. Self-awareness and reflective practice is integral and a prerequisite, both at the level of the individual practitioner and in the staff team as a whole, in order to lower destructive processes, acting out behaviours and the likelihood of what has been called 'malignant alienation'. Holmes (2002) states that

> there is evidence that difficulty in the staff-patient relationship is a significant predictor of in-patient suicide. Watts and Morgan (1994) found that, prior to suicide, there is a marked deterioration in relationships between patient and staff, characterised by increasing emotional distance and hostility, a condition that is dubbed malignant alienation. A psychotherapeutic approach can help contain and detoxify the difficult feelings that patients who are disturbed inevitably arouse in those who work with them.

In addition, an active programme of group therapy for patients is also recommended in acute settings to enable a culture of group/community mindfulness. Of course, ward staff must be actively involved in this process by facilitating or co-working these groups with appropriate professional training, supervision and consultancy provided by psychotherapists trained in group work. This should include a weekly or twice-weekly community meeting (or large group) for all patients and staff, and regular small groups for selected patients, depending on their level of functioning and diagnosis. It is important that ward groups become an integral part of ward life. These groups, whilst having a group analytic understanding underpinning the work, should be sustained by a treatment model relevant to the patient group on an acute ward. Other authors in this volume address these issues, providing examples of this type of coherent and appropriate inpatient groupwork.

Containing the staff

One way to survive the chaos and mental pain that are the raw materials of mental health work is to batten down the hatches and to retreat into a defensive world of cynicism and mild paranoia, in which exploration of feelings is considered to be disruptive and dangerous when it happens. (Holmes, 2002)

It is very important when considering therapeutic work in an acute setting to accept that objectives must necessarily be limited. This is because this patient group can have great difficulties with even the most rudimentary socialisation processes. Staff must recognise their own limitations with these patients and accept there will inevitably be failures 'containing' some of them and they will need to deal with what this brings up for them, as individuals and as team members. Staff should have realistic aspirations of what is possible and it is essential that they regularly meet to discuss and explore the impact working in such a setting can have upon themselves and their colleagues.

Psychotic individuals can evoke powerful and disturbing feelings amongst other patients and staff members, which, if unprocessed, can lead to interpersonal difficulties at work. For example, burnout, leading to unauthorised absences, psychosomatic disorders and stress related problems, will inevitably require recourse to the employment of agency staff, with a considerable disruption of continuity and consistency of approach. The best strategies and techniques for patient care are likely to founder, when applied without attention to the staff group's own needs, feelings and conflicts as they are aroused in the treatment situation. It is no use conciliating the tiger if you are devoured in the process. Therefore it is essential that adequate and appropriate staff support, training and supervision structures are put in place. If this is not given the right amount of thought and emphasis then problems will be stored up for the future with the inevitable consequences.

Powerful feelings of being overwhelmed and uncontained are all too common in an acute ward setting and staff need regular support to cope and deal with them. Staff working relationships, particularly in this setting, can release primitive emotions like rivalry or envy, which can lead to competitive and defensive impulses. When these stay underground they can be potentially very destructive. These processes must be acknowledged and worked with to enable staff to understand the impact they can have on themselves and the patients in their care. They need to be openly explored without the fear of harming one another. It cannot be emphasised strongly enough that if staff are to help patients to 'contain the uncontainable' then they must feel contained themselves and they cannot do this without appropriate support and supervision structures in place.

It is now widely recognised that the most appropriate way of working with staff groups in mental health services is by using the medium of the clinical work and organisational pressures as the focus of the work. In this way staff members are enabled to explore the difficulties of working with a particularly disturbed and disturbing group of patients and also explore how the organisational pressures that they face can affect how they function as individuals and as team members.

Team development and reflective practice groups (TDRP)

Staff teams working in an acute ward setting need a set of clear, consistent and coherent objectives linked to patient care and there should be a strong core team identity, a shared and common vision of the work together. Each team member should feel valued by the team and valuable to the team. Team members need to be prepared to participate with others collaboratively and interdependently but also feel able to work independently, when necessary. Teams work best when members address defensiveness, anxiety and avoidance within the team. It is also helpful if team members can be open and honest about here-and-now feelings. By remaining and working with feelings and actively reflecting on the relationship between what is happening in the present and has happened in past experience, individuals gain insight about (and can take responsibility for) personal defensive barriers and maladaptive behaviours. For instance, in a situation when a difficult patient is creating particular management problems and there are a variety of opinions about how to deal with this being expressed, if team members can discuss the options openly, saying what feelings are being brought up from a personal perspective as well as from a professional one, then a wider and deeper understanding of the complexity of the situation can be achieved. This not only helps the team understand why the situation evokes certain responses from different team members but can also enable a shared creative space to be opened up in which a more reflective dialogue on how to manage the situation can take place. In this way the team can learn more about each other and how powerful, personal feelings can be evoked in the interactions with patients. Also, if a safer space to look at work issues becomes available, then differences can be explored more empathically and shared, mutually agreed procedures and interventions can begin to evolve and develop in a consistent and coherent way. The recognition and acknowledgement of an individual's real experience, in the here-and-now and how this reflects their past life experiences, in relation to current working practice, is a powerful motivator both for the individual and for the group when it is shared and discussed in a relatively secure, dynamic and reciprocal group space.

Experience has shown that all teams can benefit from an outside facilitator who provides a space for a Team development and Reflective Practice group (Milton and Davison, 1997, Rifkind, 1995, Obholtzer & Roberts, 1994). When considering the personal, inter-personal and systemic impact of working with mentally ill, traumatised and excluded or alienated patients, it is essential that there is an understanding of unconscious processes, like splitting, which can involve staff members finding themselves assuming polarised or extreme positions in direct opposition to one another. Gabbard (1989) offers several salient examples of the complexity of this process and how its' impact can affect staff in an acute setting. Unconscious group, systemic, organisational and social processes have an important effect on staff-patient relationships and then ultimately on the outcomes of treatment. Better understanding of these processes can enable the staff engaging with patients with complex mental health and psycho-social problems to enhance and strengthen their working practices. This is particularly important in closed, restricted or semi-restricted environments like forensic and acute settings where organisational dynamics can be complex and intensified with high levels of anxiety (Riordan, 2008, Carlyle and Evans, 2005). In the space provided by a TDRP group, the health and well being of the whole team is considered in light of the impact of the work. The interpersonal, systemic and organisational factors that help or hinder the establishment and maintenance of effective therapeutic relationships between staff and patients can be explored and worked through. An example of this would be when staff members avoid interpersonal interactions with patients by spending too much time in the ward office doing administration work. It may well be that there is a real organisational issue here, particularly as there is an ever increasing demand placed on staff for data collection and pressure to conform with other procedural, rather than clinical, functions. However, their primary function is to work with patients and, if this is a regular occurrence, it has to be discussed by the team and its' meaning and significance should be explored by the team together. There may be a combination of organisational, structural, clinical, group and individual factors involved. The most appropriate place to do this work is in a regular TDRP group. Alternatively, if a team member is becoming overly involved with a patient and if this comes to the attention of other staff members, this too must be raised and explored, preferably in the relatively safe space provided by a TDRP group. The staff member in question may be experiencing powerful personal issues evoked by the behaviour of the patient and they can be helped understand this if a non-judgemental dialogue can be established with colleagues. All of us working clinically in a mental health context, can be affected (infected) by structural and organisational pressures and conscious and unconscious projections from patients. These intense feelings towards patients should be seen as useful material for discussion in a spirit of open communication. Once this is acknowledged and accepted the personal and team tensions and pressures involved in the work can be reflected upon, thought about and hopefully worked through, mediated and contained. This will optimise the benefits for patients and staff and also enhance therapeutic and organisational objectives.

Supporting staff teams can be complex and difficult. The context and then the process involved in working within specific settings must be fully considered. If the context is an NHS clinical service and the process is delivery of a service to the public, optimising the effectiveness of the service is crucial. It is important to understand and acknowledge that a successful, relatively effective clinical service needs training, consultation, supervision, and team development structures to help and support the staff. If we expect team members to provide a safe and containing environment for high-risk groups with whom they work, we have in turn to provide a safe and containing environment for them. Provision of staff TDRP groups can substantially improve the quality of work and also enhance the health and welfare of staff members. A space can be provided where the impact of difficult cases can be discussed and staff tensions can be explored in a safe and confidential setting. More adventurous and creative work can be facilitated and it can help to establish a more stable environment for difficult work to take place.

TDRP groups should, as a bare minimum, take place weekly or fortnightly and should be facilitated by a psychotherapist with training in group dynamics, and they should be actively supported and attended by senior staff, including consultant psychiatrists and ward managers, if possible. They should also be facilitated by someone from outside the immediate organisational structure. Dennison highlights these aspects when he comments on the regularity of his work with a staff team:

> fortnightly is a minimum practical frequency, and I would strongly recommend weekly if resources permit. It has also been important that I was independent of the team's normal line-management structures, coming in as an external facilitator to provide a safe space for team members to air whatever they choose without fear of any impact on their careers (a study of the effects of trauma on ambulance crews by Alexander and Klein, 2001, for example, noted that crews were deterred from seeking help because of just such concerns over confidentiality and career prospects' (Carson and Dennison, 2008).

The role of the staff group consultant is to facilitate communication and dialogue in the group. If there are underlying tensions and strains within the team these need to be brought to the surface and therefore enable the group to make sense of them. Staff tensions, rivalries and conflicts can inhibit the potential for developing good practice. When these are addressed in a collaborative supportive environment the members have the potential to develop the quality of their work through better understanding of interpersonal and institutional dynamics and how these can impact on everyone involved, whether they are patients or staff members. For example, when a member of the team has the impression that they get no real help from colleagues in difficult situations or declares no one can understand their particular position. It may be that they are fearful that any request for help may expose their vulnerability and will be seen pejoratively as weakness. Alternatively, they might feel, because of their own earlier experiences in life, that others will not respond positively or helpfully or even understand their position. In some circumstances, depending on our own life experiences, it can be difficult to acknowledge feeling hurt and undermined or confused and uncertain about what to do. It is often not easy to share feelings in a working context. Some people might not feel able to ask for help or trust that others would be prepared to help. Similarly, many people may feel that the difficulties they experience at work are theirs alone. We would all like to feel we are coping and doing a good job and for others to value us as such. We may be afraid that acknowledging our own vulnerability will lead to being attacked, criticised or seen to be wanting in some very personal way. It is an essential task of the staff group to be able to create a 'safe enough' environment where these vulnerable parts, shielded by our defences, can be responded to, shared and understood.

In all groups/teams the basic issue is how to manage the balance/tension between the identity and needs of the individual and the needs of the group. These tensions between the individual and group and the relationship between them are played out in the everyday life of any working organisation. The optimum configuration for the individual is to feel a separate, autonomous person with something of value to give and also be able to receive something back in a balanced relationship with the group. That is not being overwhelmed or taken over by the group and not rejected or isolated, becoming unattached from the group. Fear and anxiety result from a loss of a healthy sense of self in relation to ones' meaningful work grouping either by being taken over and subsumed by the group or left out and isolated from the group. At some time or another, all of us are capable of finding ourselves in that awful place in our working lives. Facilitators need to be sensitive to this and create a setting in which this can be explored and negotiated by open discussion and dialogue. In any group situation, conflict is inevitable. It needs to be seen as an acceptable and appropriate expression of human behaviour. Indeed we often cannot move through a difficult situation unless we get into a fight about it. The problem is not having fights – the problem is not being able to resolve or repair them. Differences need to acknowledged and valued as individual contributions, while similarities are shared as common team aims. In staff groups where team members are required to work with very disturbed or chaotic patients staff group discussions, as Dennison points out:

> …frequently become heated and the mechanisms of projection and its associated splitting ('good' versus 'bad') may occur in the group. On some occasions the group itself may 'split' into two halves seeing completely opposite views and meaning in the case being discussed, struggling to find any common ground. Or one member of the team may find their view completely at odds and not understood by the rest of the team – leaving them feeling vulnerable to scapegoating or exclusion, or feeling they themselves have gone 'mad'. If the team is a 'well-functioning family' – in contrast to the patient under discussion's own original and usually dysfunctional family – it can contain these difficult and powerful feelings and survive. In fact the 'parallel family' analogy often crops up in sessions and is found helpful, being quickly recognised and understood. Further learning takes place when in most cases links are recognised between the form of the dynamics that have played out in the team, and the particular patient's early family history. (Carson & Dennison, 2008)

In these situations facilitators must help team members and managers understand and accept that:

- conflict is inevitable and necessary for change
- not everyone or everything is going to be ok (at least not all the time)
- they must hold the group's anger and unresolved tension (often expressed through individual team members)
- the effects of scapegoating have to be minimised and that attempts to locate the 'bad' in an individual or in the group are misplaced.
- the need to bond /belong with others and to accept that the resulting tensions when faced with personal differences are inevitable and will produce tension and anxiety.
- help team members recognise and acknowledge the underlying forces and processes which may be at work.

It is important to note that most staff teams operate within a hierarchical structure and the differences in status etc. must be acknowledged and worked with. For instance, managers and staff are both 'victims and supporters' of the organisation they work in, they can be both powerful and the powerless at times. The tension of being sandwiched between the clinical work with very damaged and disturbed patients and demands from management can often lead to inappropriate responses as attempts to reconcile these demands are made without reflection or consideration of the consequences on staff members. Similarly, once a team discovers a way of managing their situation that appears to work, they can come to rely too much on always managing that way. If the only tool they have is a hammer, then every problem they face becomes a nail. In this way the team becomes caught in processes of self-limitation, which inhibit change and development. Through this type of dependency, individual team members, at all organisational levels, can limit both their ability to adapt to new situations and to bring creativity and innovations to old ones. In other words, self-limitation becomes the main subconscious task of the organisation or group.

Although their primary concerns must be with the group, there are times when a TDRP facilitator needs to hold and contain individual members when there are issues they feel unable to express freely within the context of the group. Some things cannot always be talked about openly. As an example, a member of staff comes and says that another member is not fulfilling her or his duties adequately, but will not tell the staff member in question or the team leader. The facilitator in this instance may feel that it is not appropriate to press for the issue to be raised in the group therefore risking a potentially destructive situation, which would be difficult to resolve. It may well be hoped that the issue would eventually come out in the group if the group is 'safe enough'; however, staff groups are often felt to be very unsafe places, for a number of reasons already alluded to. This situation can leave the facilitator bearing and struggling with the tensions between the needs of the individual against the needs of the group. The main priority, of course, is to act on the information and explore the issue. Facilitators have to hold a situation like this to help contain the anxiety levels in the team and enable an opportunity for working through, in the hope that the individuals will be encouraged to gradually begin to say what they need to say to each other at some point later. In effect the facilitator, at this point, has to work with a 'virtual' group. Although they may, for a period, only be working with 2 individual team members the 'virtual' group is always there in the mind of the facilitator and the other participants. Thorndycraft and McCabe (2008) acknowledge this in their work with staff groups,

> Spurling (2005) writes that 'the provision of two different settings allows for difficulties, which might arise in one treatment setting, such as powerful negative therapeutic reactions, to be addressed in the other' (p.546). This principle applies in both clinical treatment groups and staff groups. For instance, as Bateman and Fonagy (2004) point out, the patient can take refuge within individual therapy when group therapy becomes frightening or seek sanctuary in the group when individual therapy becomes too difficult (p.200). This also applies to staff groups. The provision of one-to-one sessions by the facilitator under certain circumstances can significantly contribute to the individual feeling freed up in their decision-making concerning their career and professional development, perhaps in a way that line management would not achieve, due to the limits of their role and their particular organisational status.

This notion of a 'virtual' group can be helpful when working with a team when some members are regularly absent from sessions; it is extremely rare to get a whole team at sessions. Practical issues, like shift patterns, irregularity of consultant or manager visits etc, can complicate the ideal of full team member, TDRP groups and, in reality, it is not always possible to maintain continuity of membership or inclusion of all relevant staff members in all meetings. Members are on 'more important' work, etc, the medical consultant does not attend, the administration or reception staff do not think it is appropriate, the night shift can't be there and so on. In reality we are often only working with the 'virtual' group. But this does not mean that effective or important work cannot be done; on the contrary, in the 'virtual' context the team can be 'held and contained' without everyone being present at any given time.

In the past there has been a difficulty in translating group analytic principles, suitable for psychodynamic psychotherapy groups, into a work situation (Bramley, 1990 and Hesse, 2001). An acute ward is a very different setting and although group analytic principles are the mainstay and framework, which underpin and inform TDRP groupwork, they need to be adapted to take different contexts into account. For instance, the notion that every staff member should always be present and that for optimal and effective work to take place all communication has to take place within the 'openness' of the group does not adequately account for the reality of working in a contemporary acute ward setting nor does it mean that 'sub-optimal' groupwork (Zelaskowski, 1998), is ineffective. While this may be the 'ideal' it is not practicable and adaptations are required. In the example cited above the facilitator was required to balance the needs of an individual or a couple of members of the group at the expense of group openness because the context required such an intervention. In time, perhaps the group may be able to discuss and explore these difficult issues together in an open and direct way, as safety develops and dialogue and communication improve.

Many difficulties that arise in running staff groups are often the consequences of an insufficient analysis of the motivation behind the initial request for support. Requests may come from managers whose underlying motivation for a staff group facilitator is often a reflection of their difficulties managing their team and will therefore look for external help to compensate for management deficiencies. Issues around confronting poor practice, resistance to clinical supervision and conflict in general may be part of the underlying difficulty. Often poor line management is the problem. The consequent impact on staff may lead to poor morale, absenteeism, sickness, stress or burnout. There is the hope that somehow a weekly or even monthly staff group with an outside facilitator can resolve these problems. The team may be feeling helpless and powerless and this can create a 'rescue fantasy' with a powerful and unrealistic projection on to the facilitator. This is often present in on-going TDRP work and can leave the facilitator feeling helpless and powerless. However, if this can be identified prior to any engagement it is essential that it is taken into consideration when assessing the team's needs. An outside facilitator is not there to compensate for inadequate line management. When TDRP work is considered there should be adequate preparation. A questionnaire could be circulated to all team members, exploring expectations, who is for and who is against? Similarly, a meeting with the team, perhaps with some one-to-one sessions with team members, should be arranged to check out expectations, explore the hierarchical structure, look at the differences in professional backgrounds, different ways of working, who should be in the TDRP group etc. A thorough evaluation of the team and the context within which it functions has been undertaken prior to starting TDRP work. The appropriate and relevant tasks and boundaries for the team can then be discerned and this in turn enables the facilitator to more fully understand the internal and external institutional dynamics and in turn to 'hold and contain' these in their own mind and in the minds of the team members.

The Royal College of Psychiatrists recently outlined their Standards for Acute In-Patient Wards (2007) by grading them into 3 levels of importance. These are:

* Type 1 standard – Failure to meet these standards would result in a significant threat to patient safety, rights or dignity/or would breach the law
* Type 2 standard – Standards that an accredited ward should expect to meet
* Type 3 standard – Standards that an excellent ward should meet or standards that are not the direct responsibility of the ward

Unfortunately, while there are many Type 2 standards addressing the training, supervision and welfare of staff, these are almost exclusively focussed on the interests of staff members as individuals. Although there is an acknowledgement of their 'group' context in the recommendation that 'All staff have access to a ward based reflective practice/staff support group to discuss clinical work', this is relegated to a Type 3 standard. Also, there is no acknowledgement of organisational pressures in the recommendation and again this seems to reveal a basic lack of understanding about the interrelatedness and interdependence of individual team members upon their colleagues, their managers and the structures within which they work. Unless staff welfare and support is emphasised and established as a primary concern of at least, the Type 2 standard, then the importance of all aspects of the working context remains sadly unacknowledged and undervalued.

There is no question that resources can be scarce in the modern NHS and that other services with a more immediate clinical or crisis-led nature may be prioritised over staff support. However, if the basic underpinnings of the structure, the foundation upon which it stands or falls – the staff – are not seen as primary, if their welfare is not given priority, then this raises questions about the quality of the work undertaken and highlights the all too apparent dangers evident in the high levels of staff sickness, absence and distress which currently plague many inpatient units.

References

Bateman, A and Fonagy, P. (2004) *Psychotherapy for Borderline Personality Disorder*. Oxford: Oxford University Press.

Bion, W. R. (1970) *Attention and Interpretation* London: Tavistock.

Bramley, W. (1990) Staff sensitivity groups: A conductor's field of experiences. *Group Analysis*, 23, 3, 301-16.

Carlyle, J. and Evans, C. (2005). Containing containers: Attention to the 'Innerface' and 'Outerface' of groups in secure institutions. *Group Analysis*, 38, 3, 395-408.

Carson, J. and Dennison, P. (2008) The role of groupwork in tackling organisational burnout: two contrasting perspectives. *Groupwork*, 18, 2, 18-25.

Department of Health, (2004). *The National Service Framework for Mental Health – Five Years On*. London: Department of Health.

Fagin, L. (2001) Therapeutic and counter-therapeutic factors in acute ward settings. *Psychoanalytic Psychotherapy*, 15, 99-120.

Gabbard, G.O. (1989) Splitting in hospital treatment. *American Journal of Psychotherapy*, 146, 444-451.

Hesse, N. (2001) The function and value of staff groups on a psychiatric ward. *Psychoanalytic Psychotherapy*, 15, 121-30.

Holmes, J. (2002) Acute wards: problems and solutions – Creating a psychotherapeutic culture in acute psychiatric wards. *Psychiatric Bulletin*, 26, 383-385.

Laing, R. D. (1960) The Divided Self. London: Tavistock.

May, R. (2005) *Our Acute Problem*. Mental Health Comments -Psychminded website, June 2005

Milton, J. and Davison, S. (1997) Observations of staff-support groups with time-limited external facilitation in a psychiatric institution. *Psychoanalytic Psychotherapy*, 11, 2, 135-45.

MIND (2000) *Environmentally Friendly? – Patients' Views on Conditions in Psychiatric Wards*. London: MIND.

Obholzer, A. and Roberts, V.Z. (1994) *The Unconscious at Work: Individual and Organisational Stress in the Human Services*. London: Routledge.

Pines, M., Hearst, L. E., and Behr, H. L. (1982) Group analysis (group analytic psychotherapy). In Gazda, G. M. (Ed.), *Basic Approaches to Group Psychotherapy and Group Counselling*. Springfield, IL: Thomas, 132-178.

Rifkind, G. (1995) Containing the containers: The staff consultation group. *Group Analysis*, 28, 209-22.

Riordan, D. C. (2008) Being ordinary in extraordinary places: Reflective practice of the total situation in a total institution. *Psychoanalytic Psychotherapy*, 22, 3, 196-217.

Robertson, S. and Davison, S. (1997) A survey of groups within a psychiatric hospital. *Psychoanalytic Psychotherapy*, 11, 2, 119-34

Royal College of Psychiatrists For the Healthcare Commission. (2005). *The National Audit of Violence 2003-2005*. London: Royal College of Psychiatrists.

Royal College of Psychiatrists (2007) *Accreditation for Acute InPatient Mental Health Services (AIMS): Standards for Acute InPatient Wards*. London: Royal College of Psychiatrists.

Ryle, A. and Kerr, I. (2002) *Introducing Cognitive Analytic Therapy: Principles and Practice*. Chichester: Wiley.

Sainsbury Centre for Mental Health, (2004). *Acute Care 2004: A National Survey of Adult Psychiatric Wards in England*. London: Sainsbury Centre.

Simpson, I. (1995) Group therapy within the NHS: We all know about 'Good Enough' but is it 'Safe Enough'? *Group Analysis*, 28, 223-35.

Snibbe,, J.R., Radcliffe, T., Weisberger, C., Richards, M. and Kelly, J. (1989) Burnout among primary care physicians and mental health professionals in a managed health care setting. *Psychological Reports*, 65, 775-80.

Spurling, L. (2005) Combined therapy with borderline patients. *British Journal of Psychotherapy* 21, 4, 543-58.

Thorndycraft, B. and McCabe, J. (2008) The challenge of working with staff groups in the caring professions: The importance of the 'Team Development and Reflective Practice Group' *British Journal of Psychotherapy*, 2008, 24, 2, 167-83.

Tillet, R. (2003) The patient within – Psychopathology in the helping professions. *Advances in Psychiatric Treatment*, 9, 272-79.

Watts, D. and Morgan, G. (1994) Malignant alienation. *British Journal of Psychiatry*, 164, 11-15.

Winnicott, D. (1976) *The Maturational Processes and The Facilitating Environment*. London: Hogarth Press and Institute of Psycho-Analysis.

Zelaskowski, P. (1998) The suboptimal group. *Group Analysis, 31, 491 – 504*.

7
Groupwork:
The evidence-base

Chris Evans, Nick Huband
Tom O'Reilly, and Eleanor Overton

Introduction

Twenty years ago the other chapters of this book might have been considered to be forming the 'evidence-base' for inpatient group work. In the context of politics of health-care in the 21st century the place of psychotherapy in modern healthcare has changed and we now look for a different kind of evidence-base. Twenty years ago psychotherapy was associated with private practice, and patients were interested in self-exploration as well with 'cure' or amelioration of difficulties. In most Western countries today therapy is seen as part of health-care and it is expected to show the same evidence-base as other medical interventions such as cancer treatment. At the same time, a steadily larger proportion of therapies are delivered within 'third party payer' systems, either nationalised as in the NHS, or via compulsory, subsidised insurance systems. Over the last thirty years costs have rocketed and systems have faced problems reconciling the amount of money that people are prepared to pay (through tax and insurance) with the increasing costs of treatments and the costs of providing social care for an aging population. The 'evidence-base' therefore concerns itself with both cost-efficiency and treatment quality and range.

In this climate, one particular research design, the randomised controlled trial (RCT) has become an enormously influential 'gold standard' for evaluating medical interventions. Here, particular attention has been paid to enhancing, where possible, the quality of the RCT by 'blinding' both participants and investigators from knowledge of treatment allocation (the double-blind RCT). Banks of evidence are created by aggregating results from RCTs in systematic reviews, and double-blind RCTs are generally seen as providing the highest quality evidence. Whilst this gold standard position is justifiable for treatments such as drugs for cancer, for other types of health-care interventions such as the psychotherapies and social care, the case is not so clear. There are significant problems transferring the RCT model to social and psychotherapy interventions, and in particular that it is not possible to deliver or receive psychotherapy 'blind', producing the problem of the expectancy effect, of which more later.

In this chapter we are not advocating a rebellion or revolution against accepted methods of evaluation. Instead we will attempt to tease out the complexities in evaluating evidence for group therapy against the backdrop of the need for research in the current climate. We will explore the challenges for inpatient group therapists to be able to talk about research and evidence-based practice, and the need for them to read, learn and contribute to the research literature. However, let's start from clinical experience.

Relating inpatient groups to the research context

Vignette: clinical setting

Five minutes into the inpatient group psychotherapy meeting, Jon continued to verbally attack the staff present for detaining him against his will. He was outraged by his Mental Health Act detention the previous week whilst going about his business of buying a new car. His speech was rapid and forceful as he went on to boast about his riches and his close relationship with the Prime Minister. A nurse therapist interjected and, whilst acknowledging his rage, she also remarked on the silence of the other patients present.

After a brief silence, Delphine, another patient, said that she was sick of listening to Jon going on about his wealth and his friends and she didn't believe a word of it; the sooner he accepted this the quicker he would get out of here and off his Mental Health Section. The tension increased as Jon responded aggressively. He jumped up out of his chair and waved a fist at Delphine. One of the nurse therapists interjected immediately, asked Jon to take his seat, and reminded him of the group rules which prohibited violence. Jon looked at her disdainfully, pushed his chair out of the circle, sat down but continued to mutter angrily.

Another patient, Helen, said that she hated these meetings, as she felt worse after each one of them. She added that she would rather talk to the nice male doctor. Ravi said he agreed with some of what Helen had said, adding that he didn't like it when patients shouted at each other, like they just had, but he valued the opportunity to talk about the death of his parents and several of his siblings in the recent Tsunami. He described the extreme guilt that he hadn't seen his family for several years and, on hearing of their deaths, he had wanted to die too. Helen asked Ravi how long he had been here and he replied six months. He said that he felt really anxious about going home as he liked both the staff and patients, all of whom had helped him. He added that he would miss the opportunity to talk about the loss of his family and he was frightened that he could end up trying to kill himself again. A nurse therapist acknowledged his anxiety about discharge but reminded him that he could be able to continue with psychotherapy after his discharge. Ravi said that he knew this but he didn't think it he would feel safe enough to do that with someone else that doesn't know him like people here do.

The earlier tension had given way to an overwhelming sense of sadness. Delphine noted that Anna, who was sitting next to her, appeared very agitated and upset. Anna's legs were shaking and tears ran down her face as she agitatedly twisted her long black hair around her fingers. Delphine offered her a tissue, which she grabbed angrily and began wiping away her tears. Ravi wondered what had upset her. Through tears, Anna said that she did not want to be here either; she spoke of her shame and embarrassment that, yet again, she had ended up in hospital. She said that she was very confused and asked what day it was. Delphine said it was Friday and she then told her this was an inpatient group psychotherapy meeting, which happens on a Monday, Wednesday and Friday for one hour between 9.00 and 10.00. Delphine added that the function of the meeting was to enable them (patients) to talk about their problems that may have led to admission to the ward. Anna said that she remembered it from the previous time she had been here.

This fictitious vignette is reminiscent of the challenging groups that three of us have run. In the remainder of the chapter we will consider how the three nurse therapists who support this group and other supportive members of our multidisciplinary teams might use research to address the following challenges our fictitious therapists faced:

1. a statement from the general manager and clinical director that all therapies in the service must be evidence-based and the evidence-base for the group must be

presented to the directorate management group;

2. a request from the directorate clinical governance group for the team to carry out an audit, a needs assessment or a service evaluation project that addresses the work of the group;

3. an emerging wish in the therapists to have more justification when responding to staff and patients who ask why the group should happen, and in particular to have evidence beyond their own experiences of the group.

Many requests like the first two are driven by managers' personal and organisational anxieties. Although we may need to respond to such requests by seeking out evidence, it is important to bear in mind that sometimes they can represent incomprehension and sometimes envy of the engagement with the clients. However, just as we have to respond to patients' demands for explanations without becoming arrogant or despairing, we need to do our best to respond to external requests similarly. Sometimes it is enough to say 'we don't know the answers, but will try to find out.' Handling organisational requests well is part of the new modern way in which the 'outerface' (Carlyle & Evans, 2005) of the group is constructed and held.

We will now describe the 'research world', outline some different types of evidence, and summarise three very different papers that present evidence about inpatient groups.

The research world and its language

It is a huge step from the type of 'process evidence' that therapists routinely assimilate second by second in an inpatient group, to the evidence in systematic reviews of RCTs. However, it is also long journey from first sitting in an inpatient group, to running them reasonably comfortably, week in, week out. It is vital that some therapists journey into the research world to learn what it can tell us and to be able to criticise constructively some of its sacred cows and mistakes.

Research aims to share discoveries with a general audience. This wider dissemination differentiates research from clinical practice which aims to help individual patients. Like clinical work, research involves compromises, and in particular, balancing the feasibility of carrying out the research against the confidence in the results it will produce. 'Research' isn't easy to define. The Department of Health (DoH) defines research as the adoption of 'systematic and rigorous methods':

> 1.7 .... Services must promote innovation and its benefits whilst protecting participants from risk and waste. Innovation embraces a much wider range of activities than those

managed formally as research. Research can be identified as the attempt to derive generalisable new knowledge by addressing clearly defined questions with systematic and rigorous methods.' (Department of Health, 2000)

The DoH recognises a diversity of systematic evaluative methods including routine adaptation of clinical methods to new circumstances, clinical audit, local needs assessments, routine service evaluation, but the 'research' evaluation arena is dominated by RCTs and their aggregated results summarised by systematic reviews.

The position of double blind randomised controlled trials

Double blind randomised controlled trials (DBRCTs) have a strong claim to pre-eminence in evaluation of medical interventions. They are ideal when comparing one medication against another or against a placebo, where the patients who might benefit are clearly defined (by a diagnosis or type of problem) and where there are measurable, short-term outcomes. The randomisation of patients to two or more interventions is a way of balancing extraneous influences caused by differing patient characteristics. The double-blind administration of interventions whereby neither the patients nor those carrying out treatment know which intervention is being delivered protects against psychological expectancy effects. Purely knowing what the intervention is has a powerful effect on the outcome. Statistical methods allow powerful analyses of results, providing that no single participant's results affected another's ('independence of observations'). The combination of randomisation, blindness and statistical analysis have transformed pharmaceutical medicine and led to what has become known as 'evidence-based medicine' (EBM, e.g. Sackett et al., 1996) and 'evidence-based practice' (e.g. Reynolds, 2000) and increasingly the model influences funding decisions.

One of the finest early arguments for widespread use of RCTs is the short and very readable monograph by Archie Cochrane (Cochrane, 1972). That single small book, combining with the economic and political need to bring independent regulation to a burgeoning pharmaceutical industry, brought the RCT to the fore. Cochrane was less interested in double blindness than in randomisation and he was largely uninterested in statistical niceties. However, the book is a wonderful read if one wants to understand the background to the creation of bodies like the USA Food and Drugs Administration (FDA; www.fda.gov), the UK Medicines and Healthcare products Regulatory Agency (MHRA; www.mhra.gov.uk) and the crucial UK National Institute for Health and Clinical Excellence (NICE; www.nice.org.uk). Though a decade old now, Jadad (1998) remains an excellent slim summary of the RCT by an enthusiast but one who raises wise concerns.

RCTs and other research methods

Most quantitative studies use statistical analyses to test hypotheses. Outcomes in mental health often include self-report questionnaires but other measures include rates of readmission, self-harm, return to employment and suicides. Less commonly used are 'time to event' data such as time to readmission, time to re-employment and time to death.

Qualitative studies emphasise the interpretation of non-numerical data, such as social, emotional or experiential phenomena. Such studies do not produce effect size comparisons nor lend themselves to summarisation. However, qualitative methods can produce valuable information that cannot be obtained using a purely quantitative approach. For example, participants interviewed at the end of group therapy can throw light on which aspects of the therapy they found the most helpful. Quantitative and qualitative methodologies often complement each other and 'mixed methods' studies with both quantitative and qualitative components are becoming increasingly common.

Study *design* is sometimes talked about in hallowed terms also used almost reverentially of grandmaster quality chess play or abstruse mathematics or theoretical physics. However, design of health care research is not that complicated, is certainly not just an intellectual exercise and, though it undoubtedly needs training and an apprenticeship in research to hone the skills, it is not that difficult to understand. The key issue is that methodological design determines whether information collected in the study can provide reliable answers to the questions or issues the study was intended to explore. Good design is a marker of study quality (e.g. Khan et al., 2003, p.17) and we will discuss this later in the chapter.

In general good design features of quantitative research include the use of comparison or control groups, randomisation where possible, blindness (patient does not know which interventions they are assigned to) and double-blindness (neither clinician nor patient knows which intervention). These help isolate the effect of the intervention from random effects (errors) or systematic effects (bias or confounding effects). For example, inpatients in a group may derive benefit simply from escaping their stressful lives outside hospital and from good relationships with staff and other patients; any improvements that take place will reflect these benefits in addition to the specific benefits of the group or other interventions whilst they are on the ward. Research design therefore needs to compare the effects on patients of attending the group with the effects of other patients attending a control group. Random allocation to the group or control group is needed to remove allocation bias. Double-blind conduct of psychotherapy trials is rarely possible for practical reasons but to avoid bias, ideally people evaluating outcomes should be independent of those running the groups. Because running an inpatient group on a ward will affect the ward atmosphere and hence affect, to some extent, even patients who do not attend the group, randomisation of patients to attend or not *within* a ward is 'contaminated group' design. One solution to this problem is for the patients from one ward to attend the group being evaluated and these patients' outcome to be compared with outcomes of the patients from another ward (the control), with the wards allocated randomly to either condition. Such a randomisation across wards is known as a 'cluster-randomised trial' in which wards or even whole units are randomised to implement groups or not. The cluster randomised trial, arguably with much more claim than the individual randomised RCT to be a 'gold standard' evaluation for group therapies, is described more below.

A traditionally ordered hierarchy of different types of methodological designs are summarised in Table 1. Designs lower in the table are usually easier and cheaper to carry out but are more susceptible to bias. It is important to note that the reliability and utility of any study depends not only on design but also on execution. A well-designed RCT can still be biased if outcome assessment is not blind to treatment, something that is impossible to achieve for most psychosocial interventions (see more below). In fact, a well-executed non-randomised controlled study may produce more credible results than a poorly executed RCT (Ferriter & Huband, 2005). RCTs also have other problems; they are costly, there can be ethical issues in randomizing patients, and external validity can be poor, limiting how much the intervention reflects the types of treatments that can be routinely carried out in clinical practice. However, the RCT remains a crucial reference point for evaluating affordable and effective mental health care.

Research aggregation and generalisability

One problem with research is that any single study is always embedded in a particular setting. Multiple studies across relevant settings are therefore needed to demonstrate generalisability. As the volume of research in health-care has grown, methods to summarise the evidence have become increasingly important. The leading method of summarising evidence currently is the systematic review ('sysrev'). This has become so crucial that many hierarchies of evidence now place a systematic review above any single RCT. Systematic reviews get their name because they use systematic methods both to identify and to appraise studies and to attempt to assimilate ('meta-analyse') the findings. Systematic identification of studies for inclusion in reviews use large databases of published papers and, more recently, of controlled trials. Systematic reviews make public the selection strategies by which studies are identified to be reviewed so that it should be easy to replicate or to add to earlier reviews. However, it is

Table 1

A hierarchy[1] of study designs for questions about effectiveness of healthcare interventions (adapted from Khan *et al*, *Systematic reviews to support evidence-based medicine*. London: Royal Society of Medicine Press, 2003

LEVEL 1 EVIDENCE

Randomized controlled trial ('RCT')

Study type: experimental

Control group: yes

Notes: allocations are concealed; examines differences in outcome between intervention and control groups

Example: allocation to intervention or control condition done centrally using random number tables, with researchers & caregivers 'blind' to allocation.

Pros: minimises bias because confounders that may affect outcome are usually evenly distributed between the two groups; theoretically has good internal validity

Cons: may have poor external validity (poor generalisability); may be unethical to randomize; costly; poorly suited to exploring mechanisms & processes.

LEVEL 2 EVIDENCE

Experimental study without randomisation ('quasi-randomised study')

Study type: experimental[2]

Control group: yes

Notes: method of allocation falls short of genuine randomisation

Example: allocation to intervention or control condition done using, for example, allocation by ward or by nursing team.

Pros: as for level 1.

Cons: as above; potential bias since it fails to conceal allocation from caregivers and confounds allocation to the INPATIENT group with other factors.

Cohort study

Study type: observational[3]

Control group: yes

Notes: follow-up of participants who received an intervention comparing outcomes with those of a control group that did not

Example: researcher compares sample of inpatients receiving group psychotherapy with another inpatient group that did not

Pros: no ethical issues about randomisation; may have much higher participation than experiments; allocation may be impossible (e.g. testing effects of ethnicity match between patients and therapists).

Cons: lack of allocation makes attribution of causality difficult, always uncertain and often impossible.

Case-control study

Study type: observational[3]

Control group: yes

Notes: comparison of intervention rates between participants with the outcome (cases) and those without it (controls)

Example: researcher compares group psychotherapy 'improvers' and 'non-improvers' to see if rates of attending group psychotherapy differed

Pros: no ethical issues about randomisation

Cons: again, lack of experimental allocation makes attribution of causality uncertain though such studies often either started exploration of an issue (e.g. linking lung cancer with smoking) or were sufficient to make further risk that a link was accidental unacceptable (e.g. link between consumption of Thalidomide anti-emetic by expectant mothers and meromelia (limb deformities) in children of the pregnancies.

LEVEL 3 EVIDENCE

Cross-sectional study

Study type: observational[3]

Control group: no

Notes: examination of relationship between outcomes and other variables of interest (including the intervention) as they exist in a relevant population at one particular time

Example: researcher examines characteristics of all recently discharged inpatients, and looks for relationships between level of functioning, length of stay and type of treatment received

Pros: no ethical issues about randomization

Cons: extreme difficult allocating causality as above.

Pre-post study ('before-and-after' study)

Study type: observational[3]

Control group: no

Notes: comparison of outcomes in participants before and after an intervention

Example: researcher uses questionnaire to measure clients' depression before and after a psychotherapy group, and compares mean scores.

Pros: readily conducted; no ethical issues about randomisation

Cons: susceptible to bias; participants may have improved even without the intervention, might have improved more without it.

Case series

Study type: observational[3]

Control group: no

Notes: description of a number of cases of an intervention and their outcomes

Pros: readily conducted; may provide clinically relevant material and suggest topics for higher level study

Cons: lack of generalizability to other settings or cases; participants may have improved even without the intervention

LEVEL 4 EVIDENCE

Case reports

Study type: observational[3]

Control group: no

Notes: description of a single case of an intervention and the outcomes

Pros: readily conducted; may provide clinically relevant material and suggest topics for higher level study

Cons: lack of generalizability to other settings or cases; participant may have improved even without the intervention.[1]

Notes:

1. Different types of questions may require the use of different study designs. For example, long-term outcomes may be better assessed using an observational rather than an experimental design.

2. Use of different interventions among participants is allocated by the researcher

3. Use of different interventions among participants is observed (but not allocated) by the researcher

accepted that there is a 'grey literature' of results that may be unpublished or published in journals that are not covered by the main reference databases. Systematic reviews pay close attention to study design and some such as those within the Cochrane Collaboration (www.cochrane.org), restrict themselves to 'Level 1 designs' which are RCTs. Whilst this is probably appropriate for pharmaceutical interventions, the validity of this approach for psychotherapies is uncertain and it is almost totally illogical for evaluation of inpatient groups.

Systematic reviews classify studies according to key study characteristics. The acronym PICO is often used for the four characteristics considered particularly important in this respect: Participants, Intervention, Comparator and Outcome. Table 2 provides a summary of PICO and notes some other key elements of evaluation study design.

A final challenge for a systematic review is to summarise the results from many studies where outcomes may have been obtained on different measures. The currently dominant method is to convert results to an 'effect size'. A 'consumer' of research needs to be able to think not only about what a difference on a measure, such as the Beck Depression Inventory or the CORE-OM might represent, but also understand this 'effect size'. We will not go into detail about this here, but for continuous outcome measures, effect size is usually the numerical difference between the mean scores of those who had the therapy as compared with those who had the control intervention, divided by the initial standard deviation of those scores (Cohen, 1962; Cohen, 1988). Standard deviation is an indication of the size of the 'scatter' or spread of patients' outcomes. Effect sizes allow findings from studies to be aggregated and results for patient sub-groups to be contrasted, e.g. men vs. women.

We, and the therapists in the above vignette with their managers, are fortunate that a systematic review of inpatient group psychotherapy has been carried out. This is summarised below. It will form a central plank in answering the general manager's first challenge; 'is there an 'evidence-base' for the group?'

A systematic review of 108 studies on the effectiveness of inpatient group psychotherapy

Kösters and colleagues (Kösters, Burlingame et al. 2006) attempted to condense the findings of published studies of the effectiveness of inpatient group psychotherapy carried out in a number of countries between 1980 and 2004. These studies were found by searching three electronic databases of published literature and through enquiries on an American Psychological Association online discussion list for other relevant unpublished reports ('grey literature').

As with any well-conducted systematic review, inclusion and exclusion criteria were defined prospectively and given in the report. The inclusion criteria were empirical studies with adult participants and reported in English or German and all modalities of group psychotherapy were considered. Those where participants were children, adolescents or offenders were excluded.

A total of 108 studies met the inclusion criteria. Only 24 were controlled studies (Level 1 or 2 in Table 1), whereas 46 were pre-post designs (Level 3 in Table 1). A further 38 studies were not considered in detail because they provided insufficient information to allow an effect size to be calculated.

Of the 24 studies with a control group, 23 were of CBT and one was of psychodynamic therapy. Of the 46 pre-post studies, 18 were of CBT, 17 of psychodynamic therapy, 3 of eclectic therapy, and 8 of unknown modality. The paper's authors consider that this means that Gestalt and eclectic therapies were under-represented. It also seems likely that the studies mainly reflect settings in which patients attend inpatient groups for much longer than is now common in the UK.

To summarise the studies' findings the authors first calculated an effect size for each reported outcome in each study. These were then averaged to obtain a single overall effect size for each study. Finally, these effect sizes were combined using a statistical technique (meta-analysis) which weights according to the estimated influence each study has on the overall outcome. Although there are difficulties to be overcome when attempting this procedure for pre-post data, the authors were able to split the 70 studies into sub-groups and calculate an overall effect size (Cohen's d, see definition of 'effect size' above) for each.

The authors report that *'beneficial effects were found for inpatient group therapy in controlled studies (d = 0.31) as well as in studies with pre-post data (d = 0.59)'*. Here, values of d of 0.2, 0.5 and 0.8 represent small, medium and large effect sizes, respectively. Importantly, 85% of the controlled studies used a standard or alternative inpatient treatment as the comparator. The small to medium effect size (0.31) obtained for these controlled studies may thus be interpreted as a measure of the additional benefit of group psychotherapy, and the authors suggest demonstrates *'a clear additive value for inpatient group treatment.'* A further finding was that *'greater improvement was exhibited in mood disorder patients when compared to mixed, psychosomatic, PTSD and schizophrenic patients'*.

This review is a good example of how quantitative data from disparate studies can be combined to give an estimate of the effectiveness of inpatient groups across a number of settings and the effectiveness for specific patient groups. This approach has certain limitations, for example some experts argue against using meta-analysis in pooling studies where the participants, interventions or outcome measures are heterogeneous.

Table 2
PICO and other characteristics of quantitative evaluation research

Characteristic	Example	Notes
P: Participants	Psychiatric inpatients	May sub-group by diagnosis, age, sex etc
I: Active intervention	Inpatient group psychotherapy	May sub-group by modality (e.g. CBT, psychodynamic, Gestalt)
C: Comparator intervention (comparison or control group)	If a controlled study, this may be another intervention (e.g. individual therapy or a different kind of group), it may be just being on a waiting list for the group (only usually possible in very long term inpatient care), or 'treatment-as-usual' (TAU), i.e. not receiving the group.	If an uncontrolled pre-post study, outcome scores taken at the end of treatment are compared to those taken at the start of treatment.
Allocation unit	Traditionally this is by individual patient, but that creates a high risk of cross-contamination where peers on a ward attending a group create a channel for the group to affect those allocated to the comparator intervention. Hence it may be that wards are allocated to host inpatient groups or not, or even that whole hospitals are allocated to implement inpatient groups. (Both are examples of "cluster allocation" or "cluster randomisation" if randomised.)	Designed to reduce cross-contamination between groups and create "independence of observations" in the outcome measures.
Measurement unit	Again, traditionally, by individual patient. However, if one aim of implementing inpatient groups were to improve ward atmosphere then the measurement unit might be the ward either by using ward level data (e.g. ratings from CCTV observation) or aggregated individual data (e.g. staff sickness rates, staff and patient ratings of ward climate).	Must be pertinent to the aims of the groups and the evaluation. It is perfectly possible in large cluster-randomised studies to have analyses at multiple levels so in educational interventions there may be evaluations at school, class and individual levels.

O: Outcome(s)	Whatever component(s) of a participant's clinical and functional status used to assess improvement or deterioration	Examples include Beck's Depression Inventory scores, CORE-OM scores, discharge from hospital within given period, time to readmission.
Covariates and predictors	Variables measured either to reduce bias or noise that they may introduce or to assess their possible prognostic or meditational effects. As with outcomes, may be measured at different "levels", individual, group, ward.	Typically gender, diagnosis, age, initial scores on the outcome measure (if appropriate or measurable, e.g. CORE-OM scores are generally measurable at admission, discharge and follow-up in studies of neurotic disorders but might be meaningless if the patient were psychotic at admission). Time in the group is a complex predictor/covariate and the analysis of covariate effects is statistically complex and always needs expert statistical advice.

What's wrong with the current hierarchy of evidence?

There are four main problems with the current hierarchy of evidence for group psychotherapy. Before summarising these, it is important to note the host of other problems with oversimplifying the nature of evidence. This general argument has been summarised beautifully by no less an authority than Sir Michael Rawlins, the Chair of NICE in the UK since 1999, recently reappointed until 2011. The conclusion of his lecture (the 'Harveian Oration' to the Royal College of Physicians) 'On the evidence for decisions about the use of therapeutic interventions' (Rawlins, 2008) is worth quoting in full:

> Experiment, observation and mathematics – individually and collectively – have a crucial role to play in providing the evidential basis for modern therapeutics. Arguments about the relative importance of each are an unnecessary distraction. Hierarchies of evidence should be replaced by accepting – indeed embracing – a diversity of approaches. This is not a plea to abandon RCTs and replace them with observational studies. Nor is it a claim that the Bayesian approaches to the design and analysis of experimental and observational data should supplant all other statistical methods. Rather, it is a plea to investigators to continue to develop and improve their methodologies; to decision makers to avoid adopting entrenched positions about the nature of evidence; and for both to accept that the interpretation of evidence requires judgement.
>
> I am aware that those who develop and use hierarchies of evidence are attempting to replace judgements with what, in their eyes, is a more reliable and robust approach to assessing evidence. All my experience tells me they are wrong. It is scientific judgement – conditioned, of course, by the totality of the available evidence – that lies at the heart of making decisions about the benefits and harms of therapeutic interventions.
>
> For those with lingering doubts about the nature of evidence itself, I remind them that while Gregor Mendel (1822–84) developed the monogenic theory of inheritance on the basis of experimentation, Charles Darwin (1809–82) conceived the theory of evolution as a result of close observation, and Albert Einstein's (1879–1955) special theory of relativity was a mathematical description of aspects of the world around us. William Harvey's discovery of the circulation of the blood – as he described in *De Motu Cordis* – was based on an elegant synthesis of all three forms of evidence.

Whether this represents the start of a change at NICE is unclear. The arguments to retain the hierarchy for pharmaceutical interventions will probably be successful although even there the approach is not ideal for overall evaluation as it cannot be statistically powerful enough to detect rare but crucial side-effects that often take medication off the market nor is it powered to evaluate the difficult balances between good direct desired effects and common side-effects of traditional antipsychotic medication such as akathisia and tardive dyskinesia . However, for psychotherapies and for group therapies in particular, the door appears to have been opened for arguments in favour of other evaluative methods to be heard. Above all, Rawlins's paper shows the real problems with the current healthcare evaluation idea of a 'gold standard'. Whether this idea will be abandoned, as the monetary 'gold standard' was, is unclear. The monetary gold standard was replaced by 'fiat currency' in which value of currency is defined by government diktat within a global banking system of agreements (e.g. Bretton Woods, which had a weaker link to the value of gold). The Bretton Woods agreement was broken by the U.S. in 1971, replacing the value of gold with the value of the dollar. Of course, the recent global financial changes underline that no political agreements can be guarantees of certainties and nor was a 'pure' gold standard. However, expecting an illogical overvaluing of particular forms of evidence to solve the global (or Western) health care funding crises looks as much due for a change as does our previous confidence in our banking systems.

Specific problems with RCTs and the conventional hierarchy of evidence for inpatient group psychotherapies

Coming back from the global to the issues for inpatient groups it is probably worth summarising the four specific problems for conventional RCTs for our area.

The first problem is actually fairly general to psychosocial interventions and is that double-blindness is near or completely impossible to achieve. Whilst not fatal, this weakens the claim of fully logical allocation of generalisable causal effects on the basis of an RCT or multiple RCTs, for example 'inpatient group psychotherapy using interpersonal psychotherapy techniques works better for depression than treatment as usual'. The problem is that without double-blindness it could be that the therapists' belief in the therapy inspired them to help the patients to improve. To some extent this may not matter and it may be that therapies that inspire therapists and communicating such inspiration may be all we need. However, therapies, perhaps existential or analytic, which are less new and inspiring in their theory structure, may be followed by low morale at discharge but a steady improvement in self-belief over the months that follow, and this will not be picked up in evaluation by short-term outcomes, the norm in such work. As a result, current research design risks insufficiently dissecting the issues and picking up only the placebo effect and not a sustained and useful effect. 'Dissecting studies', including studies where therapists and researchers really have balanced loyalties to the therapies compared in the study are needed given that randomisation alone does not guarantee only one interpretation of significant findings.

Another key problem with RCTs of inpatient groups is of contamination: a group in a ward is likely to have a beneficial effect on the whole ward and may affect even those who do not attend. This makes it necessary to do cluster-randomised studies. As noted above, these are a particular kind of RCT much more suited to evaluation of inpatient groups than RCTs randomising individual patients within wards or units and, as we cannot escape hierarchies of evidence, the research design which, though very costly, has most claim to a 'gold standard' for evaluation of IP groups.

In a cluster-randomised study, units (hospitals or wards) are randomised either to have properly resourced inpatient groups or not, or to try comparing groups against some other intervention, say enhanced pharmacy support, money spent on the setting, or more individual attention for patients. After a suitable period of time the predefined outcome measures for the different settings (allocation units, see Table 2) are measured and the analysis is of those measures. Those outcome measures might include measures on the individual patients in the different units or might not, for example, they might just consider numbers of violent incidents or discharge rates by ward, as opposed to individual changes.

That links to a further problem, that inpatient groups are often as much about the setting as they are about direct therapeutic action. They are sometimes considered to have more of an effect on the ward setting than on the individual participants. The differences between groups may be as much a function of anti-group dynamics in the ward or institution (Nitsun, 1996) as they are a function of the group itself. If one accepts arguments that a group's effect on the ward culture is its primary effect, and also takes into account the fact that a group can itself be crippled by, or dramatically enhanced by ward culture, then this dramatically changes the models needed to evaluate the impact of ward groups. Sociological and anthropological theories, based largely but not entirely on qualitative research suggest such concerns are valid. Taking this into account then the quantitative evaluation designs that would give power to explore this are again cluster randomisation ones but now also require evaluation of the predictive or covariate effects of ward culture for which there are not yet widely accepted measures.

The final problem is with the statistics of the usual RCT when allocation is by individual and not cluster-randomised. In this situation, all members in the group together, arguably even previous members of the group who later members have never met, have effects on the way the group functions, affecting the other and later group members. This violates the assumption of 'independence of observations' underpinning standard statistical methods of analysing differences between conditions. The model of independence of members in groups is most clearly violated in non-didactic and non-educational groups which are based on interpersonal communication, including most interpersonal, humanistic, experiential, systemic, and group analytic groups. Whilst cluster randomisation and careful analysis of individual change both at the group and the individual level go some way to help this problem, if impacts on the culture of a ward take months or even a year or so to develop following the start of a group in which patients may attend for only a few sessions on average, then we may be using the wrong time model of the group altogether even in a cluster-randomised trial as currently usually defined and funded. A full psychological model would need to take into account the fact that inpatient groups can take time to establish and reach maturity and therapeutic power, and the fact that groups may fluctuate markedly, for example with changes in ward staff, individual members' major life events or catastrophes.

We have been unable to locate a single cluster-randomised study of inpatient groups. Whilst this does not mean there are no published accounts of such studies or that any such studies are not under way, the reality is that there is little of this 'gold standard evidence-base' for or against inpatient group work. This is a problem as organisations tend, wrongly, to equate lack of evidence of utility with evidence that something has no utility. However, there is a silver cloud, which is that we can look at the evidence there is, which may not be reviews of gold standard cluster RCTs, but is not without value. It also means that we can consider how those of us delivering inpatient groups might start to develop more of an evidence-base by trading information and improving our ability to share information about such groups.

Back to the clinical setting

None of this should be used nihilistically. Although many of the RCTs that have been carried out are crying out for reanalyses, they provide a referential base against which we should evaluate our own groups where possible. We need to gather evidence and build the arguments for the development of good measures of group processes, ward culture and for cluster-randomised trials.

In this spirit the therapists in our vignette wanted to be able to say something constructive to the directorate management committee about the evidence-base for inpatient groups, and to make specific suggestions for going about this that the directorate clinical governance group might support. They felt that mixed quantitative and qualitative data collection would be most appropriate but were uncertain what might help them explore questions pertinent to them, their political situation and the group. As the therapists might have done, we scoured bibliographic databases for studies of inpatient groups that might give us models to follow or develop. We found three non-experimental studies that are summarised below to give a flavour of the range of possibilities. It must be said that we have been surprised how little work we found on inpatient groups from the enormous range of possible mixed and qualitative methods.

Non-experimental studies

Sytema and Bout (2006)

Set in the Netherlands, this study considers the outcome of an inpatient group treatment programme for couples. Treatment was intensive and followed a fixed weekly protocol for 7 weeks, 24 hours per day. Treatment aimed to improve communication and problem solving techniques. It included skills therapy and individual therapy for psychiatric problems as well as the inpatient groups. Six groups of couples were treated per year. Each group included five couples. From September 1991 to March 2001, 257 couples started treatment in 57 groups. Only five couples did not complete the entire programme. Couples were recruited on the basis of having one of the following: (1) one spouse having a psychiatric problem (29%); (2) a major marital problem (23%); or (3) a combined psychiatric and marital problem (48%). ICD-10 diagnoses were made, where appropriate, by the team psychiatrist.

Outcome was assessed using two self-report instruments: the Dutch version of the Symptom Check List (SCL-90) and the Interactional Problem Solving Inventory (IPSI). These outcome measures were completed routinely on admission, at discharge and at follow-up six and eighteen months later. The mean total scores per couple were used for analysis.

Results

Of 257 couples starting the therapy only five (2%) failed to complete it. Follow-up data were available for 67% of couples. The data showed significant improvement on both SCL-90 and IPSI from baseline to 18 months follow-up in all three groups. The three categories of initial problems (1 to 3 above) did not predict differing improvement on the SCL-90 though the largest changes were found in the group with marital problems only. It was also noted 'although the couples improve on the IPSI, they do not reach normal population levels' (p.399).

Pros/Cons of this study

This is the only inpatient couple therapy service in the Netherlands and probably in the world so all information is useful. It is clearly a very expensive therapy and achieves a very low dropout rate. Though final follow-up data were only available for 67% of couples at the 18-month follow-up, such a duration of follow-up is excellent and not widely attempted and results from 67% of couples are clearly helpful. The results show useful improvements for the majority of couples but by no means all and without a control group of any kind it is hard to evaluate the specific benefit of the complex intervention. Perhaps the most important weakness in the study is that as the authors concluded, 'We do not know which elements work and which could be omitted from the programme' (p.402). This is a disarmingly honest but disappointing conclusion for such a complex and multifaceted intervention.

Reddon et al (1999)

Reddon et al. (1999) examined the importance of Yalom's twelve Therapeutic Factors (TFs) as identified by 100 male sex offenders pre-discharge after they had been involved in an inpatient group psychotherapy programme. Each participant had been involved in 32-35 hours of group therapy per week, for a period of between 6 and 18 months. Treatment duration depended on individual progress and included groups focusing on recognising cognitive distortions and restructuring patterns of thinking to prevent re-offending. Other groups covered psychoeducational topics such as anger-management and assertiveness training. The 12 Therapeutic Factors were identified using the 60-item Yalom Card Sort. Participants were asked to sort the 60 items into seven categories ranging from 1 (most helpful) to 7 (least helpful). Rankings of factors were correlated with treatment length, offender age and IQ, and victim age and gender to see if these were associated with any factors being given particularly high or low ranking. In addition, the results were compared with Yalom's sample of psychiatric outpatients rating outpatient groups.

Results

The sex offender group ranked 'Catharsis', 'Self-Understanding' and 'Group Cohesiveness' as the top three TFs and 'Altruism', 'Guidance' and 'Identification' as the bottom three. The ranking of 'Instillation of hope' decreased as the length of treatment increased. Older offenders ranked 'Instillation of hope' higher and 'Existential factors' lower than younger offenders. 'Instillation of hope' showed significant negative correlation with IQ and 'Self-understanding' correlated positively. Victim age was not significantly related to any therapeutic factors.

The sex-offenders' rankings were similar to previously reported rankings from psychiatric outpatients for 10 of the 12 TFs. However, sex-offenders consider 'Family re-enactment' to be more important and 'Interpersonal learning' to be less important than did the psychiatric sample.

Pros/Cons of this study

On the positive side, as the study's authors note: 'the importance of various therapeutic factors in the treatment of sex offenders involved in psychotherapy had never been documented' (p.93), however, all participants had engaged in a single programme in one Canadian hospital so results might not generalise. The study had a comparison group, but this was not a control group, as the groups were not matched in any way. The correlations between TF rankings and some variables and the lack of correlations with other variables are interesting, but without a theoretical structure within which to understand any therapeutic importance of these findings it is hard to distil much that helps either clinical work or future research from this.

Sigmund Karterud (1989)

The basis for this Norwegian study (Karterud, 1989) is his statement that Bion's (Bion 1961) phenomenology and metapsychology of 'basic assumptions groups' (*BA fight/flight, BA dependency* and *BA pairing*) is probably the most cited theory in group psychotherapy literature and that identifying basic assumption phenomena is thought to be an easy task resulting in therapist considering reliability and quantitative measures unnecessary. However, Karterud is critical of earlier studies of BA states in groups challenges the validity of studies that point to BA pairing being closely associated with fight/flight than dependency. He is also critical of Bion's use of Kleinian theory to BA states and argues that Kohut's Self- Psychology model provides a more plausible frame of reference.

The study and method

Karterud observed groups as a non-participative observer and the groups were audiotaped and subsequently the speech turns coded. The data came from 75 sessions of six inpatient groups involving 91 patients. The groups had multiple group leaders, lasted for 45 minutes and were held 3 to 5 times per week. Using his 'Group Emotionality Rating System', he classified 29,850 verbal statements into categories of: dependency, fight, flight, pairing and neutrality. In addition he categorised the statements as either an isolated emotional expression or a contribution to an emotionally dominating group experience (basic assumption). At the session level he and his colleagues used group focal conflict analysis to determine identifiable group conflict, resolution and the predominant relationship expressed in the conflict. The first 24 sessions were researched co-jointly with three other researchers. On establishing adequate reliability, Karterud analysed the remaining 51 sessions. Forty-one sessions were classified as fight/flight, ten as dependency and 24 were classified as 'pseudo-groups'. None was a purely pairing group. Karterud reports inter-rater agreement on the statement categorisation (but not the session categorisation), sample patterns of rates of fight, pairing and dependency statements within a session, distributions of the numbers of statements by category across the 75 sessions and some correlations between categories.

Results

The results are hard to summarise but Karterud suggests that more than 20 fight statements per 45 minutes indicated a BA fight/flight group; that more than 15-20 pairing statements per 45 minutes indicated BA pairing and that a fight/dependency statement ratio lower than 0.50 suggests BA dependency. He noted that only ten sessions were BA dependency giving little detail on that group state and he notes that pairing statements were more frequently observed in combination with *fight/flight groups* than *dependency groups*

He argues that these findings confirm the superiority of a self psychology over Bion's own Kleinian model of group processes.

Pros/Cons of the Study

The pros were that patients were diagnosed according to DSM-III criteria, there were direct group observations, attention to reliability of categorisation and a mixed method. The cons were the small number of dependency group sessions (n=10) compared to the number of fight/flight group sessions (n=41). Also it was not at all clear that the model being applied was the only or even necessarily the best way to understand the processes in the groups, and this makes the conclusion less convincing than it might have been.

*

All three of the above studies are of forms of inpatient group therapy involving considerable resources and all the groups are far from typical of the main IP groups run in UK NHS settings. Interestingly, all three are heavily quantitative despite moving away from the experimental evaluative design. The first illustrates a collaboration between a sociologist and the psychotherapist who was the head of the couple therapy service. It has impressive duration of follow-up and detailed statistics but throws little light on the experience of the multifaceted intervention. The second has a quasi-experimental component; comparing the sex-offender patients' views with those of non-offender psychiatric outpatients and also looking at how variables within the sex-offender sample correlated with the rankings of the Therapeutic Factors. This study seems to produce few clear messages for clinicians or researchers. The last study seems clear in suggesting that more work is needed and casts doubt on the Bion basic assumptions theory of groups. Though fascinating, it begs many questions about the sufficiency of the classification and whether this really tests Bion's model.

Despite these reservations as well as because of them, we hope to encourage the therapists to carry out process and outcome research into group therapy. Since there are no clear national or general guidelines about targets for such inpatient groups any audit would have to work to a local standard. Examples of standards and targets that could be used in such an audit are the proportion of the patients who attend the group, the proportion who remain in the group for its duration, and whether patients who attended seem engaged. This last idea is an example of something that is theoretically crucial but hard to quantify, and perhaps best explored with qualitative as opposed to quantitative methods. Despite this, an audit that used agreed criteria and ratings from all therapists of all attenders, made independently immediately after the group before discussion, could be used to monitor this.

A local needs assessment might look at how many patients could attend a group but do not do so, and further it could explore patients' and ward staff's views about why some patients do not attend. Routine internal service evaluation could involve monitoring attendance against possible attendance without setting a target, in other words doing an exploration rather than a true audit. Immediate pre-discharge interviews could be carried out with patients to explore their thoughts about many aspects of their admissions including the option of the group, and this could provide new insights into people's experiences of admissions and the group. Carrying out this kind of work can help the therapists' who want to be able to say more to other staff and patients about reasons for attending the group, on top of studies such as that of Kösters et al (*op cit.*).

Although the aim of such small research projects would be to inform the ward and the directorate, such work may well be of wider interest even if not providing clear and definite 'generalisability' hence such work, done well, might be suitable for publication provided that patients' confidentiality is clearly absolutely protected or that their consent has been obtained for publication. When such work becomes formal research is another important issue. In UK health and social care and in most Western countries, formal research needs some form of research ethical clearance. Wise practitioners will get as much advice from their Trust R&D support and their managers as possible.

The argument about the limitations of RCTs that we have attempted to delineate have led to the argument that we not only need evidence-based practice (EBP) based on RCTs and other related high quality studies that may lack generalisability to routine clinical practice, but that we also need complementary 'practice-based evidence' (PBE: Margison, Barkham et al., 2000). Our suggestions for the types of studies therapists can carry out illustrates that PBE extends from small process-type research to more formal research studies. Within this emerging complementary model of EBP and PBE it is crucial to recognise that no research evaluations start without good case reports or case series (if only because these are needed in order to be able to successfully apply for funding for intensive research). Few if any RCTs of psychotherapies, even showing strong effects, will clarify which aspects of the intervention is the therapeutic element. Hence most RCTs highlight a need for qualitative work and dissection of who appears to benefit and who does not benefit in order that clinicians can make use of the findings to be able to improve their work.

Discussion

We hope this chapter will encourage inpatient group therapists to interest themselves in research, read more about it, start local practice-based evidence projects and perhaps move on to develop a thread of research in their careers.

None of the research papers described here provides definitive evaluations of inpatient group psychotherapy nor clarity about how it might achieve good effects. One reading of Kösters, Burlingame et al. 2006 is that as all but one of the controlled studies were of inpatient CBT groups, the only evidence that exists is for CBT groups. However, few of those studies were randomised, and most were of groups of longer duration than practised on NHS acute wards. Furthermore, as we hope we have convinced the reader by now, the only arguable 'gold standard' evaluation of inpatient groups is a cluster randomised trial and there seem to be none of those and even those would beg many questions. Hence it is extremely premature to close that argument and the need for much more research is clear.

Psychotherapies, and inpatient group psychotherapies, have been hampered in developing their research-base partly because in the UK and elsewhere, therapists are an informal profession made up of people from a wide variety of backgrounds. The mental health core professions (including psychiatry, psychology, nursing, occupational therapy, social work) vary markedly in the amount and style of research teaching in their trainings. Graduates with sociology or anthropology degrees may have the best core training to research inpatient group work but unless one had the kind of research training that psychologists receive (clinical, forensic or counselling), a therapist seeking a serious research component to their career is well advised to read excellent introductory books on psychotherapy research such as McLeod (2001, 2003) Cooper (2008) and the overarching review of RCTs and reviews by Roth and Fonagy (2005) and ideally find a research methods masters course and get funding to attend it.

Despite some popular fantasies, research, like most human activities is itself a group or networking activity and not an individualistic one. Support for research should be sought from employers or by joining organisations that can help connect people with other researchers. The Society for Psychotherapy Research (www.spr.org.uk) is a good starting point. Its conferences are friendly places to start networking, as are the BACP, BABCP, UKCP and BPC research conferences. One idea gaining momentum in this area is that of Practice Research Networks (e.g. Audin, Mellor-Clark et al. 1999). Art Therapists in the UK have led the way in developing their ATPRN (see www.baat.org/atprn.html). A final resource as one develops formal research ideas is the NHS network of 'Research Design Services' (see www.trentrdsu.org.uk or search for your local equivalent.)

References

Audin, K.J. Mellor-Clark, J. Barkham, M., Margison, F., McGrath, G., Lewis, S., Cann, L., Duffy, J. and Parry, G. (2001) Practice research networks for effective psychological therapies. *Journal of Mental Health*, 10, 3, 241-251.

Bion, W.R. (1961) *Experiences in groups and other papers*. London: Tavistock/Routledge.

Carlyle, J. and Evans, C. (2005) Containing containers: attention to the 'innerface' and 'outerface' of groups in secure institutions. *Group Analysis*, 38, 3, 395-408.

Cochrane, A.L. (1972) *Effectiveness and efficiency. Random reflections on health services*. London, Nuffield Provincial Hospitals Trust.

Cohen, J. (1962) The statistical power of abnormal-social psychological research: a review. *Journal of Abnormal and Social Psychology*, 65, 3, 145-153.

Cohen, J. (1988) *Statistical power analysis for the behavioral sciences*. Hillsdale, NJ, Lawrence Earlbaum Associates.

Cooper, M. (2008) *Essential research findings in Counselling and Psychotherapy: the facts are friendly*. London, SAGE.

Department of Health (2000) *Research Governance Framework for Health and Social Care*. London, Department of Health.

Ferriter, M. and Huband, N. (2005) Does the non-randomized controlled study have a place in the systematic review? A pilot study. *Criminal Behaviour and Mental Health*, 15, 2, 111-20.

Jadad, A. (1998) *Randomised controlled trials*. London, BMJ.

Karterud, S. (1989) A study of Bion's basic assumption groups. *Human Relations*, 42, 4, 315-335.

Khan, K.S., Kunz, R., Kleijnen J. and Antes, G. (2003) *Systematic reviews to support evidence-based medicine*. London: Royal Society of Medicine Press.

Kösters, M., Burlingame, G.M., Nachtigall, C. and Strauss, B. (2006) A meta-analytic review of the effectiveness of inpatient group psychotherapy. *Group Dynamics: Theory, Research, and Practice*, 10, 2, 146-163.

Margison, F.R., Barkham, M.Evans, C. McGrath, G. Mellor-Clark, J. , Audin, K., and Connell, J. (2000) Measurement and psychotherapy: Evidence-based practice and practice-based evidence. *British Journal of Psychiatry*, 177, 8, 123-130.

McLeod, J. (2001) *Qualitative research in counselling and psychotherapy*. London, SAGE.

McLeod, J. (2003) *Doing counselling research*. London, SAGE.

Nitsun, M. (1996) *The anti-group. Destructive forces in the group and their creative potential*. London, Routledge.

Rawlins, M. (2008) De testimonio: on the evidence for decisions about the use of therapeutic interventions. *Lancet*, 372, 9656, 2152-61.

Reddon, J.R., Payne, L.R., and Starzyk, K.B. (1999) Therapeutic factors in group treatment evaluated by sex offenders: a consumers' report. *Journal of Offender Rehabilitation*, 28, 3/4, 91-101.

Reynolds, S. (2000) Evidence based practice and psychotherapy research. *Journal of Mental Health*, 9, 3, 257-266.

Roth, A. and P. Fonagy (2005) *What works for whom? A critical review of psychotherapy research*. New York, Guilford.

Sackett, D. L., Rosenberg, W.M.C., Gray, J.A.M., Haynes, R.B. and Richardson, W.S. (1996) Evidence-based medicine: what it is and what is isn't. *British Medical Journal*, 312, 71-72.

Sytema, S. and Bout, J. (2006) Treatment outcome of an inpatient group therapy for couples. *Journal of Family Therapy*, 28, 392-403.

8
The single session format

Common features of groupwork in acute psychiatric wards

Oded Manor

What guidance may be offered about the practice of groupwork in acute psychiatric wards? Clearly, a variety of approaches already exists and that may be a positive sign. The question is whether it is possible to identify any common features over and above that variety. These features may necessarily be suggested only tentatively. Yet, each practitioner may find her or his way more easily bearing these possibilities in mind. This chapter will review suggestions that have been put forward in the literature. Occasionally, I shall also draw on my practice experience, and at times – propose logical connections that may be made among some disparate ideas. The focus will be on each groupwork session as a one-off opportunity when members meet together for the first time, and part without knowing whether they will meet again. Such an approach is known as 'the single session format'. It will be also suggested that, even during a single session, the working alliance may have to be handled appropriately. The metaphor of a 'systemic container' will be proposed to help with that.

The context: Groupwork on acute psychiatric wards

Working with groups seems to be helped by knowing something about what happens in groups. This knowledge has been called 'group dynamics'. The range of ideas about addressing group dynamics in the service of group psychotherapy, group counselling and groupwork is vast indeed (for just few examples, see Corey, 1995; Roberts and Northern, 1976; Shaffer and Galinsky, 1974; Manor, 1994; Manor, 1999). More specialist knowledge about applying group psychotherapy in psychiatric hospitals (Robertson and Davison 1997) and particularly with inpatients in therapeutic communities (Campling and Haigh, 1999; Norton, 2003) has been available for quite a while. Compared to these, the knowledge about specific applications of groupwork in acute psychiatric wards is perhaps somewhat less extensive. Yet, already a variety of approaches is evident. Leading texts have been published by Clarke and Wilson (2008), Kanas (1996), Rice and Rutan (1987) and Yalom (1983). In this book you can also see examples of the diversity of practice, and that is before considering non-verbal activities which were excluded because of limitation of space.

Can any guidelines be identified within this diversity? I have not carried out a systematic and comprehensive literature search to answer this question. I have only drawn on fairly well publicised sources of knowledge that seem relevant. Within these mainstay circles, many practitioners seem to bear in mind the fact that a high proportion of people who are admitted to acute psychiatric wards suffer from schizophrenia. Practitioners' general thinking seems to follow Roth and Fonagy's (1996: p.184-196) summary of outcome research, but avoid too dogmatic adherence, as some areas of practice have simply been under-researched to date.

Norton (2004) stresses that the way the ward as a whole is organised in acute psychiatric inpatient care is of paramount importance. Montgomery (2002: p.36) points out that 'Patients in acute crisis' should be excluded from psychodynamic group psychotherapy. Both Holmes (2002) as well as Rathbone and Campling (2005), seem to agree with Norton's (2004) emphasis on the ward as a whole, but break down the argument into distinct levels of analysis. The groupwork practice all these people seem to advocate stresses weekly sessions that focus on patients' 'here-and-now' experiences on the ward as well as their life outside. Many agree to avoid deliberately promoting prolonged intensification of feelings with these particular patients.

Two sources seem to offer more detailed yet generic ideas about the uses of small group sessions on acute psychiatric wards. One is Vinogradov and Yalom (1989: p.111-132) and the other is MacKenzie (1997: p.338-343). As Yalom's work is extensively discussed in this book, I shall draw more directly from that of MacKenzie.

MacKenzie suggests that groups on acute psychiatric wards 'face many unique difficulties. Patient turnover is rapid, the level of pathology is high, motivation may be low, and the mix of problems is continuously fluctuating'. (MacKenzie 1997: p.339). Therefore, the nature of groupwork he recommends stresses 'Maintaining realistic expectations by choosing *modest goals* which 'initially might involve only the next 24-hour period' of coping with immediate life situations, clarifying 'current issues and circumstances'... and promoting 'a problem-solving review of alternative strategies' (MacKenzie 1997: p.340).

The practice methods that seem viable to him are organised within a *single session format*. He explains that these groups 'are best conceived as remaining forever in the *engagement* stage. They are continually rebeginning and working to consolidate into some sense of groupness. Therefore, therapeutic factors from the supportive cluster – *acceptance, hope, universality and altruism* – should be mobilised..... The tasks include *controlled mobilization* of affect with cognitive support' (MacKenzie 1997: p.340). The practitioner's style is expected to be active: 'reinforcing mastery of affect, impulses, thoughts and daily routines' (MacKenzie 1997: p.342). Only when patients begin to settle in the ward can the range of issues be extended. Planning for patients' discharge can start as soon as it is viable.

It has to be said that many ideas are compressed by MacKenzie into the five pages allocated to the subject. In the present chapter I shall try to fill in some details related to some of these ideas, and logically expand the thinking to raise a few more possibilities. I shall suggest that the emphasis on the single session format still requires an understanding of the working alliance, and that practitioners may be helped by resorting to a systemic view of that alliance. Possible implications for practice will be raised for consideration, especially the dynamics of each session as a 'systemic container'.

Diverse practices and a common theme

It may be helpful to use the chapters in the present book as examples of the diversity we face. Here you will see staff opting for various forms of groupwork. To begin with, the goals of such groups differ. Some aim to encourage the development of problem-solving skills by the patients (Grey, 2007, and also her chapter in this book). Others aim at helping patients orientate themselves to the ward environment (Hajek, 2007, and her chapter in this book). A third type of goal is to encourage also free discussion that may help patients become conscious of unconscious issues that trouble them – sometimes also in relation to patients' past experiences (Radcliffe & Diamond, 2007, and their chapter in this book).

Not surprisingly, the practice methods differ too: from an emphasis on highly structured exercises for problem solving (Grey, 2007) to the more benign 'holding' stance of the psychodynamically informed approach (Radcliffe & Diamond, 2007). In-between, you will also find the informal yet proactive stance involved in interpersonal learning (Hajek, 2007). Yet, close reading of these accounts suggests that beyond the differences among them, they share at least one theme: all emphasise the need to encourage patients' active involvement during the group. None of the approaches seems to convey a sense of passive receptivity by patients. All pay considerable attention to issues of engagement. Therefore, it may be helpful to focus here on engagement issues first.

Issues of engagement

Groupworkers have explored the need for emotional involvement of group members for a long time (see for example, Bertcher, 1994). Macgowan (2008a) has suggested four major headings that underpin research in this area: group cohesion, group climate, group engagement and the therapeutic alliance. Each of these has been studied empirically and Macgowan (2008b) has offered reviews of the research involved in relation to outcomes of groupwork.

There is no space to discuss each of these headings here. Of these four, the heading of 'therapeutic alliance' is the one where forming shared meaning about the therapeutic endeavour is considered most vital. Indeed, the emphasis on shared meaning may be crucial to practice in the present context. The reason lies in the dynamics that seem to arise in acute psychiatric wards. These dynamics have been characterised by boredom, chaos, frightening symptoms and, quite often, lack of consistency of handling these difficult experiences (Hardcastle et al., 2007; Radcliffe & Smith, 2007; Hill, 2008). Consequently, ensuring that all those influenced by practice share the same understanding of the goals and the methods of groupwork seems particularly important on such wards. This is why the therapeutic, or simply working alliance, was chosen to be the basic framework for structuring the present discussion.

The working alliance

Systematic research into the working alliance in psychotherapy owes much to the pioneering work of Bordin (1994). Two seminal volumes have been published: that edited by Horvath and Greenberg (1994), and one with more cognitive behavioural leanings edited by Gilbert and Leahy (2007). The latter includes references to the evidence base for the relevance of the therapeutic alliance to outcomes.

In regard to a definition, it has been suggested that the working alliance can be seen as the

> collaborative aspect of the relationship between worker and client as well as other people involved with both, in pursuing agreed goals. (Manor 2000b: p.375-6)

The working alliance is an aspect of the therapeutic relationship that deals with collaboration. In groupwork, such collaboration has to develop not only between the worker and each patient, but also among all the patients who attend each group. Each patient is expected to receive help not only from the practitioner but also from his or her peers. To do this, each may have to sort out various feelings towards other group members; for example, trusting them, sharing power with them, or feeling attraction and affection towards them. The attention paid to each patient's bonds with all those who attend the same group is the hallmark of groupwork and distinguishes it from the various forms of individual help. Therefore, the working alliance in groupwork is more complex than that fostered during individual forms of help. Indeed, it has been noted by many that the systems approach is a framework that addresses such complexities. By now, a number of groupwork publications are grounded in the systems approach (Agazarian, 1997; Donigian and Malnati, 1997; Durkin, 1981; Manor, 2000a; Manor, 2008; McClure, 1998).

The 'Integrative Systems Perspective', suggested by Pinsof (1994), seems to capture many of the issues involved. The details of that framework may be further debated, but its major thrust is supported by extensive research.

The framework leads the practitioner to constantly ask how the various systems involved (the patients, the practitioner, the ward staff, the families, patients' employers and so on) influence and, in turn, are also influenced by three major issues:

+ 'goals' of groupwork,
+ 'tasks' (that is, the methods) chosen and
+ 'bonds' that develop during the sessions.

The message is that the systems formed by patients and staff, as well as those who surround them, may have a crucial impact on the nature of these three aspects of the alliance. Let us look at each separately.

Goals

Goals are the expected outcomes of the therapeutic endeavour. Examples of groupwork goals you will find in this book have already been mentioned. Compared to mainstream group psychotherapy, these are relatively *modest goals* that concern mainly the immediate lives of group members. For example, Hajek (2007) lists Yalom's (1983) goals as 'engaging the patient in the therapeutic process, reducing isolation, reducing anxiety connected with hospitalisation and providing experience of universality and of being helpful to others'. Grey (2007) sees the major goals as encouraging the development of problem-solving skills by patients. Radcliffe and Diamond (2007) identify the goals as 'a chance to talk about their (patients') experiences' and become conscious of what has landed them in hospital. Indeed, it seems very appropriate to work for relatively modest goals with people while they are struggling with such intense difficulties as the florid symptoms of psychosis (MacKenzie, 1997).

Tasks

Tasks are 'the major activities that the therapist and patient systems engage in during therapy' (Pinsof, 1994: p.181). In everyday terms, these are the 'methods and skills' – what each party is expected to do to achieve the goals; for example, to turn up on time, to suggest topics for discussion, to show that they listen, to express feelings, to help members take turns in talking and so on.

The tasks also include the ways sessions are organised. This aspect seems important as the chaos in the ward may easily spill over into the group session. In these wards patients are admitted and discharged at various rates while attempts are made, not always fully successfully, to contain their symptoms through medication.

That situation has led to accepting that these groups are likely to be 'rapid open' (Henry, 1988). In rapid open groups, membership is not only open; that is, members do not merely keep changing, but they change every week. At times, each session may be attended by different people. The structure of a 'single session format' has been recommended (MacKenzie 1997: p.340) in order to cope with rapid open groups. This structure usually means guiding the group to begin each session as if the group is meeting for the first time and to end it as if this group may not meet again. Each session is planned to be a self-contained experience.

MacKenzie (1997: p.251-267) advocates an active yet supportive stance for practitioners in such groups. He recommends pursuing what he calls 'the supportive cluster' of therapeutic factors (MacKenzie, 1997: p.340) - referring to the scheme researched by Yalom (1995). These factors are the following:

- acceptance or cohesion: as in 'Belonging and being accepted by the group',
- hope, as in 'Knowing others had solved problems similar to mine'
- universality, as in 'Learning that others have some of the same 'bad' thoughts and feelings I do' and
- altruism, as in 'Helping others has given me more self-respect'.

The question is, of course, how to bring about these experiences – what methods to use? Process oriented approaches; for example, the person-centred approach developed by Rogers (1970), often involve the practitioner in listening and waiting for the moment when her intervention may help. Yet, it is clear that most practitioners of groupwork in acute psychiatric wards tend to resort to active and often structured approaches. There is probably a sound reason for this. The rapid turn-over of patients who are struggling with psychotic symptoms, and the often unstable regime of the ward, easily make for a high level of experienced chaos. Because of the intensity of the emotional experiences involved, a high level of instability may actually exacerbate patients' symptoms. This may be the case because such levels of chaos may be experienced as demands to process more information than each can do at such times. Such an experience of 'information over-load' is easily created. The active and structured approaches to groupwork, mentioned already, aim to prevent information over-load. These approaches help by controlling the intensity and complexity of experiences that arise during the group. In particular, structured approaches involve the practitioner in taking the initiative to intervene; for example, suggest topics for conversation or impart information, before the patients do so themselves. Readers may consult various sources that account for this proactive structured stance (Caplan, 2005; Kaplan, 1988; Galinsky et al., 2007). They may then heed the advice of the latter about the most extreme of structured approaches: 'Countering the view that manuals are mechanistic, they can be employed in a way that is sensitive to group dynamics and the tenets of groupwork practice' (Galinsky et al., 2007: p.86).

Structured methods often emphasise what Middleman and Goldberg (1990) call 'Selecting communication pattern purposefully'. By this phrase, the authors mean that the groupworker openly and directly suggests to group members who will talk to whom about what. For example, many social work practitioners are accustomed to taking the initiative and resorting to sub-grouping: dividing the group into pairs or larger sub-groups, and giving each a topic for discussion; for example, their feelings about the food served on the ward. It stands to reason that dividing the group in these ways is done for a purpose: a certain quality of interaction is usually sought. The practitioner may aim at more personal exchanges, or may want to shield members from simultaneous exposure to too many people, or may merely want to save time. Whatever the aim, the communication pattern is usually selected with a certain purpose in mind.

Of course, sub-grouping is not the only purposeful pattern identified. Here are a number of other patterns:

- 'maypole'; when the practitioner talks to each member individually,
- 'round robin'; when each group member speaks in turn,
- 'hot seat'; when the issues with which one group member is concerned are the focus for everyone in the group,
- 'agenda controlled' when the practitioner identifies all the topics for discussion, and
- 'free form'; when the practitioner invites group members to raise whatever topic they wish in whatever way they wish to do this
  (Middleman and Goldberg Wood, 1990: p.53-129).

Each of these interventions is likely to have a different impact on group relationships. At the same time, all these interventions are likely to require the use of empathy, genuiness, concreteness and warmth (Egan, 1973: p.27-31). Grounded in these modes of communication, all such interventions can be considered as *generic skills of structured groupwork*.

Bonds

'*Bonds* address the affective and psychodynamic aspects of the relationships between and within the therapist and patient systems .... It deals most commonly with the extent to which the key patient system members trust, respect, care about and feel cared about by the therapist and the therapist system.' (Pinsof, 1994: p.183).

I think that, in Britain, we would use the term 'closeness' when referring to such experiences. The bonding perspective of the therapeutic alliance seems always very important, but it may be particularly problematic on acute psychiatric wards for reasons that have already been explained. MacKenzie (1997: p.251-267) stresses a number of features that may help bonding:

+ positive intentions of practitioners and members,
+ a degree of neutrality that includes explicitly expressing acceptance,
+ liking and respect for the patients,
+ resorting to a conversational style so that a real relationship emerges while being goal directed,
+ describing patterns at a behavioural, cognitive or interpersonal level,
+ directly praising every small achievement, and finally –
+ instilling hope and supporting rather than challenging defences.

In view of these guidelines it would make sense to focus on bonds related to 'holding' (Bowlby, 1979) and 'containing' (Bion, 1963; 1970). The two terms have been used interchangeably (Hinshelwood & Skogstad, 2000; Holmes, 1992) to denote the capacity to withstand patients' expression of anxiety fear and anger. Instead of suppressing difficult feelings or retaliating as a response, the containing groupworker can help the patient make wider sense of the experiences involved.

Of course, reciprocal influences appear among these aspects: each has an impact on the other two and, in turn – is affected by those two. Perhaps one of the markers of good practice is a sense of coherence among goals, tasks and bonds where the agreed goals lead to choosing relevant tasks, and the bonds that arise meaningfully support the work as a whole (Manor, 2003). Yet, these three aspects of the working alliance are susceptible to influences of the many systems surrounding the group. Brief comments about these systems will be offered now.

Systems that influence the alliance

The systems that influence the working alliance may be personal, interpersonal and social (Manor, 2000a).

At the *personal level*, different patients may struggle differently with the psychotic difficulties that have led to their admission. These difficulties are well documented in clinical textbooks (see for example, Barlow & Durand, 1995). Delusions, hallucinations, disorganised speech and at times grossly disorganised behaviour are well known 'positive' symptoms. Flattened affect, inability to initiate and persist in many important activities and limited ability to converse are 'negative' ones (Barlow & Durand, 1995: p.557-562). Miller and Mason (2002: p.52) add positive symptoms of the state of confusion, rapid thoughts that are hard to follow and inability to pay attention or concentrate. Yet, the particular combination of difficulties may vary from person to person. The individual permutation presented by each person may have an impact on their responses to the goals, the tasks and the bonds involved.

At the *interpersonal level*, the ways patients and staff understand their respective roles in the group is likely to influence their response to the group as well. Are patients to just sit there waiting to be cured or take an active part in the process? Are staff expected to talk to the patients or facilitate a shared conversation with them? These differences matter, as a mismatch of expectations may derail even the best planned group.

At the *social level*, staff morale may be subject to external influences exerted by the hospital management, the ward structure, government policies and public opinion about mental health (Hardcastle et al., 2007: p.162-202; Chiesa, 2000). In particular, the attitude about this service that prevail among policy makers of mental health (see, Department of Health, 2005; Department of Health, 2007; Hardcastle et al., 2007; Miller & Mason, 2002; Radcliffe & Smith, 2007; Hill, 2008) and among those who train and supervise staff may influence staff performance.

To achieve the aspired sense of coherence among the aspects of the working alliance, it may be useful to think first of the session as a whole – as a total experience.

The single session as a whole: Identifying the concentrated middle

A number of authors have explored the dynamics of single sessions in groupwork. Perhaps one of the most generic is the framework proposed by Birnbaum and Cicchetti (2005). These authors go through a range of goals and the skills (the tasks, in the present scheme) that may help during the beginning, the middle and the end of a single group session.

- The beginning is 'a prelude, setting the stage for the work that is to occur, clarifying and defining the direction the session will take.' (Birnbaum and Cicchetti 2005: p.27).
- The middle stage is the 'work' stage (Birnbaum and Cicchetti 2005: p.32).
- 'The ending stage completes the sessional group life cycle. It provides a natural and specific opportunity to review and evaluate the session as a whole'. (Birnbaum and Cicchetti 2005: p.38).

This framework may not be structured enough for some practitioners, as they will have to leave it to group members to identify all the topics to be discussed in each session. Also, the theory underlying the authors' framework is not explicit. Yet, the framework may be used as a skeleton around which much can be built.

Long ago, Ross and Thorpe (1988) have already drawn on the work of William Schutz in charting the order of groupwork activities during each session as a mirror. The stages would form a symmetric sequence: from the stage of Inclusion (for example, who belongs to the group), through that of Control (for example, who dominates the conversation) to the stage of Affection (for example, who is attracted to whom), and then back - through Affection, to Control and then to Inclusion again. The symmetric reversal of processes distinguishes this framework from all the rest. Typically, the middle period; that dedicated to the 'Affection' stage, is associated with working on relatively more intense and complex issues; for example - closeness, jealousy, possessiveness, sexuality and so forth, compared to those handled during the 'Control' and 'Inclusion' stages.

Within various humanistic psychology approaches to groupwork, each session is seen as a 'stand alone' experience. Here are some examples.

Manor and Dumbleton (1993) suggested a scheme derived from psychodrama. That scheme was built around the sequence of 'warm-up, action, integration' and can be found in a number of psychodramatic textbooks (for example, Blatner, 1973; Holmes, 1992). Clearly, the 'action' phase is the relatively more intense and complex one - when the psychodramatic scene is enacted. Here too the more complex and intense stage arises in the middle of the session.

Gestalt Therapy revolves around a cycle. Although the phases of that 'awareness cycle' are not always described in exactly the same way, it can be seen that the most complex and intense phases: 'action' and 'final contact', occur in the middle of that cycle (Clarkson, 1989: p.27-40).

Returning to a more general view, Lindsay and Orton (2008: p.86-88) suggest the ordering of interventions in humanistic psychology groups according to their 'emotional intensity'. They too, place the most intense intervention – the 'cathartic' one, in the middle of the session - to 'leave time for integration, insight and support'.

All these frameworks have one feature in common: they all see the more complex and/or intense stage as occurring in the middle of the sequence they describe. All suggest *a relatively simple beginning gradually building up to more complex and/or intense issues during the middle period, which is followed by a gradual decrease of these features towards the end of the session.* I suggest we see the combination of higher intensity and higher complexity as contributing to the need for *greater degree of concentration* by each group member. We may then be able to begin to talk about a 'concentrated middle' as the feature that all these schemes have in common.

In order to apply these ideas in a sensitive and enabling ways, it may be helpful to think why this 'concentrated middle' tends to appear in some forms of groupwork.

Towards an explanation: The systemic container

Why do some practitioners appreciate the need to warm up for the concentrated middle and to cool down when that period is over? It may be possible to find an answer to this within the systems approach too. In this respect, Agazarian's (1997: p.62-83) systemic understanding of the term 'boundarying' may be most helpful. Boundarying is a cognitive-emotional operation we perform when we identify some issues as 'relevant', 'appropriate', 'called for' etc.. Is politics discussed at a dinner party? Is the level of a guest's income questioned? In groupwork the results of such boundarying is that certain issues are included in the group's discussion; members feel it is legitimate to pay attention to these issues, and so - these issues begin to be regarded as part of the group's positive experiences – its approved culture. The approved culture is symbolically seen as being 'inside' the group boundaries. In the present context, examples of these issues could be the effects of medication, or the food served on the ward. Other issues are regarded as 'irrelevant', 'inappropriate', 'not really called for' etc., and these are regarded as being outside the group's legitimate concerns. Often, discussing such issues may be seen to contribute to 'problems' and negative group experiences. Examples could include forms of sexuality, or certain religious beliefs. Such issues are then excluded from the group's discussion – symbolically, these issues are put outside the group boundaries.

Groups create such boundaries in order to prioritise the investment of their energy – concentrating on some activities more than on others (Durkin, 1981). Instead of continuously exploring what should and what should not be talked about, the group creates its own norms: a ready made yard stick which is used to direct group members when choosing what to talk about. These norms are, so to speak, the cement upholding the group boundaries. Such acts of boundarying help group members mobilise *energy* they need in order to take in and *process information* (Wilden, 1980).

* *The initial warming-up period* is necessary because each group member needs

first to process the information about entering the group and becoming an active member of that group. From the environment of the often chaotic, alienating and threatening ward, each needs to move into a new role inside the new environment – that of the group. That role is likely to call for openness to feelings - fostering support and a sense of meaning. Conceptually, the beginning calls for 'Crossing from 'outside' to 'inside' a group and also entails crossing from outside social roles into one's systems–centred member role' (Agazarian, 1997: p.66-67); in our case, simply - group member role. Such information, about the differences between operating 'outside' and 'inside' the group, needs to be processed by each group member first.

- During *the middle of the session*, each member is expected to concentrate on new feelings and ideas, to show interest in other members, to convey acceptance and support and to actively participate in the exchanges. The norms of behaviour adopted for doing so may be markedly different form the ones prevailing on the ward.

- *A cooling down period is needed towards the end.* As the session draws to a close, group members need to process the information about leaving the group and, in our context, returning to the ward. Again, the norms of behaviour on the ward are likely to be different from the ones patients leave behind when the group session ends. This point seems to need a separate explanation.

Research into the outcome of psychotherapy (Lambert, 1992) has long ago looked at 'extratherapeutic change'; that is, factors that are part of the client (ego strength) and part of the environment (social support), and are *not related* to participation in therapy. Meta analysis of research findings suggested that these factors account for 40% of the improvement following involvement in various forms of therapy. This trend, for external factors to markedly influence patients, may not be very different on acute psychiatric wards. What patients find as they step outside the therapy session (incomprehensible shouting, loneliness in their room) may influence a great deal of their reactions to that session even if the session itself was warm, empathic and containing. Therefore, it would seem imperative to send patients out of the session as well equipped to deal with the chaos of the ward as we can. To achieve this, patients may need to take time and prepare themselves for the change – often for a contrasting change. In their minds, they need to locate themselves in the environment of the ward again – with its very different and often disturbing interactions. Groupworkers may need to help them do so.

The advantages of constructing a concentrated middle are probably clear. The question is how to do that.

Constructing the concentrated middle

As noted before, people admitted to acute psychiatric wards are likely to suffer 'information over-load' as the variety of psychotic and other symptoms engulf them and the rapid change of patients in each ward overwhelm them. Therefore, *pacing the amount of information* that each patient needs to process at a given moment seems vital. I would like to suggest that such pacing may be helped when experiences and topics for discussion are ordered to allow for a concentrated middle.

The question of pacing

Emotional disclosure of patients can be constructively steered by skilled facilitators. For example, if a patient brings up a very intense experience (a dream, a complex encounter on the ward) just as group members sit down in the room, the groupworker can say something like: 'This seems so important. I wonder if we could help more by waiting a little until we all settle down first.' If a patient brings up such an intense experience at the very end, perhaps the facilitator can say something quite similar; for example: 'This seems so important. I hope we can come back to it next week. Can we?' In the same vein, topics for discussion can be purposefully selected by practitioners too, and this will be discussed in the next section.

Armed with such understanding, practitioners may begin the session with issues that require relatively less concentration. Next, they may build up the level of concentration around the middle of the session by exploring relatively more intense and complex issues. They may then return to less concentrated topics at the end. How may such a cycle be achieved?

Gauging the 'depth'

The idea is to sequence the experiences and topics according to the amount of processing each may require. The amount of processing needs to be gauged in advance. It seems to me that this is likely to depend on the degree of intensity and the degree of complexity required for processing each topic or experience (Wilden, 1980). Each of these 'utterances' (topic or experience) has these two features: it can be more or less intense; for example, it raises mild or severe anxiety. The 'utterance' may also be more or less complex; depending on the number of issues that affect one another. 'Utterances' that include a greater number of issues affecting one another are more likely to be experienced as more complex. No quantitative approach is attempted here. Rather, a form of intuitive judgement is probably called for. Here is an example:

Remembering group members' names is usually not a very intense experience, and this issue mixes only two aspects: the appearance of the person and the sound of the person's name. The degree of complexity of this issue is probably relatively low. As both intensity and complexity are low, this issue may require relatively less concentration. Therefore, it makes sense to introduce the question of remembering group members' names at the beginning of the session.

However, exploring difficulties of sleeping on the ward may be a different experience. This issue is likely to invoke past memories, sexual feelings, longing for safety and many more beside. The feelings invoked by these aspects may well be rather intense. At the same time, there are many more of them – certainly more than two. Such a wide range of aspects may mix and mingle in members' minds, each influencing all the others and being influenced by them. Therefore, the complexity of this issue is also likely to be experienced as relatively high. Put together, the combination of *intensity* and *complexity* may be seen as the degree of *concentration* an issue requires. In the present example, we may say that the issue of sleeping on the ward at night is of high intensity as well as high complexity. Therefore, this issue is likely to require more concentration than the first one - remembering the names of group members. It would make sense to facilitate the exploration of such an emotive issue during the middle of the session.

However, remembering one good thing that was said during that session may be an issue that has very few aspects and one that raises only a mild sense of gratitude and warmth. Such an issue may require relatively little concentration. Therefore, it would seem appropriate to raise such an issue towards the end of the session.

Some practitioners see such a mixture of intensity and complexity as similar to the meaning of 'emotional depth'. If so, *you may visualise the cyclical design of the session as a container: it is relatively shallow at the edges, it deepens in the middle and it ends up nice and safe at the edges again. The idea is very much to prevent information over-load by dynamically pacing the degree of concentration required of patients during each session.* Because the considerations leading to the construction of this metaphor are systemic, I sometimes use the term '*systemic container*' to describe this notion.

For the present purpose, the systemic container may be constructed to promote the 'active-supportive' stance advocated by MacKenzie (1997: p.251-267). Such a stance will be enhanced by being continuously grounded in the working alliance. Therefore, practitioners may want to clarify the goals, the tasks and the bonds and also select aspects that can be shared with the systems involved before and after each session. These systems may be other staff members, external agencies or, at times, even friends and relatives of group members. Different parts of the experiences are likely to be appropriate for sharing with each of these sub-systems, but usually something constructive can be shared nevertheless.

Of course, more details are needed in order to work out all the implications of this idea. Readers interested in further intricacies related to these issues may consult Agazarian (1997: p.62-67). Larger and seminal studies of the processing of information can be found in McClure (1998), Wilden (1980: p.155-201) as well as Watzlawick et al. (1967).

All those details notwithstanding, it would be highly simplistic to expect a one off matching of the working alliance components to suffice, as some aspects of this alliance seem to change over time.

The working alliance over time

The systems involved with each group are likely to remain the same over the short duration of a single session. However, changes in the goals, the tasks and the bonds, are to be expected. Following Birnbaum and Cicchetti (2005) these changes can be charted as occurring before, during and after each group session. Let us look at these now.

Relationship before the group session

There is no space to review here the literature about preparing for groupwork (See Manor, 2000a: p.97-103). Yet, it is probably vital to remind practitioners that the goals and the methods of the groupwork project have to be planned in advance and that these will affect the nature of the relationship in the group; that is, the bonds. The initial plan has to be known to other staff members and appreciated by them if they are to support the encouragement of patients to attend the group. Arrangements for supporting the groupworkers and supervising them (Manor, 1989) can be worked out in advance too. In addition, it seems helpful to prepare each patient for the groupwork experience before joining the group. A framework for doing so out in the community has been proposed (Manor, 1988) and the details may well not apply to a psychiatric ward. Yet, the dynamics may hold: groupwork may be both incomprehensible and threatening to many people. It may help potential group members to understand its goals and its methods and to form an initial bond with the groupworker before they turn up to the group for the first time (MacKenzie, 1997: p.134-139). As part of this process, practitioners may want to find out in advance whether any minority issue may trouble potential group members.

Relationships during the session

With the preparation period complete, the session itself can be approached more comfortably.

Beginning the session

As Birnbaum and Cicchetti (2005) note, each stage has its own goals, tasks and bonds. The beginning sets the tone. The goals of the beginning stage may be to connect members to one another, agree on the purpose of the session, clarify the expectations people have in regard to norms of behaviour, set the agenda, identify the order of topics and give group members a sense of the structure of the whole session in advance. The practitioner's tasks are the skills that may help achieving these goals. Birnbaum and Cicchetti (2005: 31) are very general in listing four of these:

+ allocation of time for the various activities,
+ shaping norms for sessional contracting so everyone agrees on ways of behaving during the session,
+ inviting full participation and
+ slowing the agenda.

In addition, actively creating an initial contract among members is often considered vital, and articulating the goals of the session is often included.

During the beginning of the session it seems important to emphasise issues that need relatively little concentration; those that address 'one thing at a time'. As mentioned already, 'slowing the agenda' (Birnbaum and Cicchetti 2005: p.31) is highly relevant here as a form of pacing involvement. The aim is to allow patients to enter the roles of group members slowly and gently. If one or two try to raise more concentrated issues at the beginning, it may be better to slow them down by suggesting that those issues would be addressed a little later 'when we settle down a little'. Resorting to the generic skills of structured groupwork mentioned before, may help too.

In addition, there are many sources that describe further skills in details. Here are some examples: Bertcher, 1994; Kennard et al.,1993; Manor, 2000a: p.104-109; MacKenzie, 1997: p.151-179; Middleman and Goldberg Wood, 1990; Ross, 1991.

A reassuring and undemanding level of bonding, not necessarily very intense, seems to be helpful. A level of bonding is called for that is close enough to be engaging and interesting, and distant enough to assure members that the whole experience is going to be unprovocative, containing, safe and nourishing.

Middle of the session

Once the members begin to feel contained, the session may move to the middle stage. This is the time for 'work'; that is, for focusing on the goals agreed for that session. Birnbaum and Cicchetti (2005: p.31) point out that 'For most groups, problem solving is the framework in the middle stage'. The major goal is to enable group members to engage in some form of problem solving, however generally understood, and do so constructively. Birnbaum and Cicchetti (2005: p.32) break down that goal to:

+ 'maintaining continuity between the beginning and the middle stage,
+ working with obstacles,
+ use of group problem solving and
+ attention to the here and now'.

Of course, these goals will vary to some extent depending on the initial choices made with each group. Many skills have been recorded as helpful for such work. Birnbaum and Cicchetti (2005: p.36) mention:

+ 'shaping norms for problem solving,
+ making demand for work,
+ illuminating group process,
+ keeping the focus on the work and
+ identifying obstacles to the work'.

The account offered by Middleman and Goldberg Wood (1990) includes clear definitions and examples of many other skills. In particular; 'Continuous group skills' and 'Skills for building groups' (Middleman and Goldberg Wood, 1990: p.96-114) seem very relevant to this part of the session. Another well established source of such skills is the book by Bertcher (1994) already cited. The generic skills for this work were already discussed, and these may well permeate practice during each of the stages, including the middle one.

Again, a certain level of closeness (bonding) may be optimal during this stage. During the middle stage a relatively higher level of concentration may be possible compared to the beginning. Yet, it may help remembering that, in groups offered on acute psychiatric wards, even that level should probably remain rather limited. Examples of appropriate issues may be memories of compulsory admission, family members' reactions to the admission or any other issues where stronger feelings may arise and a relatively greater number of aspects may affect one another. These issues need to be pitched at the appropriate emotional level in view of patients' vulnerabilities on the day. Examples of doing so have already been discussed. The logic of the knowledge summarised by MacKenzie (1997: p.251-267) may lead practitioners to seek a benign holding climate – not necessarily equal to the intense intimate atmosphere of psychodynamic or humanistic group psychotherapy. Although engaged in some form of emotional work, group members should continue to feel contained by the experience, secure in the knowledge that a worker is there - continuously taking care of their well being all the time.

Ending the session

Around ten minutes before the agreed end of the session, the practitioner needs to see to it that termination issues are taken care of. This is the time for completing the cycle. Birnbaum and Cicchetti (2005: p.38-40) identify five goals for this period:

+ Reflection,
+ transition between sessions,
+ sessional closure,
+ empowerment and
+ a sense of satisfaction and accomplishment'.

The same authors (Birnbaum and Cicchetti, 2005: p.40-42) also offer five skills they consider relevant:

+ allocation of time for termination work,
+ developing norms about the value of reflection,
+ soliciting feedback from each member,
+ reaching for discrepant points of view and
+ attending to both group contents and process.

A script of just one example demonstrating such work is available (Manor, 2000a: p.185-189) and practitioners may want to choose those skills that are appropriate; for example, a review of the main themes discussed during the session, identifying any lesson learned, expressing appreciation of members' efforts or eliciting 'a nice thing' each member can do when they leave the session. Other last session skills may be relevant too; for example, Summarising (Bertcher, 1994: p.102-113), and some form of ritual at the end (Ross, 1991: p.63-65) that enhances a sense of closure; for example, each member identifies the colour they like most at this stage. Then the groupworker points out to the emerging rainbow effect. Of course, the generic skills that facilitate the supportive therapeutic factors should not be abandoned.

Perhaps the nature of closeness (bonding) during termination deserves special attention. Agazarian explains that 'The boundary at the end of each ... group (session) marks the transition from apprehensive to comprehensive experience and prepares people to change out of their (group) member role and back into their everyday social roles.' (Agazarian, 1997: p.72). The same logic that has led to pacing the entrance of members into the role of group members may lead to helping them exit these roles and re-enter the roles they assume on the ward. To do so, group members may need to create a greater distance between themselves and other members of the group, let alone the workers. The relative openness of the middle stage may not be appropriate anymore. The point is to prepare group members for re-entering the roles of patients on the ward through handling topics that require less concentration while inspiring in each member faith and hope. The idea is to send group members out into the ward 'well wrapped up'; sensing they take with them something valuable - something they want to remember, feeling warm about the experience and looking forward to another one if appropriate.

Relationship after the session

Having suggested that much can be borrowed from existing literature about sustaining the working alliance before and during the session, suggestions about relationships after such a session ends are probably not as articulate (yet, see – MacKenzie, 1997: p.343). Other systems with which patients are involved may well take over now. As already mentioned, group members have to return to the unpredictable dynamics of the ward where chaos, loneliness and sometimes aggression arise. In some wards coping with such dynamics may be a daunting task, not necessarily similar to going back home or even returning to a hostel in the open community. Are there ways in which groupworkers can increase patients' resilience of coping with the ward dynamics after each session? Clearly, the environment to which group members return after the session matters a great deal. Can the groupworker find ways of increasing the support offered there? Far more research is needed about this, and some possibilities present themselves for exploration. For example, Cognitive Behavioural groupwork (Free, 1999; Scott & Stradling, 1998) has excelled in devising homework tasks that group members can carry out in between sessions and these may be considered. Practitioners in day centres sometimes contact the carers of certain group members after the session to ensure that extra emotional support is offered to distressed members in between sessions. Perhaps this form of bonding may be explored in an acute psychiatric ward too by contacting an appropriate member of staff; perhaps nurses, on the ward.

Summary

This chapter began by asking whether any guidelines, however general, may be derived from sources of groupwork knowledge that may enhance groupwork in acute psychiatric wards. The question was not put forward with the intention of narrowing the range of practice methods on such wards. Rather, it was hoped that various pools of knowledge may serve as generic guidelines within which each practitioner could find the form of practice specifically appropriate to her place of practice.

First, the context of groupwork in psychiatric wards was briefly reviewed. Major features for groupwork practice in such wards were identified. These were summarised as:

+ stressing *modest goals*,
+ adopting active and *structured methods* within the *single session format* of rapid open groups, and
+ fostering closeness (bonds) characterised by *containing*.

Then current practices were considered. The diversity of practice was evident and also a common theme: the need to actively engage patients in this form of groupwork was suggested. That need led to looking at the working alliance in groupwork – noting that because the alliance is among group members as well as between each member and the groupworker, this alliance was likely to be particularly complex. A systems perspective was suggested in order to account for the complexity, which led to seeing the working alliance as a question: how the various systems involved influenced and, in turn, were influenced by - the goals, the tasks and the bonds involved in each form of groupwork. A fairly detailed analysis of the possibilities was pursued, particularly in relation to goals, tasks and bonds.

With a clearer view of the working alliance in mind, five single session formats, practiced mainly in humanistic psychology groups, were cited. That review led to realising that in all five formats the more intense and complex experiences were offered in the middle of the session. A rationale was then sought for the appearance of that 'concentrated middle'. That feature was explained as stemming from the need to prevent information over-load by resorting to Boundarying. The metaphor of a 'systemic container' was then introduced as an easy-to-remember description of the session dynamics: relatively shallow at the edges, deeper in the middle, ending nice and safe at the edges again.

The chapter ended with a discussion of the changes in the goals, the tasks and the bonds over time. These three aspects of the working alliance were examined as emerging within the framework of 'the systemic container' developed earlier. In that way, the work of conducting a group was seen as taking care of the systemic container before, during and after the session.

All that remains now is to stress yet again that the knowledge explored here has been derived from groupwork knowledge practiced in many different contexts – not only that of inpatient acute psychiatric wards. Therefore, each and every idea suggested in this chapter is meant only as a possibility that may be explored and modified by others as we all continue to learn from each other about this vitally important form of practice.

References

Agazarian, Y.M. (1997) *Systems-Centred Therapy for Groups*. London: The Guilford Press.

Barlow, D.H. and Durand, V.M (1995) *Abnormal Psychology: An integrative approach*. Pacific Grove: Brooks/Cole Pub. Co.

Bertcher, H.J. (1994) *Group Participation: Techniques for leaders and members*. London: Sage

Bion, W. (1963) *Elements of Psychoanalysis*. London: Heineman.

Bion, W.R. (1970) *Attention and Interpretation: Container and contained*. New York: Basic Books.

Birnbaum, M.L. and Cicchetti, A. (2005) A model for working with the group life cycle in each group session across the life span of the group. *Groupwork*, 15(3), 23-43.

Blatner, H.A. (1973) *Acting In: Practical application of psychodramatic methods*. New York: Springer.

Bordin, E.S. (1994) Theory and Research on the Therapeutic Working Alliance: New directions. In: A.O. Horvath and L.S. Greenberg (Eds.) *The Working Alliance: Theory, research and practice*. New York: John Wiley. Pp.13-37

Bowlby, J. (1979) *The Making and Breaking of Affectional Bonds*. London: Tavistock/Routledge

Campling, P. and Haigh, R. (1999) *Therapeutic Communities: Past, present and future*. London: Jessica Kingsley

Caplan, T. (2005) Active or passive interventions in groups: The group leader's dilemma. *Groupwork*, 15(1) 24-41.

Chiesa, M. (2000) At the cross-road between institutional and community psychiatry: An acute psychiatric admission ward. In: R.D. Hinshelwood and W. Skogstad (Eds.) *Observing Organisations*. London: Routledge.Pp.54-67.

Clarke, I. and Wilson, H. (2008) *Cognitive Behaviour Therapy for Acute Inpatient Mental Health Units*. London: Routledge.

Clarkson, P. (1989) *Gestalt Counselling in Action*. London: Sage Pub

Corey, G. (1995) *Theory and Practice of Group Counselling*. Pacific Grove, CA: Brooks/Cole Pub, 4th edition.

Department of Health (2005) *NIMHE Guiding Statement on Recovery*. London: Department of Health.

Department of Health (2007) *Star Wards: Practical ideas for improving the daily experiences and treatment outcomes of adult mental health inpatients*. London: Department of Health.

Donigian, J. and Malnati, R. (1997) *Systemic Group Therapy: A triadic model*. Pacific Grove: Brooks/Cole Pub.

Durkin, J.E. (1981) *Living Groups: Psychotherapy and General Systems Theory*. New York: Brunner/Mazel, pp.172-198

Egan, G (1973) *Face to Face: The small group experience and interpersonal growth*. Monterey, CA: Brooks/Cole.

Free, M.L. (1999) *Cognitive Therapy in Groups*. Chichester: John Wiley & Sons.

Galinsky, M.J., Terzian, M.A. and Fraser, M. (2007) The art of groupwork practice with manualized curricula. *Groupwork*, 17(2), 74-92.

Gilbert, P. and Leahy, R.L. (2007) *The Therapeutic Relationship in the Cognitive Behavioral Psychotherapies.* London: Routledge, Taylor and Francis Group.

Grey, S.J. (2007) A structured problem-solving group for psychiatric in-patients. *Groupwork*, 17(1), 20-33.

Hajek, K. (2007) Interpersonal group therapy on acute inpatient wards. *Groupwork*,17(1), 7-19.

Hardcastle, M., Kennard, D., Grandison S. and Fagin, L. (eds.) (2007) *Experiences of Mental Health In-Patient Care: Narratives from service users, carers and professionals.* Hove: Routledge.

Henry, M. (1988) Revisiting open groups. *Groupwork*, 1(2), 215-228.

Hill (2008) The mental health units that shame the NHS. *The Observer*, 29 June 2008, pp.14-15.

Hinshelwood, R.D. and Skogstad, W. (2000) *Observing Organisations: Anxiety, defence and culture in health care.* London: Routledge.

Holmes, J. (2002) Acute wards: problems and solutions. *Psychiatric Bulletin*, 26, 383-385

Holmes, P. (1992) The Inner World Outside: Object relations theory and psychodrama. London: Tavistock/Routledge.

Horvath, A.O., and L.S. Greenberg, L.S. (eds.) (1994) *The Working Alliance: Theory, research and practice.* New York: John Wiley.

Kanas, N. (1996) *Group Therapy for Schizophrenic Patients.* Washington, DC: American Psychiatric Press.

Kaplan, K.L. (1988) *Directive Group Therapy: Innovative mental health treatment.* Thorofare, NJ: SLACK Inc.

Kennard, D., Roberts, J. and Winter, D.A. (1993) *A Work Book of Group-Analytic Interventions.* London: Routledge.

Lambert, M.J. (1992) *Psychotherapy outcome research: Implications for integrative and eclectic therapists.* In J.C. Norcross and M.R. Goldfried, (eds.) Handbook of Psychotherapy Integration. Basic Books (pp.94-129).

Lindsay, T. and Orton, S. (2008) *Groupwork Practice in Social Work.* Exeter: Learning Matters.

Macgowan, M.J. (2008a) Personal communication.

Macgowan, M.J. (2008b) *A guide to evidence-based group work.* Oxford: Oxford University Press.

MacKenzie, K.R. (1997) *Time-Managed Group Psychotherapy.* London: American Psychiatric Press

Manor, O. (1988) Preparing the client for social groupwork: an illustrated framework. *Groupwork* 1(2),100-114.

Manor, O. (1989) Organising accountability for social groupwork: More choices. *Groupwork*, 2(1), 108-122.

Manor, O. and Dumbleton, M. (1993) Combining activities and growth games: A systemic approach. *Groupwork*, 6(3), 248-265.

Manor, O. (1994) Group psychotherapy. In: P. Clarkson and M. Pokorney (eds.) (1994) *The Handbook of Psychotherapy*. London: Routledge, pp.249-266.

Manor, O. (1999) Help as mutual aid: Groupwork in mental health. *Groupwork*, 11(3), 30-49.

Manor, O. (2000a) *Choosing a Groupwork Approach: An inclusive stance*. London: Jessica Kingsley.

Manor, O. (2000b) The Working Alliance. In: M. Davis (Ed.) *The Blackwell Encyclopaedia of Social Work*. Oxford: Blackwell, Pp.375-376.

Manor, O. (2003) Groupwork fit for purpose? An inclusive framework for mental health. *Groupwork*, 13(3), 101-128.

Manor, O. (2009) Systemic Groupwork. In: A. Gitterman and R. Salmon (Eds.) *The Encyclopedia of Social Work with Groups*. New York: Routledge (pp.99-101).

McClure, B.A. (1998) *Putting a New Spin on Groups: The science of chaos*. London: Lawrence Elbaum Associates.

Middleman, R. R. and Goldberg Wood, G. (1990) *Skills for Direct Practice in Social Work*. New York: Columbia Press

Miller, R. and Mason, S. (2002) *Diagnosis Schizophrenia: A comprehensive resources for patients, families and helping professionals*. New York: Columbia Press.

Montgomery, C. (2002) Role of dynamic group therapy in psychiatry. *Advances in Psychiatric Treatment*, 8, 34-41.

Norton, K. (2003) Henderson hospital: Greater than the sum of its sub-groups. *Groupwork*, 13(3), 65-100.

Norton, K. (2004) Re-thinking acute psychiatric inpatient care. *International Journal of Social Psychiatry*, 50(3), 274-284.

Pinsof, W.M. (1994) An Integrative Systems Perspective on the Therapeutic Alliance: Theoretical, clinical and research implications. In: A.O. Horvath and L.S. Greenberg (Eds.) *The Working Alliance: Theory, research and practice*. New York: John Wiley. Pp.173-198.

Radcliffe, J. and Diamond, D. (2007) Psychodynamically-informed discussion groups on acute inpatient wards. *Groupwork*, 17(1), 34-44.

Radcliffe J. and Smith, R. (2007) Acute in-patient psychiatry: how patients spend their time on acute psychiatric wards. *Psychiatric Bulletin*, 31, 167-170.

Rathbone, G. and Campling, P. (2005) Psychotherapeutic approaches on acute wards. *Psychiatry*, 4(5) 14-18.

Rice, C.A. and Rutan, J.S. (1987) *Inpatient Group Psychotherapy: A dynamic perspective*. New York: Macmillan.

Roberts, R.W. and Northern, H. (eds.) (1976) *Theories of Social Work with Groups*. New York: Columbia University Press.

Robertson, S.J. and Davison, S. (1997) A survey of groups within a psychiatric hospital. *Psychoanalytic Psychotherapy*, 11(2), 119-134.

Rogers, C.R. (1970) *Encounter Groups*. New York: Harper and Row.

Ross, S. and Thorpe, A. (1988) Programming skills in social groupwork. *Groupwork*, 1(2), 135-146.

Ross, S. (1991) The termination phase in groupwork. *Groupwork* 4(1), 57-70.

Roth, A. and Fonagy , P. (1996) *What Works for Whom? A critical review of psychotherapy research*. London: The Guilford Press

Scott, M. J. and Stradling, S.G. *Brief Group Counselling: Integrating individual and group cognitive-behavioural approaches*. Chichester: John Wiley & Sons.

Shaffer, J.B.P. and Galinsky, M.D. (1974) *Models of Group Therapy and Sensitivity Training*. New Jersey: Prentice-Hall.

Vinogradov, S. and Yalom, I. (1989) *Concise Guide to Group Psychotherapy*. Washington, DC: American Psychiatric Publishers.

Watzlawick, P., Beavin, J.H. and Jackson, D.D. (1967) *Pragmatics of Human Communication*. New York: W.W. Norton & Co.

Wilden, A. (1980) *System and Structure: Essays in communication and exchange*. London: Tavistock Pub, 2nd edition.

Yalom, I.D. (1983) *Inpatient Group Therapy*. New York: Basic Books.

Yalom, I.D. (1995) *The Theory and Practice of Group Psychotherapy*. New York: Basic Books, 4th edition.

9

Interpersonal group therapy on an acute inpatient ward based on Yalom's model

Katja Hajek

Introduction

In this chapter I will describe an approach to inpatient group therapy which is based on the interpersonal model proposed by Irvin Yalom (1983). Firstly, I will outline the interpersonal theory which forms the theoretical underpinnings of this model, together with the main therapeutic factors and the principles used in running such a group. I will then talk about the differences between outpatient and inpatient groups and the way the model adapts to the environment and client group. The practical part of the chapter covers the goals of the inpatient group and the use of tasks during sessions together with examples of this work. Finally, our experience with using the model on an inpatient ward will be evaluated.

Yalom's Interpersonal Model

Our behaviour, adaptive and maladaptive, is formed in a social context and is influenced by interpersonal relationships with parents, friends, peers, teachers, partners and other people. To understand a person's behaviour we need to look at a wider picture of their relationships with others. People live in groups, and groups are fundamental to a person's development or even survival. There are many different types of family groups – large, small, one parent etc, but there will always be particular dynamics (how people relate to each other) that will be specific to that group. (Yalom, 1995). There is also a fundamental need to belong to groups throughout our lives – family, religious groups, ethnic groups, supporters of football teams, etc. Personality, motivation, behaviour and development are influenced by relationships with others.

Our mental health is strongly influenced by interpersonal relationships. People with mental health problems very often have a history of difficult past relationships with their parents and other family members – sometimes characterized by abusive or violent relationships with one of the parents, dysfunctional family dynamics, loss of a parent, etc. Such experiences can be expected to influence a person in a negative way, but the manifestations of this can be varied. A typical consequence however which affects many people with mental health problems are difficulties in creating and maintaining satisfying and lasting interpersonal relationships. This often creates a vicious circle of disturbed relationships or loneliness and isolation.

A number of theories have recognized the importance of relationships in mental health. More information about the background to interpersonal approaches can be found in Brabender and Fallon (1993, pp.115-176). Yalom's approach is particularly close to Harry Stack Sullivan's interpersonal theory (cited in Yalom & Leszcz, 2005). The need to be closely related to others is a basic human need. Sullivan saw interpersonal processes as the key focus of psychiatric research. Mental disorder should be 'translated' into interpersonal terms, and treated accordingly. Treatment should concentrate on correcting distortions within interpersonal relationships. Yalom's group therapy model follows the same principles.

Therapeutic factors in group therapy

The goal of any therapeutic process is to help people change the behaviour which is troubling them or is maladaptive, to a behaviour which will be more beneficial to them and help them to get along with others better. A person who has poor impulse control and gets angry quickly can benefit from learning how to control their anger and react in a way which does not lead to antagonism and isolation. Another person who is too shy and unwilling to take interpersonal risks and as a consequence feels lonely needs to learn how to create new relationships. Any change in social behaviour is obviously a complex process that takes place over a period of time. The experiences that people have in any type of psychological treatment which assist this change are called 'the therapeutic factors'. What are those crucial factors that help people change? Yalom describes eleven factors but we will mention just some of those that play a role in inpatient group therapy:

1. Instillation of hope
2. Universality
3. Altruism
4. Interpersonal learning
5. Group cohesiveness

Instillation of hope

De Chavez et al, (2000) compared the therapeutic factors in the inpatient therapy group for patients with schizophrenia with an outpatient group. Findings suggested factors found to be most important in the inpatient setting were installation of hope, cohesiveness and altruism (Emer, 2003).

High expectation of help before the start of therapy is significantly correlated with positive outcome. When people believe that the therapy will be helpful, it is more likely to turn out as expected. Patients who attend the group are in different stages of their illness- some may be recently admitted and feel desperate, hopeless and suicidal; others may be just before discharge and are much improved. As Yalom suggested in his earlier writings:

> One of the most important functions of an inpatient psychotherapy group may be that it allows patients who feel desperate to observe the improvement and success of others with similar symptoms (Yalom, 1983).

Universality

Several patients in the same therapy group may feel that they are the only person so depressed and hopeless that they want to end their life and that nobody else can understand them as nobody else has had similar feelings. Some people are burdened by 'terrible secrets' which they cannot share with other people because they would be instantly rejected, or have experiences they want to share but never had an opportunity or dared to do so. In the interpersonal group, people can share feelings and disclose personal information in a safe and supportive environment. Disclosure and sharing of deep feelings is usually accompanied by a feeling of relief as people discover that other members of the group have had similar experiences. This therapeutic factor is called universality. On a typical inpatient ward, this has yet another dimension; the group membership comprises people from different ethnic and cultural backgrounds. The interpersonal group focuses on universal experiences (eg a person who lost a loved one will be bereaved and sad irrespective of their religion or ethnicity) and encourages members to relate to each other on this level. The therapist must help the group to move past a focus on concrete cultural differences to transcultural and universal responses to human situations and tragedies (Tsui & Schultz, 1988).

Altruism

Many patients on an inpatient ward feel that they have nothing to offer to others, they see themselves as useless, and may feel they are a burden to others. In group therapy people share experiences and offer advice to others. People not only receive help, but also give help to others. Most people feel better when they can be useful to others. 'Being helpful to others' appears very often on their list of things they enjoy or regard as important. In a typical group clients discover that they can be very useful to each other. They offer each other support, feedback, advice, they share problems and feelings. Being altruistic also improves self-confidence.

Groups on acute inpatient wards

Groups on acute inpatient wards are notoriously difficult to run and the topic receives scant attention in writings on group therapy (Aveline & Dryden, 1988; Burlingame, MacKenzie & Strauss, 2004). There are several reasons for this. Patients stay in hospital for relatively short periods of time and the patient turnover is high; patients are acutely ill and some are heavily medicated which makes therapeutic engagement a challenge; and it is usually difficult to motivate patients to attend a group. At the same time groups can provide an important socialising influence, make a substantial contribution to the therapeutic environment of the ward, and can be used to add structure, purpose, and therapeutic elements to the hospital stay which can sometimes be empty and unproductive.

Yalom's model of group treatment was designed to be practicable and useful in the inpatient environment. In this section I will first briefly describe his approach and elaborate on the differences between outpatient and inpatient groups. I will then talk about my experience with running such groups on an all male acute inpatient ward in Lambeth, South London.

The group as a social microcosm

The group is a 'microcosm' of society. It is very likely that people in the therapy group will be from different ethnic and cultural backgrounds, from different professions and social classes, they will have different attitudes and different belief systems. This provides an opportunity to be confronted with views, ideas and behaviour patterns which may be different from one's own, and helps a person to consider their own behaviour and relationships.

Members will interact with the other members in the group as they interact outside – in their community. The clients will, over a period of time, display the same adaptive and maladaptive behaviours. These behaviours are, in the view of the interpersonal model, the core data for group work. Each member's style or habits will eventually appear in the group and will generate a specific dynamic. So, for example individuals who are too angry or too sensitive or too critical will generate a specific response from the others in the group. It is the facilitator's task to observe and recognize these behaviours, identify the maladaptive behaviours and use them therapeutically – e.g. start bringing these to the attention of the individual and exploring if the individual is aware of what impact these behaviours have on the others. Sometimes it is difficult to recognize these maladaptive behaviours as they may be hidden or unclear. The therapist needs to pay attention to things such as the emotional response of the other members – these responses can serve as data. For example, members can feel exploited, intimidated or dominated by a group member. If this is not an individual response, but a response from several people (possibly including the therapist), then the therapist will explore what behaviour elicited this. This is the advantage of group therapy – the observations and feedback are not just from one person – the therapist, but from several people – the group members.

Focus on 'here and now'

One of the key elements of the interpersonal model is the focus on the 'here and now.' The 'here and now' principle refers to a focus on what is happening in the immediate therapy session. Patients are not encouraged to talk about their past life experiences (although it is acknowledged that these are important). The rationale for this is that according to interpersonal theory, there is always an interpersonal component in the patient's symptomatology/psychopathology. The therapist is supposed to treat (or help with) the underlying interpersonal pathology. This will manifest itself in the way a patient reacts and behaves in the group. (e.g various maladaptive behaviours such as aggressiveness, dependency, egotism etc. will become apparent during the group interaction). These behaviours will serve as 'data' for the therapist, and it will be the therapist's task to help the patient see himself/herself as other see them. The here and now focus also provides the opportunity to experiment with different types of behaviour. The therapist may ask the patient to try a different behaviour in the group setting. Patients are also discouraged from talking about impersonal issues such as the political situation or football. As people will talk about these things, the therapist has to try to bring these topics back to the here and now – how is this impacting on you personally?

The differences between the outpatient and inpatient groups

Outpatient groups usually have between 6-10 members who meet regularly over a period of weeks or months. There is a stable membership and a lot of time to get to know each other well. Members of outpatient group are not acutely ill, or at least are functioning adequately in the outside world.

   Inpatient groups on the other hand have a high turnover of patients (some patients may only stay on the ward for a few days, others may stay for several months). Some patients may attend only one or two group sessions, other might attend six or seven. Patients are acutely mentally ill and have a wide variety of symptoms. Some people may be uncomfortable or suspicious about attending the group. The acute psychiatric ward is a radically different clinical setting and demands a radical modification of therapeutic goals and techniques (Yalom, 1983; 1995).

The single session time frame

As stated above, the inpatient group differs radically from the outpatient group in many ways. Probably the most radical difference is that the membership changes from group to group and some patients may only attend one session. Length of admission differs greatly from patient to patient, and as we said some patients will stay in the hospital for weeks, others will be discharged within days. In the inpatient setting, most patients will be able to attend a few group sessions, but some will only attend one. The 'one session time frame' determines the therapist's working style and leadership. To quote Yalom, 'there is no place in inpatient group therapy for the passive, inactive therapist' (Yalom, 1983, p107). The therapist needs to provide a firm structure for the group. Most patients on an acute unit feel confused, disorganized and frightened. A clear structure of the session helps them to feel safe and facilitates their engagement.

Formulation of goals

A set of goals needs to be established which are clear to the therapist and to the patients. It is often the case that inexperienced therapists start running a group without thinking through the model, the format, and what the group is trying to achieve. They hope that when patients come together they will be able to talk about their feelings or find themes to discuss. Such a group can generate silence, tension, disintegrate quickly, and end up with feelings of failure.

The goals of the group should be limited, achievable and tailored to the capacity and potential of group members. A group needs to provide a positive experience for the patients to want to attend again. For some, it may be an achievement just to attend a group and listen to others for 45 minutes. It is up to the facilitator to make sure that every involvement, no matter how small, is appreciated and patients associate the completion of each group session with feelings of achievement and success.

Goals of inpatient group therapy

The group on an inpatient ward can help to engage the patient in a therapeutic process and become the main vehicle of improving the therapeutic environment on the ward. On many acute inpatient wards the therapeutic environment suffers as other priorities (dealing with crises, close observations, carrying out risk and other assessments, recording activities, administrative tasks, etc) take over. Some wards may appear rather chaotic. Patients may feel they are not understood or even listened to. They may feel staff have other much more important things to do than talking to them. There may be no structure to the day and patients spend most of the time sitting about and waiting for the few structured events such as clinical rounds, meeting with their doctor, leave from the ward etc. The main principles of the therapeutic environment are structure, involvement, containment and support, (Lecuyer, 1992; Walker, 1994; Thomas, Shattel and Martin, 2002; Emer, 2003). All of these can be promoted by running a well structured and well functioning group.

1. *Engaging the patient in the therapeutic process.* In the group the patient will have an opportunity to talk about their personal issues, their treatment and any difficulties, to obtain feedback from other group members and from the group facilitator. This allows patients to become more active participants in their treatment.
2. *Reducing isolation.* Patients who are normally quite isolated will get involved in

the discussion and will be rewarded for sharing their ideas. Attending the group helps patients to form relationships and social networks in an environment which can otherwise be impersonal and alienating.

3. *Reducing anxiety connected with hospitalisation*: Many patients will feel anxious about being in the hospital. For some it may be their first admission and they are frightened by the new environment and by being among mentally ill people. Many patients will be in hospital on an involuntary basis (under the Mental Health Act) and perceive their stay as coerced punishment. The group can provide an outlet for discussing such feelings and it can substantially ameliorate such anxieties and fears.

4. *Providing experience of universality and of being helpful to others*: Among the number of different therapeutic factors present in groups, realising that other people have similar experiences and being helpful to others can play a special role in this particular setting. Being able to offer help to another is normally highly rewarding and group sessions can be geared specifically to providing such experience.

Working style

Interpersonal groups are structured and the facilitators are active and directive. They bring in a clear agenda. Once the group gets started, the proceedings will follow members' leads, but the clinician should always be ready to offer guidance and structure if needed.

Yalom in his textbook (Yalom, 1983) talks about two levels of inpatient group therapy: The Higher level inpatient therapy and the Lower level inpatient therapy. The higher level is generally for better functioning patients who are over the most severe phase of their illness, the lower level functioning group is for those who are still acutely ill. The main difference in those two groups is that in the higher functioning group the therapist asks patients to form 'an agenda' they would like to work on in this session. This has to be something regarding their relationships with others, a trait they would like to change etc. The therapist helps each patient to select the right topic. The inpatient groups I have been running in Lambeth are those described as the lower level functioning group and they do not use the 'agenda-go-round'.

A group session normally starts with an introduction and explanation of rules and aims in terms that patients find easy to understand. Then a task is set and members work either individually or in pairs. After the task is completed, there is a group discussion which comprises the main part of the session. Each member presents their contribution in turn. If somebody refuses to join in, this is accepted and such members are simply encouraged to listen to others and to join in when they want to do so.

Following the round of presentations responding to the group task, members are asked to comment and share with the group their reactions to what was presented, to give feedback to one another, compare notes, etc. The therapist is transparent and personal. Unlike in the psychodynamic group, where it would be thought inappropriate to reveal any personal information or answer personal questions, in the interpersonal group the therapist will be ready to discuss personal information where appropriate, or answer questions about his/her feelings and reactions.

The focus is on here and now; what is happening in the immediate session at the present time. Group members are discouraged from dwelling on events from distant past, (although they may talk about what happened to them in the past if this is relevant to the present topic). They are encouraged to concentrate on current experiences with the aid of tasks. The facilitator helps members to relate to one another, look at one another, direct comments to one another and address each other by their name. The task of the therapist is to guide from abstract statements to concrete statements and from impersonal to personal. Example: Patient: 'People make me angry'. Facilitator: 'Look around the room and say who makes you angry here.' This can then be used for giving and receiving feedback. Feedback is the core element of the interpersonal/interactional approach. As feedback does not happen automatically, it is the facilitator's task to initiate it and to teach members of the group to give constructive feedback, and to establish group norms which will allow people to give and receive feedback in a supportive atmosphere.

Working with tasks

The clinician's task is to help the group stay focused and to avoid raising anxiety levels by ambiguity or by allowing silences to develop. This is different from outpatient group work where lack of structure and occasional silence and tension are among the usual therapeutic tools. In the inpatient group setting an important priority is for patients to feel safe, to know what is expected and to feel that they can master the task.

The group tasks are designed to facilitate Disclosure, Acceptance, Feedback and Personal change.

Disclosure

For the inpatient group to work, members need to feel that the discussion is about something relevant to them and to their immediate situation. The tasks usually require each member to say something about themselves. This generates a discussion of their problems and facilitates thinking about possible solutions. It is the clinician's task to make this as safe as possible. Although self disclosure can be perceived as threatening, in my long experience with groups on inpatient wards, I have found very few patients who object to engaging with the tasks or are unable to join in.

Acceptance

It is important for group members to feel that once they have disclosed some personal information, especially if this includes issues which they may perceive as unattractive to others, they are still accepted by the group. This is another powerful therapeutic factor which the clinician needs to look out for and utilise.

Feedback

All the tasks and exercises are designed to encourage interaction between group members which can generate useful feedback. For instance members make comments such as: 'I know what you mean', 'This happened to me also', 'I have been in the same situation', providing the experience of universality. Sometimes the feedback can generate a new perception of one's behaviour and contribute to behaviour change. For example a patient became agitated in the group session and shouted at another patient. At the next meeting two members he liked discussed how this affected them, saying things like 'I did not like it when you shouted last week. I felt frightened'. This led the patient to think about the impact his behaviour had on others, and to consider ways of dealing with his anger.

Personal change

Ultimately, the aim of therapy is to help group members to change patterns of their behaviour which are causing problems in their day to day life and in their dealing with other people. The example above concerned controlling anger. On the other hand, someone who finds it difficult to ask for help can learn how to approach others and receive assistance, a subdued passive person can learn to be more assertive etc.

The nature of tasks

There are a number of tasks that can be used. Tasks can be short statements or incomplete sentences the patient is asked to complete, for example;

1. *One thing I would like to change about myself is.......*
2. *One of my strengths/weaknesses is.............*
3. *The person who inspired me the most was.............*
4. *The person who is most like me in the group is................*

To demonstrate how we work with tasks, here are some examples of discussions in our group when some of the above tasks were used.

One thing I would like to change about myself is ....

(this group was attended by seven patients, all men as this is an all male ward)

George started the discussion by saying that he would like to become a non-smoker. He said that he was doing an Allen Carr course and talked about his experience. Few other members were very interested and asked George questions about the course. Tom said he also tried to stop smoking but found it very difficult, especially when he was in the hospital. George said that there is a book by Allen Carr and recommended it to Tom. Mike said that he would like to be less anxious and have more self-confidence. The group then talked about what things make you anxious and what gives you more self-confidence.

Comment: Members of this group, all acutely ill, shared two common problems (smoking and how to quit)- (universality) and offered each other advice and help (altruism). They were finding commonalities and building relationships with each other which were likely to make their stay on the ward less anxious and less lonely.

The person who inspired me the most was....

(This is quite a difficult task as it can be understood on different levels including political or religious. This was the case in this group which was attended by five men.)

Vernon said that the person who inspired him most was Thabo Mbeki – the president of South Africa. When the group asked why, he explained that he was inspired by his speeches and because he united South Africa. He then shared some personal memories he had of his home country. Nigel said that the person who inspired him the most was his foster mother as she 'has given him a second chance in life'. He then talked about her and said that she was a very kind and understanding person. Liam said that the person who inspired him the most was Peter, a Roman Catholic priest who was teaching him about religion.

Comment: The task generated a range of responses with sharing experience of role models from personal to political. It demonstrated that patients are typically keen to talk about personal issues if the atmosphere is accepting and supportive and if they feel safe. The task is a natural 'opener' after which the facilitator can follow leads from the patients.

We sometimes use unfinished sentences to elicit a discussion about people's thoughts and feelings. This task was:

I am …., I feel …., I like …., I want …., I can …., I think …., I believe …., I wish ….

This was a small group with 4 patients

Ben was first to go: He read out what he wrote: I am flat, I feel flat, I like nothing, I want nothing, I can feel nothing, I think of nothing, I believe in nothing, I wish for nothing. There was a short silence after his reading. The group was struggling with the impact of this statement. Jim said that this sounded very depressing, and others agreed. Ben then said that he has been feeling like this for several years ever since his mother died. As Ben is in his fifties, one member asked what did his mother represent for him, and Ben said she represented love and security and he felt that that is what he lost. He has not found love and security since she has gone. He then talked about his brother and his sister and said he is not in touch with them because there were some conflicts in the past and he cannot forgive them. There was some discussion about this and how to 'repair' old conflicts.

Comment: Although the group was depressive and quite emotional, there was also a lot of disclosure and sharing.

Some tasks may involve pairing patients and asking them to discuss a given personal topic for 5 minutes. The members of the pair are encouraged to ask questions and find out as much as possible in the time provided. After this we re-join in the large group and members of each pair are asked to say everything they remember about the other person. The first person is then asked if the information was related correctly. This is also an exercise in listening skills.

An exercise may be organised around a theme which may be important for the group on that day. For example the therapist knows that a separation is an important issue for several patients, or because several members of the group are ready for discharge, and will soon be leaving. A set of questions related to separation may be used, such as

1. Someone I really miss is...........
2. I handle separation by...................

If, for example the ward is unsettled as some patients have been shouting and aggressive, the facilitator may decide to prepare a task relating to anger. For example:

1. When I get angry I ....
2. When someone is aggressive towards me, I feel....................
3. The best way to deal with anger is.................

Advantages of tasks

Tasks provide structure and minimize anxiety, as it is clear from the outset what the group is going to do. The first part of the session resembles a classroom model with the facilitator being the teacher. I have found that patients respond to this well, and are quite keen to work on the task.

Beginning therapists sometimes believe that an open group without an agenda would elicit patients' feelings and ideas. However, they usually find that if they start the group with an opening such as 'What would you like to talk about today?' or 'Does anybody want to talk about their problems?', there will be silence, uncertainty and discomfort. While in an outpatient setting such emotions may later prove to be productive 'data', on an acute ward this is unproductive and will increase anxiety and confusion. I have also found in my clinical practice that new staff may also feel the task would 'restrict' patients, that patients would find the tasks difficult, or would be reluctant to work with them. This however seems to reflect the anxieties of the staff raher than the patients.

Tasks promote interest in each other. Once the group gets going, patients listen to others and are usually keen to speak. By sharing ideas and feelings the group develops cohesiveness and provides mutual support. There is an opportunity to learn from one another and to give each other feedback.

Selection of patients for group treatment

All patients on the acute admission ward are severely mentally ill, but their mental state fluctuates and so does their functioning. Some patients have been on the ward for weeks or even months, others have only just been admitted. Some patients may be manic, very thought disordered, or aggressive and therefore disruptive to the group, and so not suitable for inclusion. If the group therapist is not a full time member of staff familiar with all the patients on the ward, they need the co-operation of either an assistant psychologist or nursing staff who can advise on participation. If the therapist is coming on to the ward just half an hour before the start of the group, they will need a handover from ward staff.

It is important that the therapist explains the rationale behind selecting patients. On some wards, there is a feeling that the group should be open to ALL patients, as staff do not want to exclude anyone from activities on the ward. It is important to make sure that staff understand what the aims of the group are, that the group has to be able to 'work' on patients' issues, and that this is not possible when there are a few (or just one) patient who would disrupt the proceedings.

Practical experience with inpatient groups on an acute admission ward

We have been running groups based on Yalom's interpersonal model on one of the Lambeth acute admission wards for the past two years. The ward is an all male, 22 bedded unit which caters for severely mentally ill clients from the London Borough of Lambeth. This is located in an inner city area and is one of the most socially deprived parts of Britain. In 2005-2006 a total of 106 patients attended the group (this is about 50% of all patients admitted to the ward). A total of 48% of clients had a diagnosis of schizophrenia or psychosis, 20% bipolar affective disorder, 8% depression, 7% dual diagnosis and 17% had other diagnoses. Groups are run weekly by a clinical psychologist and an assistant psychologist. The total of 84% of patients who joined the group treatment attended between 1-3 sessions, 12% attended between 4-6 sessions, and 4% attended more then 6 sessions.

To provide an illustration of this work, below is a brief example of a recent session:

Example: John

John had attended the group in the past, but he did not come for several weeks. He decided to attend again today. He has a problem with anger and used to become very angry and aggressive on the ward. He also became aggressive during his last group session and as it was not possible to reason with him at the time, he had to be asked to leave. Today's group task was: The person who has influenced me most in my life is………
One member of the group talked about his mother, another talked about Mohammed Ali and then it was John's turn. John said that the person who influenced him most was his father. He always did things with him and John was very close to him. Then John said that his father died about a year ago and he became tearful saying that he missed him. The group listened, and then Peter turned to John and told him that he could see a new side to him now. He found him confrontational and aggressive in the past which for him was off-putting, but could see him in a different and engaging light now. The group was invited to give feedback to John and they shared Peter's views and gave support and encouragement to John. John appeared reflective and appreciative of this feedback.

The example also shows how patients who are not well enough to attend the group one week, may benefit from attending later.

At the end of each session we ask patients to express their views about the session. Typical examples of patients' feedback include e.g. 'It is good to hear other people's experiences, to realize you are not on your own'; 'It helps you to think about things'; 'In the group people listen'; 'You get to know the others'; 'You learn to understand other people's views'. Patient feedback is generally gratifyingly positive.

Some logistics and practical issues

There are some issues that should be considered before embarking on running a group on an inpatient ward. Amongst these are the frequency of the sessions, arrangements to make sure patients are invited to attend, division of labour in organising and running groups, and arrangements for data and feedback collection. It is essential that the group sessions are backed by ward staff and the ward manager. There is little chance that the group will succeed if it is not approved of by all staff and especially by the ward management.

Evaluation

There is some evaluative research that supports the usefulness of groups on inpatient wards. Leszcz, Yalom, and Norden (1985) found that inpatients consistently reported group psychotherapy to be among the most useful treatments they received. Also group therapy on inpatient wards is viewed as an important addition to psychopharmacotherapy (Pollack, 1995).

Locally we have also tried to evaluate the usefulness of inpatient groups. Recently an extensive audit of patient satisfaction was implemented on three Lambeth acute adult admission wards (Hajek & DeReuck, 2007). One part of the audit asked about satisfaction with activities including group sessions on the ward. The ward offering this type of group treatment was part of this audit, and the results were encouraging. One of the questions was: Do you find the ward activities which you attend helpful? On the ward where interpersonal group was offered 100% of patients replied yes while only 50% and 90% respectively replied yes to the same question on the two other wards which offer different type of groups.

Evaluation of the interpersonal group

To evaluate the interpersonal group locally, we devised a short questionnaire to ask participants about various aspects of the group. The questions were related to the aims of the group. One of the aims is to get to know other members of the group better: Question: Did you get to know the other members of the group better?; Another aim of the group is to involve patients in their therapy – Question was: Did you feel involved in the group? , Aim: to listen to patients views – Question – Did you feel listened to?

We have evaluated ten groups run on one of the Lambeth wards between February 2008 and May 2008. Thirty five responses were collected. Some patients attended more then one group session but each session had a different membership and a different task, and was treated separately.

The results showed that 89% of respondents indicated that they enjoyed attending the group, 74% found the group helpful, and 51% said that they have learnt something about themselves. On the whole patients did not find it difficult to work with tasks. (See summary of results in appendix 1)

The results of this small preliminary evaluation are encouraging. They suggest that the group meets the expectations/goals that it sets out to achieve, i.e. to be supportive (77% of respondents felt supported), to make sure that people feel listened to (89% said yes), to be involved in their treatment (86% felt involved) and to get to know the other members better (83%).

Conclusions

Yalom's interpersonal model of group therapy tailored to inpatient wards proved a useful and well received addition to the ward's therapeutic activities. The group is tailored to patients' needs and to the environment of the ward. Each group can stand 'alone' and patients can attend as many or as few groups as they want which is vital on a ward where length of admission can vary from a few days to a few months. The clear structure of the sessions and the use of tasks have proved productive. Even patients with severe mental health problems are able to use the group and relate well to the tasks.

A small scale evaluation showed that the group helped to engage patients in their treatment, made them feel supported and listened to, and that they found the group useful. Group sessions have an important role to play in contributing to therapeutic environment on the ward, to a supportive atmosphere, and to a reduction of anxiety connected with hospitalization. They also contribute to creating a cohesive patient group and a supportive networks amongst patients. Group therapy can be usefully adapted to the challenging environment of an acute inpatient psychiatric ward.

References:

Aveline, M. and Dryden, W. (Eds.) (1988) *Group Therapy in Britain*. Milton Keynes: Open University Press.

Brabender, V. and Fallon, A. (1993) Models of Inpatient Group Psychotherapy. Washingtoon DC:American Psychological Association.

Burlingame, G., MacKenzie, K., and Strauss, B. (2004) Small-group treatment: Evidence for effectiveness and mechanisms of change. In Lambert, M. (Ed.) *Bergin and Garfield's Handbook of Psychotherapy and Behaviour Change*. New York: Wiley.

De Chavez, M.G., Gutierrez, M., Ducaju, M., and Fraile, J.C. (2000). Comparative study of the therapeutic factors of group therapy in schizophrenic inpatients. *American Journal of Art Therapy*, 39, 108-112

Emer, D. (2003) The use of groups in inpatient facilities: needs, focus, successes, and remaining dilemmas. In DeLucia–Waack, J., Gerrity, D., Kalodner, C, and Riva, M.. (Eds) *Handbook of Group Counselling and Psychotherapy*. London: Sage (pp 351-365).

Hajek, K. and DeReuck, T. (2007) *Patient Satisfaction Audit*. Lambeth Directorate. London: South London and Maudsley NHS Foundation Trust. Unpublished Document. Copies available on request to the first author.

Lecuyer, E. (1992) Milieu therapy for short term units: A transformed practise theory. *Archives of Psychiatric Nursing*, 6, 108-116

Leszcz, M., Yalom, I.D., and Norden,M (1985) The value of inpatient group psychotherapy; Patients' perceptions. *International Journal of Group Psychotherapy*, 35, 411- 433

Pollack, L.E (1995) Informational needs of patients hospitalized for bipolar disorder. *Psychiatric Services*, 46, 1191-1194

Thomas, S.P., Shattel.M and Martin,T. (2002) What's therapeutic about the therapeutic milieu? *Archives of Psychiatric Nursing*, 16, 3, 99-107

Tsui, P. and Schultz, G.L. (1988) Ethnic factors in group process: cultural dynamics in multi-ethnic groups. *American Journal of Orthopsychiatry*, 58, 1, 136-142

Walker, M. (1994) Principles of a therapeutic milieu: an overview. *Perspectives in Psychiatric Care*, 30, 3, 5-8

Yalom, I.D. (1983) *Inpatient Group Therapy*. New York: Basic Books.

Yalom, I D. (1995) *The Theory and Practice of Group Therapy*. New York; Basic Books

Yalom, I.D. and Leszcz, M. (2005) *The Theory and Practice of Group Psychotherapy*. New York: Basic Books

Appendix 1
Evaluation of interpersonal group

		Frequency	%
Q1. Did you enjoy the group?	Yes	31	88
	No	2	6
	Unanswered	2	6
Q2. Did you get to know the other members better?	Yes	29	83
	No	5	14
	Unanswered	1	3
Q3. Did you learn anything new about yourself?	Yes	18	51
	No	16	46
	Unanswered	1	3
Q4. Did you feel the group was supportive?	Yes	27	77
	No	5	14
	Unanswered	3	9
Q5. Did you feel you were able to express your views?	Yes	31	89
	No	4	11
	Unanswered	0	0
Q6. Did you feel listened to?	Yes	31	89
	No	2	6
	Unanswered	2	6
Q7. Did you find using the task difficult?	Yes	8	23
	No	25	71
	Unanswered	2	6
Q8. Did you feel you were involved in the group?	Yes	30	86
	No	3	9
	Unanswered	2	5
Q9. Did you find the group helpful?	Yes	26	74
	No	7	20
	Unanswered	2	6

The Communication Group

Reflections on the setting up, running and supervision of an inpatient group

Adam Jefford, Alistair Grandison
and Bhupinderjit Pharwaha

Introduction

Inner city acute psychiatric wards are well recognised to be under ever increasing pressure with rapid turn over of patients, shorter lengths of stay and increasingly unwell patients being admitted. (Dratcu, 2002). In such an environment, medication is normally the first line of treatment. It can act quickly for some patients, offering them relief from their symptoms as well as allowing them to be contained and managed more safely. It may also prevent patients' conditions deteriorating and reduces the risk they pose to both themselves and others.

Once patients are beginning to show signs of improvement there is pressure to move them on and with the development of home treatment teams (Johnson et al, 2005, Smith, 2003) this occurs increasingly early. Psychological treatments should play a crucial part in mental health care but they are not always accessible to those admitted to in-patient units, where patients are at their most needy (NICE, 2005) In such a high-pressured environment psychotherapeutic interventions, and in particular group psychotherapy, may be seen as having little relevance. However, this is not the case and group therapy in a modified form can have a valuable role to play even in such a setting, if it is specifically tailored to the acute inpatient environment.

We describe the experience of setting up and running a weekly psychotherapeutic group on an acute adult inner-city ward, and discuss in depth issues arising in supervising such a group which has now been running weekly over a four year period.

Background and setting

John Dickson Ward at Guys Hospital is an inner London 18-bed male acute psychiatric ward. This service has previously been described (Dratcu et al, 2003). In the interim the ward has changed from a mixed sex ward to a male-only ward. As with most acute inpatient psychiatric wards, it is a busy place with bed-occupancy rates consistently exceeding 100% and admitting over 200 patients each year.

Although the ward's occupational therapist provides a number of activities ranging from community and educational groups to physical activities, before the communication group there were no formal psychological interventions. With a view to promoting a better therapeutic milieu on the ward and further improving the patients' standards of care, in 2005 it was proposed to implement a more formal model of psychological care that was compatible with the setting. As no extra staffing resources were available, this was planned from existing resources.

Group psychotherapy has in many places been virtually abandoned in the acute inpatient setting. Increased work pressure, changes in working practices and financial constraints may all be in part to blame. As well as this, there is often a reluctance amongst senior medical and nursing staff to support group therapy partly because they may think it has little to offer in such a setting or they have little knowledge or experience of it.

The model of group therapy that is carried out in the outpatient setting with neurotic and personality disordered patients receiving therapy in a closed group for an agreed number of sessions, does not fit with the acute inpatient setting. In the outpatient setting patients usually undergo careful selection procedures and are less likely to have psychotic illnesses. On acute wards the psychopathology encountered is much more varied. Patients are admitted who typically are suffering from acute and chronic schizophrenia, major affective disorders, borderline and severe neurotic disorders, situational reactions, dual diagnosis with substance misuse, and organic disorders. All patients tend to be severely ill. Many may initially appear too unwell to engage in a group. Others may appear unmotivated, be thought to lack sufficient psychological sophistication, be detained in hospital against their wishes often stating they do not need any help. These are all likely exclusion criteria in the conventional outpatient group therapy setting. Group therapy, to be effective in the ward setting, needs to address two issues in particular; rapid turnover of patients with the result that rarely if ever will there be the same members in a group on two consecutive sessions, and the heterogeneity of psychopathology.

Yalom's Model

When planning our group we looked at models of in-patient group therapy and found Yalom's model (1983, 1985) to be the most relevant. Models that are based on specific diagnostic categories (e.g. schizophrenia) such as Kanas's (1996, 2000), address the need for patients with these diagnoses but are not designed for heterogeneous groups. As Yalom's model is described in detail in another chapter in this book (see Katja Hajek's chapter) we will not describe this again here in any depth. Instead, our intention is to describe the aspects of Yalom's model that we have adopted, and to then also make clear where, and why, we have deviated from his approach in order to suit our particular setting and its needs.

We have incorporated the following ideas from Yalom's model of inpatient group therapy into our approach:

> The idea that each individual group session be treated as a stand-alone 'one-off' event. Even if patients attend more that one session, they are not assumed to be able to hold in mind the way the group works. The staff need to explain clearly the way the group works each time, as if it were a new event. This is particularly important when the group meets weekly rather than daily, and when there is a turnover of both staff facilitators and patients between sessions.

The aim is that the group should be a safe and supportive experience. This is also the case for group therapy in other settings. However, in traditional outpatient group psychotherapy there can also be a place for more challenging interpersonal exploration, such as giving difficult feedback or expressing interpersonal conflicts. In the inpatient setting it is important that the group feels safe, supportive and constructive, and avoids too much conflict or tension. The facilitators aim to reduce anxiety and avoid directly challenging patients. They provide clear focus and structure, and take an active and supportive stance rather than a more passive, reflective role. For example, anxiety provoking silences are avoided, and facilitators will intervene to try to assist patients who are finding it difficult to stay in the room.

Yalom (1983, 1985) reminds us that the role of acute inpatient group therapy is not to resolve patients' symptoms. He describes six basic achievable goals for inpatient group therapy.

- Engaging patients in the therapeutic process
- Demonstrating that talking helps
- Problem spotting
- Decreasing isolation
- Being helpful to others
- Alleviating hospital-related anxiety

The overall aim is to help patients to make more sense of their experience of being on the ward. The group aims to help interpersonal interactions between patients and between patients and staff. It can also help patients to make more sense of their current difficulties in the ward setting and in their lives outside.

The main differences and adaptations between our group approach and that of Yalom's model are described in the following sections on setting up the group, and on how the group operates.

Setting up the group

The idea of setting up a group on the ward was initially suggested by the ward manager, who was an enthusiastic supporter of the project, as was the Associate Specialist, one of the senior medical staff. Other interested staff from the ward team were recruited to plan the project, including nursing staff and the ward's occupational therapist. The senior manager of the local therapeutic community day service, a group analyst (first author), agreed to provide supervision. There were initially a core team of six ward staff who would go on to facilitate the groups. One of the differences between this group and some other inpatient groups was in deciding early in the process that the ward staff themselves would develop the skills to facilitate the group. The expertise in groupwork would be provided by the supervisor and over time by the staff's developing their own skills through experience and reflective practice. This is in contrast to some other in-patient groups where the 'experts' come in to conduct the group sessions, sometimes alongside ward staff.

In the course of several preparatory meetings between the supervisor and the facilitators, Yalom's model was discussed and adaptations were agreed, one being that we would run the once a week instead of every week day as Yalom recommends. One reason for this was the presence of other programmed activities in the weekly ward timetable, another was a pragmatic sense of what could be realistically set up without a far greater reorganisation of the whole ward and staff routine.

The weekly model also affected the choice of whether to follow Yalom's suggestion of a 'lower' and a 'higher' functioning group, based on the patients' capacity to function and levels of disturbance. The initial decision taken was to try to be as inclusive as possible, and to invite as many patients as possible to attend each group session. There are pros and cons to this approach. Yalom's main point in regard to this is that the more acutely disturbed patients can exhibit behaviour that is agitated and confused, and too disruptive to the meeting. His model for the 'lower functioning' group caters more for the needs of these more acutely unwell patients. Our solution has been to be as inclusive as possible with some exclusion criteria - for those patients considered unlikely to be able to tolerate the sessions, or thought likely to be too disruptive to others. Thus selection and preparation before the group sessions becomes an important task. The hope is that patients unable to attend one week may be more able to attend and benefit from later group sessions as they recover.

In preparatory meetings close consideration was given to practical issues such as where and when it would happen, and how staff could arrange to be reliably available given shift rotas and ward timetables. This planning would be critical if the group were to be successfully established and accepted by ward staff and patients. From the pool of available staff, facilitators would change each week to give all the facilitators a chance to be involved and develop their skills. Once the group was established, two facilitators would participate in each therapy session. One and a half hour supervision sessions were run fortnightly with as many of the facilitator team present as possible.

There was much debate about what name to give the group and we eventually settled upon 'the Communication Group'. This reflects some of the aims of the group, to improve communication between patients and between patients and staff. It was interesting to note how much energy went into discussing the name of the group. This could be seen as a useful container for staff to express initial anxiety about what the group experience would be like, and their own role in it.

How the Group operates?

The group takes place once a week at the same time for fifty minutes in a large activities room on the ward. This gives a secure setting that is part of the ward but separate from the main areas. Patients have to be let through a door to the room by staff, but are able to leave if they wish. This gives the advantages that patients do not feel trapped in the group as they can leave, but also that the staff can control whether anyone should be readmitted to the group having left.

Patients are encouraged to participate in the group as early as possible after they have been admitted, some within the first twenty-four hours. The ward has a daily morning planning meeting where patients are told about the group. Patients who are considered suitable are seen by a member of the nursing staff on the day of the group, are told what is involved, and encouraged to attend. It is explained that they will only have to speak if they want to, and although it is preferable for them to remain for the duration of the group, they are allowed to leave before the end.

The aim is for between four and ten patients per session, and typically six to eight attend. In addition to the two group facilitators, an additional staff member is often present in the room as an observer. This may be for example, a member of staff who plans to join the group as a new facilitator, or a student nurse.

Patients and facilitators sit in circle. If an observer is present then they sit outside the circle. Once the group starts then no new patients are allowed to enter the session. Patients who leave are usually allowed to return, unless their behaviour is considered too disruptive.

Each group starts with one of the facilitators introducing themselves, explaining the purpose of the group and saying how long it will last. Patients are then asked to introduce themselves in a round, and to say whether there is anything that they would like to use the group to talk about today. After that the facilitators return to one of the members who has said that there is something that they wish to talk about and invite them to do so. The group discussion lasts for approximately forty-five minutes. Shortly before the group is due to end the facilitators inform the group that it will soon be finishing and invite the members to again say their names and briefly state how they have found today's session. The reason for asking names to be repeated is to reinforce the helpful 'icebreaking' social aspect of the group being a place where some patients first talk to each other and start to get to know each other. Often a group member who has been largely silent during a session will at least volunteer their name by the end.

The facilitators hold a fifteen minute debriefing session after each group, followed by supervision every other week.

Some examples of group material

Some very common recurrent themes from the group material include the following:

Going on leave from the ward

In one of the early supervision sessions the psychiatrist expressed surprise and interest in the way group members talked about leave from the ward. In contrast to the usual encounter in the ward rounds where patients would focus on arguing their case for more leave, in the group members were talking about their anxieties; *'I get anxious about going on leave … this place turns in to your home'; 'I know what you mean, this place is safe. It's the outside you don't know about'; ' I start to sweat about it you know'.*

The experiences of coming into hospital, being unwell and having problems

Patients often give each other advice and support as well as sometimes challenge each other.

How do you cope with being unwell on the ward? Three responses in one session:

'Listen to music, or change rooms as sometimes there are stray souls that linger in between the walls.'

'Read the paper or go have a chat with someone in the smoking room. If you're not well you know it for yourself and know how bad it is. You should be aware of your mental state, your behaviour and dress.'

'If you have your arm cut off etc you know that it's gone and something's not right. If you don't know you're mentally unwell then maybe you aren't that bad or mentally unwell in the first place.'

The pros and cons of using alcohol, drugs and prescribed medication.

These are frequent topics of discussion. The group is often divided over whether illegal drugs or alcohol help or exacerbate problems. Similarly members share experiences of prescribed medications; their side-effects and whether they are helping.

The ward as a repressive place where freedoms are restricted, and things do not work as they should, versus the ward as a safe and protective environment

These two viewpoints are usually present in some way. It is rare to hear negative comments about the staff or the ward without some balancing positive comments from other people. We could relate this to Melanie Klein's psychoanalytic concepts of the division and projection of experiences into 'good' and 'bad'. For most people being a patient in any hospital ward involves a degree of regression and dependency. This consequently stirs up strong feelings about authority and being dependent – being cared for but also being controlled in some way.

Asking staff for rationales about why things happen or do not happen on the ward

This is very common. Usually it is helpful for staff to give rationales. However there is a risk of the group turning into a 'complaints session' and therefore skill is needed on the part of the facilitators in turning this around to more personal concerns, or useful dialogue.

Supervision

Staff facilitating the group have widely varying experience of delivering therapy, and supervision has been an essential part of helping them develop their skills, confidence and a way of working. The ward staff have developed a sense of ownership of the group over time. It is worth noting that they spend time with the same patients on the ward outside the group sessions. This means that care needs to be taken over how to manage being in a different role and relationship with patients inside and outside the sessions, and this is one area discussed in the supervision. As the staff are not trained to run groups but are learning 'on the job' there is an element of trying things out without the opportunity to work alongside an experienced group therapy specialist. In each supervision session staff present the last group session as it happened over the course of the session. This includes who was present, what patients said in the introductory round, and the material raised and in what sequence and finishes with the ending 'feedback round'. It is striking just how difficult it can be to present the material chronologically. We understand this as reflecting how chaotic, fragmented and often psychotic the material can be, and how this can flood or disrupt thinking for staff and patients. As the supervision meeting directly follows a group session, staff have limited time to process what has happened beforehand and there is a 'ripple' effect from the group which carries the emotional tone of the session as well as some of the disturbed thought processes. An example is an encounter with staff just before the supervision session. Staff were laughing and joking, making silly comments and enjoying quick and witty banter. Soon afterwards in the supervision session it was reported that two manic and competing patients had dominated the group. Similarly, finding a supervision session itself to be chaotic or sleep-inducing gives clues to what the patients may have been experiencing and projecting into staff. Such parallel processes carrying into supervision have long been recognised in the analytic tradition (e.g. Searles, 1955). Remembering and describing a session is particularly difficult when the ward is disturbed. This shows the challenges and efforts involved for staff and patients to meet together and manage to be thoughtful and reflective in the face of internal and external disturbance.

Having an observer taking notes in the session has helped us to convey what has happened in supervision. Despite the risk that this may disturb some patients, we have found that the group accepts this when we explain it to them. The difficulties in thinking described above also emphasise the need for post group discussions, and time in supervision to make sense of the group experience.

Staff who take the lead facilitator role in the group often express concern about whether they have got the introduction 'right'. It is an important intervention, in order to set the aims and establish a structure. However, it can feel like there is a lot of pressure to magically unlock the group and make the conversation flow easily. There are many variables that determine whether a useful dialogue will take place. Much can depend on which patient speaks first in the introductory round in setting the tone. If the first person says little about themselves or their current concerns, then the rest tend to follow suit. Where possible we therefore choose a patient who is more confident and who has been to the group before.

We often discuss in supervision whether the facilitators should introduce topics rather than developing whatever the group members raise spontaneously. Ideally, patients will raise concerns during the introductory round that can form the basis for dialogue and exploration in which case patients may start talking to each other spontaneously. This is not typically the case, and there is a danger of the group becoming silent, stuck, withdrawn and anxious, or alternatively lively, but chaotic and fragmented. We try wherever possible to draw on the concerns raised by the patients. When the topic is likely to have some relevance to other group members, this is usually successful in getting dialogue going. Yalom emphasises drawing attention to what is happening in the 'here and now'. Sometimes this focused attention from staff on what is happening in the group can feel like too much pressure and the group shuts down again. The group sometimes seems to need to find a safe way to begin dialogue by focusing on something outside the group. In outpatient group psychotherapy one might point this out to the group as a group defence. In the inpatient setting, the 'here and now' focus can usefully be extended to what has been happening on the ward. If the group appears 'stuck' then staff might introduce topics about life on the ward which are likely to be relevant for most group members. Equally, for a particularly anxious group, discussions about football or TV programmes for example are seen as a way to begin a safe dialogue which will then be gently steered around towards more personal concerns. A light or playful dialogue between people can lead the way to a more meaningful and therapeutic dialogue. As Winnicott points out – '...playing leads into group relationships' (Winnicott, 1971, p48).

The staff group facilitators also face a dilemma when group members are demanding an explanation for staff behaviour on the ward, outside the group itself. Often this is related to the restrictions and dissatisfactions of ward life, and group members take the opportunity to challenge the staff present in the session to provide answers. When this is about individual treatment plans, group members are usually advised to discuss this with staff outside the group or at the ward round. When the subject is practical ward issues, it may be appropriate to redirect member's concerns to the ward community meeting. In other cases the group provides a valuable opportunity for dialogue between staff and group members and a chance to address both personal concerns and issues affecting many group members. It can then be useful for group facilitators to give clear and direct rationales for their actions. While it can be difficult for staff to be challenged in this way at times, and they may be concerned that the session will become about their answering complaints, the results of giving direct rationales are usually positive.

The following example is taken from a group session presented in supervision and illustrates how even quite difficult interpersonal encounters between staff and patients can be tackled. In this vignette Alan is one of the patients while Paul and Brian are the staff members (not their real names).

Example: Alan

The group had been talking about various negative experiences of ward life when Alan, said he had been forcibly restrained by staff and given medication against his will; 'Why did that have to happen? It was painful having my arms pressed down.' Most of the other group members challenged the staff facilitators to give answers. Paul, one of the group facilitators, began talking about the different reasons for having to use physical restraint, especially when there is a danger to self or others. Alan angrily demanded to know why this was done to him. Paul said 'OK I'll explain it to you before the end of the group, but I want to let everyone here know why we have to do that.' He turned to the others and continued to explain how the use of restraint is about making the ward safe for everybody –it depends on what has happened before, and meant trying other alternatives first. He returned to Alan, 'Can you remember what was happening before the restraint?' Alan responded, 'You wanted to give me medication and said I had to calm down.' Paul asked 'And before that?' Alan said 'you mean when I was trying to hit that guy? He was pissing me off.'

Alan was fairly calm at this point. There was further discussion about the circumstances, how the situation could have been handled safely and whether an alternative solution could have been found. Another patient, Brian, said that the ward had been particularly busy and stressful for everyone in the previous week and perhaps the staff had needed to react more quickly than they might usually have done in order to keep the ward safe. The atmosphere of the session seemed to change to one where staff and patients became closer, being curious together about what had been going on. Most group members agreed in the closing round that this had been a useful session and were observed to leave the room in animated conversations.

It can be a relief for patients to hear explanations from staff who can demonstrate that they are thinking about the patients and the safe running of the ward, and can also provide corrective reality orientation to counter confusion or fear about staff motives.

Other points of technique discussed in the supervision include strategies for dealing with group members who monopolise the session, or who bring delusional or confusing material which may be hard for others to understand. While the goal can never be for all group members to take absolutely equal space in the session, there are good reasons not to allow anyone to monopolise in a way that loses the rest of the members or prevents any meaningful dialogue (see Yalom 1983, p134-5). There is a balance to be struck between the need for each individual to express themselves and to be heard respectfully and the needs of the wider group to remain interested and involved. The suggested approach to the monopoliser is for staff to intervene to limit what others may experience as a 'rant' or 'ramble', where sense is lost and other people lose interest. At the same time, by listening carefully to what is being said by the individual it should be possible to understand something of their experience that can be acknowledged and validated. Other group members can then be invited to respond to what has been said.

One area that supervision has helped the group facilitators become increasingly aware of is the effects that events on the ward have on a session. The idea of events in the wider ward setting being played out in any group held within it, is familiar from the therapeutic community literature (e.g. Hinshelwood, 1987). However, it is not easy at first to make these connections or see the relevance. One example is the effect of a violent incident, or particularly aggressive patient on the ward affecting the whole ward atmosphere. This might affect a group session in various ways, from either it being talked about directly, to a situation where the group seems preoccupied with something that might later be understood, through reflection in supervision, as expressing anxiety about safety on the ward.

Another example was the puzzlement when the patients suddenly began to struggle much more than usual with the group structure. On one occasion the group members kept bringing up practical problems with the ward environment such as a broken shower. It turned out to be connected to the re-introduction of ward patient business meetings and the confusion for some patients about what should happen in which meeting. In another session it was very hard to encourage anybody to speak in the group. Of course this can happen anyway from time to time, and when it does one tries to understand what might be going on e.g. are there particular anxieties for patients within the group itself or in the overall ward context? In this particular session, where patients seemed especially unwilling to speak, it was discovered later in the supervision session that several of the patients in the group had also been to a 'relaxation/chill-out' group that week which was all about relaxing and *not* talking. Such confusion about how to use the group underlines the importance of stating the aims and structure each time the group meets.

In addition to discussing issues arising during the group in supervision sessions, in the early stages of the life of the group much work was done on practical and organisational issues, such as making sure that the relevant staff and patients were available to attend each session. The staff who chose to be involved in running the group, were highly motivated and enthusiastic and some staff even came in to facilitate the group and attend supervision on their days off. This resulted in the group becoming quickly established as an important event in the week of the ward. It quickly became apparent that it was vital to identify in advance which staff members would facilitate the group rather than relying on whoever was on shift to do so. An initial team of six facilitators was only just enough to ensure two facilitators were available each week once shift patterns and staff absences were taken into account. We therefore recruited two more people to create a pool of eight. When a member of the facilitation team leaves it has been important to replace them as quickly as possible and to provide training for the new member. There is limited opportunity on a busy ward for the staff involved to meet and think about the group and so organisational issues are discussed during supervision. At times, pressures and forces at work on a ward can disrupt the group sessions in various ways and these need to be understood and worked through. The rest of the staff not directly involved in the project need to value and support the group. Otherwise there are so many competing demands and priorities on a ward that can sabotage the sessions (Simpson, 2002). For example making sure that staff members are really free to run the sessions and that other staff can respond to alarms etc during sessions, or that patients expected to attend the group are not called away for other reasons. After approximately two months the group began to become an established event for both staff and patients in the wards therapeutic programme. Over the course of the first year of the group, the balance of time spent in supervision on organisational concerns and on the group material shifted markedly in favour of the group material, compared with the starting point.

Facilitators' experience of being involved in the group

All the staff who have been involved have found it a rewarding and valuable experience. Some of the benefits were common to staff of different disciplines, whereas others were specific to each profession.

Nurses

1. Nurses said that they gained a richer understanding of patients' experiences, such as how they perceived their conditions. An example of this was a patient with a diagnosis of bipolar affective disorder who explained that he viewed his illness as a reaction to the lack of sun in this country, which he found 'stifling.' He said this with sadness, highlighting the contrast with Barbados, his country of origin, where there was enough sun to maintain his well-being. Another example was when patients talked about access to their medical notes. Some patients said they did not want to see their notes and were content for professionals to keep the files because they did not want to think about what they 'have' (i.e. a diagnosis, or a sense of themselves as unwell).

2. Often staff can feel they do not have time to stop and think about events affecting functioning and communication with each other. They can be left feeling desensitised, sidelining important issues and focusing instead on the practical task of running the ward. As well as the group allowing patients a chance to reflect on issues they raise in the group, it also allows facilitators a chance to reflect the same issues from their own perspective.

3. Nurses felt the group helped break down the barriers between them and patients, the 'us versus them'. They valued the opportunity to play a less custodial role and to be able to demonstrate empathy and interest in a more therapeutic context. Although nurses sometimes felt uncomfortable when challenged in the group they felt able to deal with these challenges constructively.

4. Nurses found it uplifting to observe patients who did not talk to each other on the ward giving advice and support to others in the group. Although this advice was not always conventional, it was good to see these patients sharing experiences and trying to help others.

5. There was often a 'rolling over' after the group. For example patients who were together in the group would be sitting with each other in the dining room and sometimes even conversing. This was in contrast to the regular set-up of supper where people would sit with established comrades or in isolation. Despite being a small ward with many people, the ward can be an isolating place. Patients seemed to feel a little closer and familiar with each other after the group even for a small moment in time during supper.

6. The opportunity to develop skills and knowledge of an area, especially for newcomers, which it is unlikely they would have had elsewhere. It encouraged the development of skills and awareness in team group dynamics and staff reported that the supportive supervision was valued in reflecting upon these processes.

7. The focus being patient led. Patients found it was genuine in its aims with facilitators coming from a non-expert stance seeking to just understand one another better. This helped them appreciate more difficult groups with disruptive behaviour or where people did not talk.

Doctors

1. It allowed them to develop additional skills that it may not have been possible to elsewhere in their training.

2. Patients seemed to appreciate having extra time to spend with medical staff particularly as in the group they felt the agenda was set by themselves rather than the doctor as is the case in the usual clinical interaction. As a result, this helped in fostering therapeutic relationships and often resulted in patients talking more openly in subsequent clinical interactions.

3. It allowed an opportunity to observe patients' behaviour, within a less formal setting rather than relying on patients' own or nurses' reports. All doctors who have taken part in the project have remarked on how it led them to realise that patients who were very unwell, and difficult to engage in a formal interview, were often more aware and able to express themselves than previously thought.

4. It led to a greater sense of bonding with other members of the multidisciplinary team and especially those involved in the group, as in a busy high pressured environment there could be a tendency to withdraw in to professional groupings.

5. Overall doctors reported that it resulted in them thinking more about patients' difficulties and strengths and gave more of an understanding of how they see them.

Conclusions

It was found that a weekly inpatient group based on Yalom's model of highly modified group therapy, and using only ward staff as facilitators, could be introduced on an adult acute inpatient ward. However, for this to be done successfully and run smoothly, it required careful planning, regular high quality supervision as well as a large number of highly motivated staff. Given a sufficiently supporting framework, the group although not formally evaluated appears to have a valuable role to play in patients' care as well as impacting positively on staff skills and morale.

It is well recognised that inpatients on adult acute psychiatric wards often feel frightened of each other, isolated by their symptoms, disturbed and regressed to some degree. The regular structure, and opportunity for communication that the group allows, helps to provide a 'safe' environment for all patients where dialogue can occur which appears to help patients overcome these problems. Our experience shows that the group helped patients to move from a position of isolation to one of a better understanding of their own and each other's problems. It therefore appears that the group helps to improve patients' overall experience during their time spent as an inpatient and improves the overall psychotherapeutic culture of the ward and complements the reliance on drug based treatments.

References

Dratcu, L. (2002) Acute hospital care: the beauty and the beast of psychiatry. *Psychiatric Bulletin*, 26, 81-82.

Dratcu, L, Grandison, A. and Adkin. A. (2003) Acute hospital care in inner London: splitting from mental health services in the community. *Psychiatric Bulletin*, 27, 83-86.

Hinshelwood, R.D. (1987) *What Happens in Groups: Psychoanalysis, the individual and the community?* London: Free Association Books.

Johnson, S., Nolan, F., Hoult, J., White, I.R. Bebbington, P, Sandor, A, McKenzie, N, Patel, S,N, and Pilling, S (2005) Outcomes of crises before and after introduction of a crisis team. *British Journal of Psychiatry* , 187, 68-75

Kanas, N. (1996) *Group psychotherapy for schizophrenic patients*. Washington DC: American Psychiatric Press.

Kanas, N. (2000) Group therapy and schizophrenia: an integrative model. In B Martindale, A Bateman, M Crowe and F Margison (Eds.) *Psychosis: psychological approaches and their effectiveness*. London: Gaskell pp. 120-133.

National Institute for Clinical Excellence (2005). *Violence. The short-term management of disturbed/violent behaviour in psychiatric in-patient settings and emergency departments.* Clinical Guideline 25. London, National Institute for Clinical Excellence

Searles, H.F. (1955) *The Informational Value of the Supervisor's Emotional Experience. Collected papers on schizophrenia and related subjects*. London: Hogarth Press.

Simpson, I. (2002) Inpatient group work for patients with psychosis. *Nursing Times*, 98, 41, 33-35.

Smith, M.G. (2003) Crisis resolution/home treatment and in-patient care. *Psychiatric Bulletin*, 27, 44-47

Yalom, I.D. (1983) *Inpatient Group Psychotherapy.* New York: Basic Books.

Yalom, I.D. (1985) *Theory and Practice of Group Psychotherapy.* New York: Basic Books.

Winnicott, D.W. (1971) *Playing and Reality.* London: Pelican.

11
Problem Solving Groups for Psychiatric Inpatients: A practical guide

Susan Grey

Introduction

In this chapter, the development of a protocol for running problem-solving groups on an 18-bedded male acute inpatient ward is described. The aim was to provide a therapeutic activity for all patients, to teach basic problem-solving skills as well as providing stimulation and social contact, and helping improve concentration and reasoning. Preparation was of great importance, both in terms of the materials used and encouragement of patients to attend. Each session lasted 30 minutes and followed the same format. Patients were given a written problem scenario and asked to first identify the problem, then generate possible solutions, and then discuss the advantages and disadvantages of the solutions. Two group facilitators were necessary to help keep to the format, encourage participation and deal with any problems that arose. The group was accepted well by patients and attendance varied with up to eight patients at any one session.

Providing psychological therapy for psychiatric inpatients is a challenge to ward staff for many reasons. Since most patients can be adequately looked after in the community, inpatient treatment is only used for those with the most acute or intractable problems. On the average ward, patients with any combination of complex problems are likely to be found, including schizophrenia, bipolar disorder, personality problems, forensic issues, drug dependency or alcohol problems, and a substantial proportion of individuals will be in the acute phase of illness. Furthermore, wards are likely to be locked at most times, with many patients confined to the ward and left with little more than the television and fellow patients for company.

Many acute psychiatric wards are staffed primarily by nursing and medical staff with limited time for planning and running therapy groups with inpatients, and in some cases the expertise is also lacking. Even when the expertise is there, unexpected crises and changes in shift patterns can make it difficult to maintain a reliable programme of group therapy activity. Wards with dedicated staff working normal hours, such as clinical psychologists or occupational therapists, or nursing or psychiatric staff with an official brief to carry out therapy activities, are more likely to be successful in providing a regular programme of group work. Some hospitals have dedicated therapy centres staffed by occupational therapists or clinical psychologists. These provide much needed therapy for those patients who are well enough to leave the ward, but increase the problem of how to help those who stay behind.

So for many reasons it is difficult to provide therapeutic groups to that rather varied group of often quite distressed patients who are confined to the acute inpatient ward. The Problem Solving Group is one example of a group activity that can be offered to almost all patients, if facilitated by an experienced staff member. This chapter describes how the group was used on an acute male ward, and offers guidance on some of the common difficulties encountered.

Rationale

The social difficulties experienced by people with a diagnosis of schizophrenia are well-documented. For example, Bellack et al (1994) describe deficits in all aspects of social problem solving skills. These include being less assertive and less persistent, less able to negotiate conflicts, less able to construct clear arguments, less fluent, less skilled at using non-verbal communication, and finally, having diminished affect and interest. There are a number of possible reasons for these deficits. People with schizophrenia commonly experience repeated episodes of loss of control over their thoughts, social isolation and social failure. This is likely to lead to a gradual erosion of cognitive and behavioural abilities, diminished expectations and discinclination to persist with complex social situations. Other research suggests that people with schizophrenia have frontal and hippocampal dysfunction which may cause poor processing of complex tasks. Also, poor perceptual skills may cause errors in judgement of negative affect in others, leading to difficulties in responding to feedback from others.

The impact of the illness across perceptual, cognitive, emotional and behavioural domains requires a multimodal approach, comprising medication for the psychobiological aspects; training in social problem-solving to strengthen protection against stress and case management to compensate for residual symptoms and deficits

(Kopelowicz et al 2003). Group approaches have been used for various psychological treatments for outpatients with psychosis, including skills training and CBT (Randall and Walker, 1988; Cwikel and Oron, 1991; Mason, 2000; Philips and Corcoran, 2000). Some of these have been shown to have some beneficial effects (eg Wykes et al, 2005, Barrowclough et al, 2006, Kern et al, 2005, Combs et al, 2007).

There has also been research into therapy packages specifically including problem solving training for patients with serious mental illness. This training is often based loosely on D'Zurilla & Goldfried's (1971) early model of social problem solving. For example, Falloon et al. (1984) were early advocates of training in problem solving for families of people with a diagnosis of schizophrenia. He suggests that problem solving is most effective when integrated in a broader package of mental health education and also suggest that therapy sessions in the patients' home can be useful (Falloon et al., 1999). Other clinicians have included problem solving training in multiple-family or single family group education, but its contribution to the effectiveness of the whole package has been disputed. For example, Bellack *et al* (2000) reported no differences in patients' subsequent problem solving skills or in clinical outcomes after a family management intervention that included training in communication, problem solving, goal-setting and multiple family group follow-up, in comparison with a multiple family supportive group intervention. They also questioned the cost-effectiveness of home treatment sessions (Bellack & Schooler, 2001). Falloon (2001) argues that multiple family group approaches are not always effective if they do not include a problem solving component. More recently he describes several promising pilot studies using problem solving training within a package including psycho-education, dealing with interpersonal problems, and strategies for analysing and coping with residual psychotic symptoms (Falloon *et al*, 2007). In general it would seem that problem solving can be helpful as part of a family intervention package, but the precise contribution of different components of therapy is still not clear. Furthermore, there is very little research on the use of problem solving training with patients away from their families in acute in-patient settings.

Aims of the group

The present project used a simplified version of the classic model, emphasizing just three steps, namely, identifying the problem, thinking of solutions, and evaluating the solutions.

The major aim was to encourage the development of problem solving skills in inpatients, but participation in the group was expected to have some additional general benefits, such as facilitating collaborative working, encouraging analytical skills, encouraging awareness of other people's point of view and improving concentration.

Setting

The setting was an 18 bed acute admission ward for men living in an inner London borough with a mixture of both socially deprived and well-off communities. There were patients with a variety of problems over the two years the group was running; predominantly psychosis or bipolar disorder, but also including drug or alcohol dependence, personality problems, affective disorders or any combination of these.

The room used for group sessions was located in a central corridor in sight of both the ward entrance and the patients' lounge. Bedrooms, bathrooms, staff offices and the dining area were located in wings running off this corridor. The central corridor also had a few chairs where patients sometimes sat and watched people coming and going on the ward. This corridor was a focal point for general activity and any preparations for organised events in the group room were very visible to everyone on the ward. Interestingly, the ward on the floor above in the same building had a similar layout, except the group room was located at the far end of one of the wings, out of sight of the entrance and the main lounge. Audits of the group activities in the ward upstairs showed that attendance was relatively poor in the more remote group room unless loud music was used to attract participants.

Staffing

The problem solving group sessions were offered to the ward as a service from clinical psychology staff, following discussion with the ward manager and consultant psychiatrist. The basic principles were explained to ward staff and opportunities were offered for observing or helping run sessions. A consultant clinical psychologist led the group initially, with a trainee clinical psychologist in attendance. After a number of practice sessions to establish the format, the lead role alternated weekly between these two staff. After a few months several volunteer assistant psychologists starting participating and, after supervised practice, later took turns at leading the group. These were mainly graduate psychologists employed elsewhere in research posts who had obtained permission from their employer to take half a day off each week to gain additional clinical experience. Undergraduate psychologists on work experience placements were also available at times to participate in the group. Eventually the running of the group became the responsibility of the trainee clinical psychologist. At times there were also nursing staff present. The group was always led from start to finish by the same staff member, but it was helpful to have one or two other staff present to facilitate discussion. In general, psychology assistants were more likely than nursing staff to contribute to the discussion. On the other hand, the presence of nursing staff was very helpful when group participants were disruptive or disturbed. There were usually a minimum of two staff members in the group sessions, but we took care to ensure that staff did not outnumber patients, except on one or two very rare occasions when we only had one patient participating. Great importance was attached to the reliability of the group, so we made sure it always took place, even if only one patient was available. This would have been difficult to achieve without the help of the volunteer psychology assistants

Format of the group sessions

An important aspect of the group was that it was intended to teach a general methodology for problem solving, and not to solve any individual's current problem. For this reason we worked on a hypothetical problem scenario in each session. These scenarios were prepared in advance and described problems relevant to the patients on the ward. The group sessions ran for 30 minutes and the format included ground rules, introductions, explanation, reading the problem scenario, identifying the problem, generating possible solutions and evaluating the solutions. However, we also found it essential to spend at least 20 minutes preparing for every session.

The scenarios described a variety of problem situations experienced by patients during a hospital admission or after discharge to the community. The problem scenarios were written by the author and colleagues, using ideas from patients' reported experiences. The problems were deliberately chosen to reflect the day-to-day hassles of psychiatric patients no matter how prosaic. For example, drug use and debts were regular themes, as were fights and the fears and frustrations of being locked up. Several scenarios were also created using experiences of patients living in the community. Again, these covered common issues such as money problems, friction with neighbours or friends, coping with employment or housework, as well as some more complicated difficulties related to family roles or religion. Seven scenarios are shown in the appendix, together with the problem lists and solution lists generated in the sessions. The marks showing how the solutions were evaluated are also shown, together with some of the comments that were made during the discussion. Seventeen more scenarios are included without this information.

Preparation

This is probably the most important and most easily neglected part of the group process, as most patients needed encouragement to attend. We advertised each group session in advance, using notice boards and listings of ward activities and ensuring that shift coordinators were aware of the day and time of the group. The group was timetabled for 3.30 in the afternoon, towards the end of visiting time, when patients can sometimes feel bored if they have no other appointments with staff and are not permitted to leave the ward. The group would always be led by a psychologist, together with an additional staff member to help facilitate discussion. We always arrived on the ward about half an hour before the group was due to start and used this time to tidy the room, remove dirty crockery, papers etc., arrange the chairs in a semi-circle, and switch off the TV and noisy vending machine. A few basic items of equipment were needed, namely about eight copies of a written problem scenario (which we selected at random from a set of 30 prepared in advance), a felt-tipped pen, three sheets of flip-chart paper, a notice board and drawing pins. The sheets of paper were pinned side by side on the notice board, with the heading 'Problems' on the first and 'Solutions' on the second. Setting up the room was often a useful way of generating interest among any patients who may have been loitering nearby. About 15 minutes before the start, we visited all communal areas and knocked on bedroom doors to let everyone know the duration and the start time of the group. There would usually be a few patients in bed at this point, but a few words of encouragement might be enough for them to decide to come along. Occasionally another patient would take it on themselves to go round the ward asking others to join in.

Running the group

Group attendance was variable, with anything from one to eight people present. Before beginning everyone was asked to introduce themselves just by giving their name. Ground rules and explanations were given every session, regardless of whether patients had attended before or not, as this helped established the procedure clearly. Patients were reminded to take it in turns to speak, to respect one another's opinions, and to stay for the whole 30 minutes if possible. We explained the purpose of the group, which was to learn a method of solving problems in three steps, first by defining the problems, then thinking of solutions and finally choosing the best solution. Finally, we gave out copies of the written problem scenario and asked someone to read it out loud.

Step 1 Identify the problem

We asked participants to identify the main problem, which the facilitator then wrote on the first sheet of paper. If more than one problem was identified they were included as long as they were relevant, we tried not to have more than three or four problems on the list. If anyone jumped ahead to suggest solutions, we would say 'ok, that might be a solution, but first we need to be clear what the problem is'

Step 2 Finding solutions

We asked the group to think of as many possible solutions as they could. We wrote all suggestions on the board, regardless of whether they were practical or not and explained that we do not make judgements about the solutions at this stage. If one person dominated, we would try to quickly paraphrase their suggestions and ask others for ideas. Two sheets of paper were usually needed for this list.

Step 3 Identify best solutions

We then asked the group to look at the list of solutions and think about whether any were particularly good and whether they could see any disadvantages to any of them. We encouraged discussion of the reasons why some solutions might be particularly good or problematic, and where possible discussed the difference between suggestions that got to the nub of the problem and those that might be generally good things to do without being specific to the problem. Finally we summarised which solutions were agreed to be most useful and put a tick by those on the list. Solutions that had potential but also posed practical problems or required further information were marked with a question mark. Solutions that were agreed to be impractical, irrelevant or likely to cause further problems were left unmarked. Seven scenarios and everything written on the flipcharts during the session are shown in the Appendix.

How patients responded

There were a number of common issues arising from each step. For scenario 1, Step 1, the most pertinent problems identified were 'he can't go to the shop', 'he can't buy his batteries', and 'he's angry and frustrated'. Other suggestions made were really explanations for the problem ('he's lost his trust in staff'), possible consequences of the problem ('staff might sedate him'), non-specific ('he's got mental health problems'), or not included in the scenario ('he's got no friends'). Highly speculative ideas or problems not actually shown in the scenario were not usually written down in the problem list, but other ideas were included if they were at all relevant, in order to encourage participation. It was usually helpful to move the discussion along as soon as the most relevant problem had been identified, since too many items on the problem list can be confusing for the next step.

When generating solutions in Step 2, there were usually one or two patients who could make some relevant suggestions, but a number of common errors required guidance to remind the participants of what sort of solutions to look for. Several issues were important to emphasise, as follows.

First, thinking of what the character in the scenario could do, rather than what other people could do. For example, in Scenario 1, if someone suggested that 'the nurses should be better organised' or 'his friend should help him' these suggestions would be acknowledged briefly, but the patient would be prompted to think of things Ron could do himself to make that happen - such as 'he could raise the issue at a ward community meeting' or 'he could contact his friends and ask them to bring him some batteries'. Second, encouraging patients to focus on the problem described on the sheet, not on their own problems. So if the patient said 'Someone stole my CD player' or 'I've got problems – I don't like my medication', this would be acknowledged briefly as an annoying experience, and the facilitator would remind the patient to think about what someone in Ron's position could do to get his batteries. A third issue was the importance of seeing the problem from the point of view of the person in the scenario. Derogatory remarks like 'he's a loser', 'he's mental' could be difficult to deal with as patients who made such remarks usually were reluctant to put themselves in the position of the person in the scenario. In these cases it was often helpful to have a brief discussion of how everyone has different problems and what seems easy to solve for some people might be hard to solve for others. Once patients accepted the general idea of trying to be helpful to the person in the scenario, rather than condemning them, discussion of solutions could usually proceed. Finally, the strategy for dealing with unrealistic or unusual solutions (eg 'he should get a Bosch-breaker etc.') was usually to include them on the list but to discuss their possible disadvantages later in the evaluation phase. Extreme solutions were suggested from time to time, such as those in Scenario 2, eg. 'take out a contract on the dealer', 'go to Picadilly and be a rent boy'. Writing these on the list sometimes caused hilarity, but were useful to illustrate the principle of not censoring solutions during the brainstorming stage. Taking these suggestions seriously was also a useful was of drawing in and disarming those patients who made jokes and might otherwise have disrupted the discussion.

After producing a list of solutions the group then discusses their advantages and disadvantages. The easiest way to do this was usually to ask people which solutions they think are the best and which solutions may not work so well. This discussion could result in a simple conclusion that one or two good solutions might be suitable, or could evolve into a more detailed discussion of the relative strengths of each solution, the difference between short term and long term solutions, and the difference between solutions that were highly relevant to the problem and those that might be good things to do without actually dealing with the nub of the problem. During these discussions the favoure*d solutions were marked as either definitely helpful or possibly helpful. Some of the comments made during discussion of possible solutions are shown for each scenario.

Other issues

Overall the format and purpose of the group seemed acceptable to the patients and many were intrigued by the scenarios, especially as they were realistic examples of the kind of problems they faced themselves. The group was open to all patients, regardless of mental state, so their contributions to discussions were variable, depending in part on how well they were. For example, one patient often left the room after a few minutes and returned later, possibly because he found it too stimulating to remain in the room for more than five or ten minutes at a time. Some patients remained silent throughout the group and were unable to think of anything to say despite being asked. Other patients grasped the point of the task immediately and were able to make helpful suggestions and encourage others to participate. Patients who found it difficult to participate at the beginning of their stay in hospital often became more responsive later on as their mental state improved. Having a mixture of patients did cause some problems, but might have been helpful to those patients who were too unwell to contribute meaningfully, but who might benefit from hearing others' suggestions or having some social contact. Among newly admitted patients, those with alcohol problems or depression tended to find it easier to stay focused and make relevant points than those with a diagnosis of schizophrenia.

We generally encouraged all contributions, selectively reinforcing elements that were relevant to the task, giving lots of eye contact and trying to ensure that everyone had at least one of their contributions included on the board. If one person was doing most of the talking we would usually thank him for his contributions and ask him to wait while we asked others to contribute. Sometimes patients did not contribute even if prompted, and this may have been because of hearing voices or difficulty controlling thoughts. In these cases we did not put further pressure on them, but included them by making eye contact and checking that they understood the discussion. It was often helpful to have a second facilitator sitting in the group and contributing to the discussion, this could provide prompts and examples of how to think of imaginative solutions. This also provided some extra assistance in encouraging patients to stay focussed on the task and avoid dominance by any individual.

Future options

There are a number of possibilities for running this group in other settings. For example, it could be offered to discharged patients, or it could take place in the Occupational Therapy Centre and include participants from other wards. Other possibilities might be to invite relatives into the groups to help key family members to learn the skills collaboratively with the patients. However, these options would move the activity away from the original target group, the most acutely ill and most restricted patients.

Within the existing setting there may be possibilities for some improvements, for example by using errorless learning. This approach is used with neuropsychological problems and assumes that learning in the absence of errors is more durable. It begins with simple tasks with a greater likelihood of success and uses overlearning of successful practice. The method has been piloted in an outpatient population of people with a diagnosis of schizophrenia (Kern et al, 2005) with a very systematic course of training over a period of several group sessions. For our 'stand-alone' ward based group it might be helpful to use simpler scenarios with a more easily identifiable main problem and to give more explicit coaching in the solution generation stage. Other variations to the procedure might improve participation, depending on local circumstances. For example, provision of tea and biscuits at the beginning of the session might encourage engagement. Running the group more than once a week could help patient retain what they had learned of the basic procedure. Whatever variations are introduced to the basic procedure, the main goal will still be to provide structure, stimulation and support within the ward environment that is accessible to all patients regardless of diagnosis.

Conclusions

The problem solving group described in this chapter offers a simple method for groupwork in an acute inpatient setting, that has high face validity for patients. The scenarios utilised in the groups are all derived from clinical experience with patients from this ward. Groupworkers require skills to keep such groups focused and to deal with the unpredictable mix of patients attending each session. This is mainly achieved by the setting of clear ground rules, using a very structured format and actively reinforcing all relevant contributions to the problem solving process. Further work would be needed to evaluate the clinical effectiveness of these problem solving groups.

References

Barrowclough, C., Haddock, G., Lobban, F., Jones, S., Siddle, R., Roberts, C., and Gregg, L. (2006) Group cognitive behaviour therapy for schizophrenia: randomised controlled trial. *British Journal of Psychiatry*, 189, 527-532.

Bellack, A.S, Haas, G. L. , Schooler, N.R., & Flory, J.D. (2000) Effects of behavioural family management on family communication and patient outcomes in schizophrenia. *British Journal of Psychiatry, 177,* 434-439.

Bellack, A. Sayers, M. Mueser, K., and Bennett, M. (1994) Evaluation of social problem-solving in schizophrenia. *Journal of Abnormal Psychology*, 103, 371-378.

Bellack, A.S. and Schooler, N.R. (2001) Correspondence: Authors' reply. *British Journal of Psychiatry,179,* 76-77.

Combs, D.R., Adams, S.D., Penn, D.L., Roberts, D., Tiegreen, J., and Stem, P. (2007) Social Cognition and Interaction Training (SCIT) for inpatients with schizophrenia spectrum disorders: Preliminary findings. *Schizophrenia Research.* 91, 112-116.

Cwikel, J. and Oron, A. (1991) A long-term support group for chronic schizophrenic outpatients: a qualitiative and quantitative evaluation. *Groupwork*, 4, 2, 163-177

D'Zurilla, T. and Goldfried, M. (1971) Problem-solving and behaviour modification. *Journal of Abnormal Psychology*, 78, 107-126.

Falloon, I.R.H., Boyd, J.L., and McGill, C.W. (1984) *Family care of Schizophrenia: A Problem-Solving Approach to the Treatment of Mental Illness.* New York: Guildford Press.

Falloon, I.R.H., Held, T., Coverdale, J. *et al* (1999) Family Interventions for schizophrenia: a review of long-term benefits of international studies. *Psychiatric Rehabilitation Skills, 3,* 268-290

Falloon, I.R.H. (2001) Correspondence: Stress management and schizophrenia. *British Journal of Psychiatry,179,* 76-77.

Falloon, I.R.H., Barbieri, L., Boggian, I., and Lamonaca, D. (2007) Problem-solving training for schizophrenia: Rationale and review. Journal of Mental Health, 16, 553-568.

Kern, R.S., Green, M.F., Mitchell, S., Kopelowicz, A, Mintz, J., and Liberman, RP. (2005) Extensions of errorless learning to social problem-solving deficits in schizophrenia. *American Journal of Psychiatry*, 162, 513-519.

Kopelowicz, A., Liberman, R,. and Wallace, C. (2003) Psychiatric rehabilitation for schizophrenia. *International Journal of Psychology and Psychological Therapy.* 3, 283-298.

Mason, S. (2000) Groupwork with schizophrenia: clinical aspects. *Groupwork*, 12, 2, 27-44

Phillips, J. and Corcoran, J. (2000) Multi-family group interventions with schizophrenia. *Groupwork*, 12, 2, 45-63

Randall, L. and Walker, W. (1988) Supporting voices: groupwork with people suffering from schizophrenia. *Groupwork*, 1, 1, 60-66

Wykes, T., Hayward, P., Thomas, N., Green, N., Surguladze, S. Fannon, D., and Landau, S. (2005) What are the effects of group cognitive therapy for voices? *Schizophrenia Research*, 77, 201-210.

Appendix
Sample scenarios, plus solutions and conclusions generated by the group.

Scenario 1

Ron is an inpatient on a section of the Mental Health Act. He has been given leave to go to the shops accompanied by nursing staff. He needs to buy some batteries. Every afternoon, when he asks the nurses to go out, they tell him that other patients have already asked to go out and he will need to wait for them to come back. This upsets Ron and causes him to become angry. He shouts and kicks at the exit doors. Then nursing staff say that he is too aggressive and angry to use his pass. So Ron doesn't get to go to the shops.

Problem	Possible solutions		
He can't go to the shop	He needs to learn how to be patient	?	Useful – but he'd still like to get his batteries
He can't buy his batteries	He could attend an anger management group	√	Helpful longer term, but doesn't get the batteries
Staff might sedate him because of his angry behaviour	He could talk to staff about his feelings	√	
He is upset/angry/	He could ask staff to go to the shops for him	√	
frustrated	He could fix a time with staff to go out tomorrow	√	Very practical
He might have lost his trust in the staff	He could get a Bosch-breaker with a 2/10 transformer and an angle grinder and could dig his way out.	?	Not very practical – staff would stop him
He's got mental health problems			
He's got no friends			

Scenario 2

Ben was discharged from a ward like this one a while ago. He is living in his own flat in the community. He is often having mates round and they usually listen to music and use cannabis and crack. Ben is obtaining his drugs from a local dealer. He is on benefits and using quite a lot of money for buying his drugs. He is not always able to pay the dealer and has built up debts with him. He also has trouble paying all his bills and his rent. The dealer has recently been on his back about the money and is threatening him that something will happen to him if he doesn't pay it back soon. Ben is feeling very pressured and anxious about these financial problems

The Problem

Drug addiction	Paying his bills
May be in danger from the dealer	May lose his property
His health	He is anxious

Possible solutions:

Call the police and shop the dealer	?	The dealer might get angry and seek revenge – Ben would need protection
Switch from crack to cannabis	?	
Admit himself to hospital		Might not be possible, if not unwell
He could ask someone for money (eg parents)	?	
Contact the housing department and communicate a plan for paying back his arrears	√	
He could get help for his addiction	?	Helpful in the longer term
Go to Picadilly and be a rent boy	?	Could cause new problems
He could get financial advice (from his care-coordinator, the community agencies)	√	
He could talk to friends/relatives	√	
He could stay with friends/relatives and sort out the problem from a safe environment		
Kill himself		
Negotiate a deadline for paying back the money to the dealer		Possibly
Take out a contract on the dealer		Might end up in prison
Run away and hide		Would have to give everything up and might end up a vagrant
Change friends		Might be difficult to do, but maybe a good longer term solution

Scenario 3

Dan is on a ward like this. He has never been in hospital before, and it is a really frightening experience for him. He feels so nervous around all the patients and staff, he does not know who to trust. He has even started worrying that some of the patients might start a fight with him. Because of this, he is spending a lot of time in his room, and does not even like coming out at meal times. In his room he is just getting more and more lonely and frightened

He is isolated He is frightened and anxious	He could ask for an induction - a one-to-one session with a member of staff - somebody he can relate to	√	
	He could ask his care- coordinator to visit	?	(this might not be practical)
	He could join a group (e.g. OT group)	√	
	He can keep a diary	?	
	He can introduce himself to the others	√	
	He could ask relatives to visit him	√	
	He could try to make friends with somebody his own age	√	

Scenario 4

Jason is on a ward like this. He can sometimes feel paranoid about other people, feeling like they are laughing at him or trying to play games with him. He does not feel that there are many people he can trust. However, there are some patients on the ward that Jason is friendly with. These other patients have got hold of a load of cannabis and have been smoking joints with him. However, when he smokes cannabis, he feels more paranoid, and he has ended up getting into fights with people who seem to have been saying things about him. Because of a recent fight, he is stuck on the ward and not allowed to go out on a pass.

The problem:

He is stuck on the ward

He is smoking cannabis, which might make him paranoid

He gets into fights

Possible solutions:

He could go on a detox-programme	?	Depends what's available through the ward
To take his minds of the drugs he could occupy himself (e.g. by taking part in OT groups, etc.)	√	Might help him find other friends
He could get a befriender to give him advice and support him	√	
He could stay away from the bad influence	?	BUT: they are his friends
He could tell his friends that he does not want cannabis.	√	Might need help from staff to achieve this
Ask a member of staff what he needs to do to get his pass back	√	
Watch his behaviour – like avoiding fights	?	Might need extra help with this

Scenario 5

Victor has just been admitted to a ward like this. He does not understand why he is here. He does not believe there is anything wrong with him. He certainly does not think he has a mental illness. He has had a few problems with his neighbours recently, but this did not seem to justify the police being called and bringing him into hospital. He is very angry about being in hospital, because he has been told he is on a Section and is not allowed to leave. He keeps looking for ways to get out of the unit, but staff have not given him a pass to go around the grounds, because they are worried he will run away.

Problem:

He has been sectioned	He is restricted
He upset his neighbours	He is known to the police now
He doesn't know why he is in hospital	He is angry

Possible solutions

Stay cool and calm (for example, occupy his mind by reading a book)	√	Better state of mind for discussing the issue
Ask for an explanation about why he is in hospital - ask a psychologist, doctor, his primary nurse or friends.	√	
Ask for a housing transfer to a different area	?	Long term – and might have the same problems in the new place
Get in touch with the Prime Minister		Unlikely that they would do anything
Find out what upset his neighbours and come to an agreement with them	√	Useful for the future
Pay £10,000 to a hitman to take his neighbours out.		Unrealistic - Might get caught
Try and negotiate with staff to obtain a pass	√	
Appeal against his section	?	Maybe later
Talk to people on the ward, they might be able to advise something	√	
Negotiate with staff for things to be done differently next time	√	Good idea for the longer term

Scenario 6

John is on a ward like this. He is on a section under the Mental Health Act. He does not have a pass to go to the shops at present. He is running out of cigarettes and only has one left. He puts this in a drawer in his bedroom and leaves to attend an appointment with one of the ward doctors. When he comes back, the cigarette has gone. John gets very upset about this. He thinks he knows who might have taken the cigarette.

Problem

He is on section with no pass

Somebody stole from him

He's got no cigarettes

He is upset/angry

He could ask a member of staff to buy him more cigarettes from the shop	√	Might help him think things through more rationally
He could report the theft to a member of staff	√	
He could contact the police		Would they respond for one cigarette?
He could ask a friend for a roll-up	?	Short term
He could pick up dog-ends and roll them up		Not healthy
He should calm down by drinking water, listening to music, using mental strategies	?	
He could talk to the person who he believes stole the cigarette	?	Important not to be confrontational
He could pray for cigarettes	?	Might not necessarily get him any

Scenario 7

Adam has recently been admitted to hospital. He has had very little money recently, and has come into hospital with no money on him at all. He does not have his benefits book with him, and does not know where it is: he was unable to find it when he was at home. He is particularly concerned, because he is a smoker and only has a little tobacco left. He is worried that he will run out of tobacco. Apart from a little supervised time in the garden he is not allowed to leave the ward.

Problem

He hasn't got any money and he hasn't got his benefit books

He needs tobacco

He is not allowed off the ward

Contact his family to help him find his books	√	
Apply for more DLA	?	May take time
Borrow money from a friend	?	Could cause friction later if the friends wants his money back but Adam can't pay him
Give a member of staff some money and ask them to go to the shops for him	?	Good idea, but not until he's got some money
Ask ward staff if there is money available	√	
Use other strategies to deal with craving tobacco eg Relaxation, O.T, Cutting down on cigarettes	√	Longer term

Additional scenarios

1

Clare has been discharged from a ward like this a while ago and has managed to get a job at MacDonald's, which she was very pleased about. However, lately things have not been going well for her. Her line manager, Bob, gives her a lot of work and watches everything she does. When Clare can't finish the work on time, Bob tells her she is stupid and hopeless at the job. He also blames Clare for things that go wrong and makes jokes about her in front of his colleagues. As a result, Clare is starting to lose faith in herself. She feels anxious about going in to work and constantly feels stressed. She thinks this is having a bad effect on her mental health.

2

Tony has been discharged from a ward like this a few months ago. He is now back at his flat. He is seen regularly by his community nurse. Over the last few weeks he has been feeling increasingly lonely and bored. He has one friend, Daniel, whom he sees once a week. He also visits his parents, who live half an hour away by bus once a week. The rest of the time he spends doing errands (shopping, doing a bit of cleaning and cooking) or in front of the TV. He does not have a job at the moment. He is starting to feel that life is pointless.

3

Mary has been on a ward like this one for a couple of weeks. Before she came in she felt lonely and isolated, and she heard a lot of voices, which she found difficult to cope with. She also had some anger problems. She has got steadily better on the ward. She found it helpful to talk to other people about her experiences and she also liked having some quiet time on her own to relax. Recently, some new patients have been admitted to the ward, who are not very well. They are shouting a lot, running up and down the corridor and can be aggressive at times. Mary finds this difficult to cope with, because it is disrupting her conversations and spoiling her quiet time. She is getting very stressed and angry about this.

4

Sam has recently been discharged from the ward and is now living in his own flat again. In the past, he has had problems looking after his money. In hospital, he drew up a budget plan with his occupational therapist and has managed to stick to it so far. One evening, his friend Tim comes round who needs to make an urgent phone call. He cannot do this from his own place because his phone has been disconnected. Sam agrees to let Tim use his phone. Two evenings later, Tim is back, asking for the phone again. Since Sam doesn't want to annoy him, he lets him use his phone another time. This pattern continues and Tim calls almost every day to use Sam's phone. He is running up a substantial phone bill, which interferes with Sam's budget plan. Sam finds it very hard to deal with the situation, as he has difficulties saying "no" to his friend.

5

Tom is on a ward like this. He has found it very difficult to settle in, because he keeps getting really angry. This happens, for example, if he doesn't like lunch, if someone switches the TV to a different channel, or if he runs out of cigarettes. Tom then shouts at people, bangs his fists against the wall, kicks doors, and on one occasion he smashed the furniture in his room. As a consequence, staff have said he can't have a pass to go out on leave and the other patients are trying to keep away from him. This leads to Tom feeling even angrier.

6

Karim is living in his own flat in South London. He has had mental health problems for about 10 years now. A year ago his mother, who he used to see nearly every day, died suddenly of a heart attack. Karim does not have any contact with his father and only sees his brother, who lives a long way away, about once a month. Since his mother's death he has been feeling increasingly lonely and isolated. He would like to make some new friends but generally feels uncomfortable approaching people he doesn't know. He thinks they might stigmatise him because of his mental health problems.

7

Simon is renting a flat in South London. He is living with his partner Mary. Both of them were diagnosed with schizophrenia a long time ago, but they haven't been in hospital for a few years. Recently, Simon went to a meeting with his housing officer, who told him that the neighbours had complained about noise coming from their flat. Simon is very worried about this. He likes to play his music for most of the day, and he does not think that it has been turned up too loud. Also Mary often shouts when she thinks people are spying on her, although this is in her imagination because of her mental illness and Simon does not think she will be able to stop. He thinks they are being treated unfairly but is getting very worried that they might get into trouble.

8

Yanni lives in a one-bedroomed flat in Peckham. He used to have a job in a warehouse, but hasn't worked for 15 years, since developing mental health problems. Until recently he used to visit his mother in Camberwell three times a week and have dinner with her. He also used to go to a local café and play cards with other local Cypriots. His mother died recently and since then he has become very isolated and has stopped going to the café to see his friends. He's started to think that people are looking at him when he goes out in the street. This makes him reluctant to go out, so he doesn't get any shopping in and isn't eating properly. He feels low and frightened about what will become of him.

9

Errol is on a psychiatric ward. He is attending a ward round with the consultant psychiatrists, his care-coordinator, and some other professionals. He is feeling increasingly stuck and claustrophobic on the ward and needs some time outside. Therefore he asks whether he can have a pass to go home and see his family. The consultant psychiatrist says he is not well enough yet and refuses. Errol gets upset and angry about this and storms out of the ward round slamming the door.

10

Jane is on a ward like this. She has a pass to go home for the weekend and on Sunday night she decides to stay out for a few days longer. Since she is on a section and was supposed to come back on Sunday night, the Ward staff tell the police that she is 'Absent without leave'. The police start looking for her and eventually find her and bring her back onto the ward. Previously, Jane had an unescorted pass to the shops. The day after her return to the ward she asks to go out, but she finds out that her pass has been cancelled. She gets very angry and upset. She returns to her room and tries to cut herself with an old drinks can.

11

Dave is on a ward like this. He's been in hospital for four weeks and is running out of clean clothes. He usually lives with his mum and dad. His mum usually takes care of his laundry. Dave doesn't know how to use the washing machine on the ward and he feels embarrassed about asking the nursing staff. His father has always said that washing is women's work, but his sister says this is rubbish. The nursing staff have pointed out that he needs to take more care of his personal hygiene, and yesterday Dave overheard a patient saying that he was smelly.

12

Jim has recently been discharged from a ward like this one. He lives in a hostel with five other people. He likes the local area which is close to the shops and he usually gets on well with the other people in the hostel. However, recently he has had a few arguments with Alan who has the room next door, because Alan says he plays his music too loud. Jim doesn't think his music is too loud at all, but he worries that the other residents might turn against him because of Alan's complaints. Jim doesn't have many hobbies and music is the main thing he enjoys doing.

13

Olwyn is on a ward like this. She spends a lot of time just hanging around the ward smoking cigarettes and has put on a lot of weight. She thinks this is due to her medication, which makes her more hungry. She doesn't like the hospital food and often eats take-aways but they probably make her put on weight too. The doctor has advised her to take more exercise, but she doesn't always feel like doing anything. The Occupational Therapist has referred her to the hospital gym, but she keeps forgetting the times of the sessions.

14

Ali has been on the ward for four weeks. In two weeks time it will be his daughter's 6th birthday. Ali is in hospital under a Section and hasn't been allowed out since he arrived. He wants to give his daughter a present on her birthday and knows she will be disappointed if he isn't there. However, he hasn't been able to buy anything because he's not allowed off the ward. He worries that he won't get the chance to buy a present in time for the birthday. Also, Ali thinks that the hospital ward isn't a suitable place for his partner and daughter to visit, as he thinks it's sometimes depressing and not suitable for children.

15

Salim has lived in England since he was 10yrs old. His father is a devout Muslim, but he knows that Salim is less religious. Salim has had serious mental health problems and was discharged a year ago after a short stay in psychiatric hospital. He has been visiting a Mormon church, where they are very friendly and encourage him to take part in their activities. They have films and discussions groups and sometimes go for picnics in the park. Recently the Mormon ministers have suggested that he might join their church, since he has been attending so often. Salim likes the activities but feels that his father would be upset if he joined the Mormons. He would prefer to just attend the activities without joining, but feels under a bit of pressure.

16

Kende has been on a ward like this for just over a month. While on the ward he has started some new medication and has not been able to leave the ward very often. Since being on the ward he feels he is not as fit as he was and he has put on weight. He eats the meals on the ward, although he doesn't like the food very much, and sometimes he also has extra food when patients send out for take-aways. Kende is expecting to go home in about a month's time and has been given a pass to go out for an hour a day. Kende's twin brother is always very fit and popular and is looking forward to seeing him again. However, Kende is worried that he doesn't look good and might not be fit enough to play football with his brother and friends.

17

Linda was discharged from a psychiatric ward like this a while ago. She enjoyed improving her computer skills when she was on the ward and became skilled at word processing and using the internet. Now she is thinking about starting a computer course at college as she would like to return to work. However, she is worried that she won't be able to complete assignments on time as she sometimes becomes anxious and paranoid and needs several days rest to calm down. She has also found out that the nearest college is half an hour's bus ride away and has worked out that travelling to college several times a week will cost her a large portion of her weekly money.

Cognitive behaviour therapy groups for psychosis in acute inpatient settings

Steven Livingstone and Til Wykes

Introduction

Psychological therapies for the treatment of psychosis have gained momentum in the last three decades. This can be attributed to two main factors. Firstly, there is a growing recognition of the importance of psychological processes in psychosis, both as contributors to onset and persistence, and in terms of the negative psychological impact of a diagnosis of 'schizophrenia'. Secondly, although pharmacological interventions have been the mainstay of treatment since their introduction in the 1950s, they have a number of limitations. These include the high incidence of disabling side-effects and poor adherence to medications. Despite high doses of medication, a significant number of people still experience persistent and distressing symptoms. These not only affect the quality of their lives but are instrumental in maintaining depression and low self-esteem.

The updated *NICE guideline on Schizophrenia* (2009) recommends that Cognitive Behaviour Therapy (CBT) should be offered to people with a diagnosis of schizophrenia to assist in promoting recovery, both for those with persisting positive and negative symptoms and for those in remission. The guideline development committee found consistent evidence that compared with standard care, CBT was effective in reducing hospitalisation rates up to 18 months following the end of treatment. They found robust evidence indicating that duration of hospital stay is reduced (by 8.26 days on average). This data comes from 31 randomised controlled trials (RCTs) of CBT versus any control, where in some studies CBT was conducted in hospital and in others in an outpatient setting. CBT was shown to be effective in reducing symptom severity at both the end of treatment and at follow-up. There was limited but consistent evidence for symptom specific measures including voice compliance, frequency of voices and believability, all of which demonstrated large effect sizes at both end of treatment and follow-up. The effects of CBT should not, however, be exaggerated as there is evidence that methods of data collection affect how much of an effect there will be. Wykes et al (2008) found that the effects of CBT reduced considerably when those collecting efficacy data did not know which group the participant was allocated to. This is commonly known as being blind to group allocation. However, there is still an effect of CBT on positive symptoms even in the most methodologically rigorous studies, although the estimated effect size is reduced to 0.22.

CBT for psychosis is not a single type of therapy: it can vary in expression and rarely is the therapeutic process the same as that adopted for other difficulties like depression. In fact Tarrier and Wykes (2004) coined a new term, CBTp, to define the CBT-type therapies which are adopted in work with psychosis. Here too CBTp varies in its expression with some therapies concentrating on distal factors and some more on proximal ones, such as situations in which people find themselves today. The data seems to suggest some marginal advantage to concentrating on proximal or here and now factors (Tarrier & Wykes, 2004). There is of course variation in the way that CBTp is provided to individuals such that some spend much time at the early engagement phases and some complete the whole course of therapy. Clearly effect sizes cited for individual studies do not take individual doses into account although some efforts have begun to identify if individuals are affected by the dose of treatment.

The shortage of trained therapists and the length of treatment required are likely to mean that widespread individual CBT for psychosis will be difficult to implement. An alternative is to present the therapy in a group format, which offers the possibility of a more general availability of a CBTp therapy at a lower cost. To date, there have been no RCTs directly comparing group CBTp with individual CBTp (NICE guidelines, 2009), although there are non-RCT studies which explore this question. Morrison (2001) presented a review of group format CBT for a number of disorders (although not inpatients with psychosis), and reported encouraging results. Wykes *et al.* (2008) carried out a meta-analysis which found no evidence of any difference in effect size between individual and group CBTp. In general, the outcome studies reviewed support the efficacy of CBT delivered in a group format and for the most part do not suggest a particular advantage for either individual or group CBT. Morrison concluded that while group work may have less concentrated benefits for individuals this is offset by the increased cost effectiveness of the group format.

Group CBT with inpatients

One advantage of individual CBT is that it provides the flexibility to respond to a wide variety of idiosyncratic symptoms. Groups may be able to replicate this by ensuring that there is some homogeneity of experience within the group. Individual formulation which guides treatment is one of the strengths of CBT, but this becomes less of a focus in group work and hence the need for relatively homogenous groups in terms of difficulties experienced. It also suggests that current CBTp would need to be adapted to rely mainly on here and now issues rather than the more distal focus of some of the CBTps. Although CBT was developed primarily as an individual therapy, some would argue that what group therapy lacks in depth it makes up for in the advantages offered by the group format. These advantages (some of which are not unique to CBT groups), would include:

Problem solving element

When a person is admitted to a general hospital ward, there is an implication that treatment will be received by the patient in passive way. The same type of reaction can occur in a psychiatric inpatient service. The process of being admitted to hospital can leave people feeling bewildered, overwhelmed and helpless. In this position they may develop the belief that something should be done 'for' or 'to' them. Group CBTp offers the opportunity to challenge this assumption. Effective collaboration between the therapist and service user is one of the central features of CBT, and this can be utilised in the group setting through procedures like agenda setting, role play, and self-help exercises. The problem solving element of CBT encourages service users to feel like active participants in their own treatment rather than passive recipients. For further information on running structured CBT problem solving groups see Susan Grey's chapter.

Information for formulation

The usual admission procedure in a psychiatric inpatient unit involves a period of assessment, and the group experience provides an added dimension to this process. By directly observing the service user's interactions with others, the clinician gains insight into their social abilities and interpersonal style. Service users who appear to be quite high functioning in a one-to-one interview can struggle in a group setting. Conversely, personal strengths such as empathy and listening skills that may not be apparent in individual therapy may be drawn out in a group context.

Normalisation

Sharing perceptions and experiences normalises difficulties, and allows service users to hear accounts from people who can empathise. As noted by Katja Hajek in her chapter on Yalom's Interpersonal Model, this sense of universality can be therapeutic. A form of resistance can arise in individual therapy whereby the therapist's viewpoint is disregarded by the service user, who states that the therapist is not able to understand what they are going through. It is more difficult to apply this to other service users who do share similar experiences, one of which is that of being a hospital inpatient.

Peer support

The group format can foster a sense of support for people who may otherwise be quite socially isolated. This is something that service users consistently report that they like about group work, and can hold true even in the absence of other benefits. In one report, a service user who, according to psychometric measures, benefitted least from the group, commented:

> I did not find anything particularly useful, but I really enjoyed coming to meet people who have had similar experiences. (Gledhill et al., 1998)

The group can provide a safe environment to practice social skills, and the opportunity to test out the hypotheses that voices have led to a reduction in social functioning. There is evidence that group CBTp leads to an improvement in social functioning, and that this benefit was maintained at six month follow-up (Wykes et al, 2005). Social functioning effects are particularly important in this socially isolated group.

Peer feedback

The group provides what is often the first opportunity for many service users to obtain constructive feedback from peers. Service users often assume that they are perceived in certain ways and make (usually negative) assumptions about how others see them. This positive aspect applies to those giving the feedback as well as those receiving it. Some service users will realise that they have previously unrecognised abilities to be helpful to someone else and this results in an increased sense of self-worth.

A group approach is an efficient way to deliver psychoeducation

The group can be used as a forum to provide good quality information as part of standard care, for example, about medication. It can also be a forum for service users to exchange coping skills, providing psychoeducation for each other in the process.

The group can be a safe environment to test new behaviours

The group can be a forum for a range of cognitive and behavioural experiments. However, it is worth pointing out that it also has the potential to be a venue for repeating dysfunctional behaviours or expressing and acting on unhelpful cognitions. For example, a client we worked with tended to lie on the floor to avoid being seen by hidden cameras. During the group, she was encouraged to gradually adopt a more upright posture, moving towards sitting in her chair, and exploring whether she experienced any negative consequences.

Service users can model the skills of the therapist and other group members

Service users often model the behaviours of other members of the group or the therapist, and in the process, they can learn effective coping strategies. Social skills can be taught, modelled and discussed in the group.

Procedures

Group selection

It is recommended that between six to eight members is the optimum number of participants for CBTp groups. Three would be the minimum, and it may prove difficult to get more than three people to attend on a regular basis, given that most wards have only about eighteen to twenty inpatients at any given time.

Inclusion and exclusion criteria would depend entirely on the type of CBTp group being proposed. For example, in a group focussing on hearing voices, it would be necessary to include only those with a diagnosis of schizophrenia and with long term experience of distressing auditory hallucinations. In general, a degree of homogeneity is preferred. This makes it easier to focus on problems relevant to everyone in the group, and enhances empathy and identification within the group.

People with organic brain damage acquired through head injury would usually be excluded. People currently experiencing acute psychosis or mania may be disruptive and hence unable to take part. Similarly, severely disruptive people with a personality disorders may need to be excluded from inpatient CBTp groups. Linehan (1993) has described an effective dialectic behavioural approach for borderline personality disorder in an outpatient setting. However, the inpatient setting typically does not allow the time for the limit setting and redirection that would be required.

Format

The average length of stay in a mental health inpatient ward varies enormously from service to service, but may be somewhere between twenty-five to forty days. Clearly this poses problems for programmed groups where each session builds on the last, since it is difficult for the same members to attend all sessions in order. This has led some practitioners to adopt an open-ended, open-to-all approach, whereby whoever happens to be an inpatient on the ward at the time is welcome to attend, and the focus depends on what the people who attend would like to discuss. Because there is no predefined programme, this avoids the problem of ensuring service users complete each session during their time as an inpatient, and makes it easy for as many service users as possible to attend. However, this type of group poses its own problems. The open-ended approach lacks focus since there is no adherence to a particular evidence-based protocol. If service users with very different presenting problems attend, it makes it impossible to focus on difficulties that would be relevant to everyone. It also makes it difficult to measure any outcomes and it is not clear what such a group would seek to achieve.

CBTp groups that focus on different aspects of the inpatient experience are discussed below. However, all of these groups share key CBTp principles in that they are guided by a clear focus on a specific problem and the intended outcome is predefined. Each of the groups proposed involves a limited number of sessions that should be possible for most service users to complete during their stay on the ward. Because each session builds on the last, it is intended that they would be run as 'closed groups', i.e. it is not possible for service users to join after session one. The groups also share the time-limited, goal-oriented, 'here and now' focus that is a feature of most forms of CBTp. There is not enough time within the group for each member to discuss the details of childhood experiences and make links with how this impacts on their lives currently. Historical issues may repeat themselves in the here and now through the influence of core schemas, and this may be addressed by cognitive-behavioural schema work. However, this type of work would be more appropriately carried out in one-to-one longer term therapy post discharge.

Number and type of group facilitators

Group therapists who are not familiar with CBT, or CBT therapists who are not familiar with group work, should first serve as a co-therapist. The main facilitator would need to be highly trained and receive regular supervision. The group leader could be any type of mental health professional, or service user facilitator, provided they satisfy the above criteria. The effectiveness of individual therapy using less highly trained facilitators has produced variable results (Turkington et al, 2002; Durham et al, 2003). For group CBTp treatment, the effects of therapist training and experience are extremely important in producing effective therapy across all participants within a group. Wykes et al. (2005) found that service users in groups with less experienced therapists did also improve, but these improvements were in fewer participants. Services that depend on short training programmes with staff who only see a few clients a year are unlikely to be as successful as those who have longer training and more massed practice with the same client group.

Experience as a co-therapist can be a very good learning opportunity for therapists in training, as it offers the chance to experience the therapeutic process *in vivo*. The co-therapist can also assist with role-play or modelling during the session. Two or even three staff facilitating and learning through observation is possible and can even be helpful, but the number of staff in the room should never exceed the number of service users. It is also recommended that the main therapist should remain constant from the beginning to the end.

CBT techniques

One of the primary objectives of cognitive behavioural therapy for depression is to help service users to identify the negative automatic thoughts that occur in problem situations, and the emotions these lead to. Identifying negative automatic thoughts and their effects is the first step towards challenging dysfunctional cognitions, and is a substantial part of CBT group work for depression. When undertaking CBTp group work with inpatients, the focus shifts to exploring the meanings and explanations people attribute to their experiences, rather than directly challenging those thoughts (for more on this issue see Kingdon & Turkington, 2002). The therapist adopts the stance of 'suspending disbelief'. It is important to note that this is not the same as collusion, which would be where the therapist confirms the service user's delusions by agreeing with them. Instead, the therapist uses their natural curiosity to explore with the service user the reasons why they have come to a particular conclusion, which involves exploring the evidence for why it might be true, as well as the reasons why it might not be true. This may include the therapist agreeing to help check out the facts underlying a belief, and discussing a delusion within the service user's belief system. The therapist may be asked directly whether they believe what the service user says is true, in which case they may introduce the idea of 'agreeing to disagree' – this means that they do not share the explanation or idea, but that this does not invalidate the other person's perspective. It is important to bear in mind that the goals of CBTp are to reduce distress, to improve the quality of daily life, and provide hope for the future. Within this framework, it would not be considered appropriate to attempt to modify a belief that does not interfere negatively with the person's life. Many CBT techniques that will be familiar to therapists can be adapted to the group setting. Cognitive techniques would include:

- Socratic questioning
- Labelling distortions
- Verbalising the internal dialogue (automatic thoughts)
- Questioning the evidence
- Decastrophising
- Advantages and disadvantages of actions
- Constructing adaptive self statements
- Reframing
- Examining options and alternatives

Behavioural techniques would include:

- Activity scheduling
- Graded task assignment
- Behavioural rehearsal

Further details and clinical examples of these techniques can be found in Fowler et al, (1995), Kingdon & Turkington (2008), or Morrison (2002).

Types of CBT groups

Hearing voices group

Twenty to fifty percent of people with a diagnosis of schizophrenia continue to hear voices despite taking appropriate medication (Newton *et al.*, 2005). Group treatment for voices is not new and consumer groups such as the Hearing Voices Network have been providing this type of advice and support in the UK for many years (Hearing Voices Network, 2001).

The now famous study by Romme and Escher (1989) has been particularly influential. Romme and a patient who experienced disabling auditory hallucinations appeared on a Dutch television programme, and invited people with similar experiences to contact them. This revealed a surprisingly high number of voice hearers in the population, many of whom had never been in contact with psychiatric services. Of the 450 respondents who heard voices, 300 reported being unable to cope with voices and 150 said they were able to handle them. This initiated the normalisation approach to the phenomenon: the experience of hearing voices is widespread and is not in itself synonymous with a diagnosis of schizophrenia. Instead, the way in which people make sense of unusual experiences and the distress caused is the decisive factor in determining whether they come to the attention of mental health services. Romme also compared the way in which different people coped with their voices, and this work became a core principle of the Hearing Voices Network in the UK: meeting other people who hear voices normalises the experience and also provides the opportunity to share coping strategies. This approach adopted by the Hearing Voices Network is not necessarily explicitly CBTp, however, there is a similarity in that CBTp groups would also seek to emphasise the normalisation and sharing coping skills approach.

There is also evidence for the efficacy of the approach in terms of an improvement in social functioning (Wykes, *et al.*, 2005). This improvement was maintained at six month follow-up, and the social functioning benefit was felt to be particularly important given the social isolation often experienced by service users who hear voices.

As part of a study looking at improving therapeutic interventions for acute inpatients, a 'Hearing Voices' group for inpatients was implemented in several sites in South London. This was based on the model developed by Kimberley Ehntholt and Til Wykes, and the protocol can be found in Appendix 1. This group was designed for people who experience persistent and distressing auditory hallucinations, and was not open to service users with other types of difficulty. The groups here were run by experienced facilitators as well as by nurses who were trained to carry out the therapy. The nurse therapists were able to stick to the protocol, in a fact did so more often than the experienced facilitators, who were perhaps more skilled at being responsive to individual concerns. The study was small and there did not appear to be differences between the people treated by different therapists. There was evidence of an improved symptom level at the end of this short therapy window but the differences disappeared at follow-up. This is likely to be the case in most inpatient CBTp studies as inpatients with acute symptoms are all likely to improve through a combination of medication, the ward milieu and any specific psychological therapy. There therefore needs to be much longer follow-up studies in large samples to identify the effects of therapy in the long term. However, what this study showed was that there was an appetite for such groups both for staff as well as service users and the feedback from both was positive.

Some service users said that they had never had the opportunity to discuss with others their experience of voices and were relieved to discover that their experience were very similar to those of others.

A more general group approach for service users who experience unusual perceptual experiences or recurrent, strong beliefs not shared by others, has been developed by Graham Hill, Isabel Clarke and Hannah Wilson. This group is known as the 'What Is Real and What Is Not Group', and is described in Clarke and Wilson (2009).

Evaluations of CBTp group treatment for voice hearers invariably report a high degree of satisfaction in service users. For example, Wykes et al (1998), found that among the most frequently reported benefits were the educational aspects of therapy, particularly with regard to medication, and learning of new coping skills (such as confronting voices or asking them to come back later). Talking about voices with other people who had similar experiences was also reported as being particularly beneficial, and many service users commented on how easily they were able to communicate within the group. Many service users said they were 'comforted' by the fact that they were not alone in their experiences. Newton et al (2007) found that participants also commented on the positive role played by facilitators. In particular, they recognised the importance of strategies used to let 'everyone have their say' and 'to make everyone feel special'. One participant also described clearly the facilitators' use of CBTp techniques (such as those described above) which enabled him to try new coping strategies and to have more control over his distressing experiences.

Case Example

Ken is a 35 year old man with a diagnosis of schizophrenia. He first came into contact with psychiatric services at the age of 21. At the time, he was training with the Royal Artillery Regiment. However, he began to experience problems with concentration, and failed to qualify for active service. He began to isolate himself from his colleagues, saying that he felt overwhelmed by social contact and preferred to spend time alone. His increasing isolation and chaotic behaviour led to him being dismissed from the army. He lost touch with many of the friends he had made through the military, and also split with his girlfriend. Shortly afterwards he was admitted to psychiatric hospital claiming that he was not only involved in global politics and military actions, but that he was the rightful president of America. His medical notes stated that he was ultimately stabilised on antipsychotic medication and discharged. His mother explained that he had been well on depot medication for a number of years, before moving away from his family to work in Scotland, where he again began to act on his delusions.

He was admitted for the second time under the Mental Health Act as he was considered a danger to the community. He was acting on the delusional belief that he was highly involved in world politics and also in top-level military decision making. At the time of admission his self care had deteriorated and he had begun to be violent towards his mother, who had been very tolerant of his threatening behaviour for some time. He had also been sending a voluminous correspondence to leading politicians and military personnel. He held the belief that references were made to him in newspapers as well as books about the military and secret service, such as Bravo Two Zero and Open Secret, the autobiography of the former MI-5 Director General, Stella Rimington. He believed that leading figures communicated with him directly through a top-secret, high tech device, through which he received their instructions in the form of spoken commands. When initially admitted to the ward, his behaviour was based mainly on acting on these commands, for example, by carefully reading newspapers and highlighting specific sections, and writing letters to politicians. He was occasionally agitated and angry about his detention, but over a period of a few weeks he was stabilised on antipsychotic medication. It was reported that he seemed less preoccupied by his delusions and engaged more with the staff and other service users. He also began to change in his interpretation of his experiences, and his level of conviction in his beliefs shifted from 100% at the time of admission to 50 – 70%. The frequency and severity of his voices remained unaltered however, and he began to complain about the stress being placed on him by their unreasonable demands. He expressed a desire to 'resign his commission'.

Ken was recruited to the Hearing Voices Group, with the aim of reducing the distress caused by his voices rather than altering his beliefs about their source. In the first session, he said very little, but with the encouragement of the facilitator he did volunteer that he was 'amazed' to hear about people with similar experiences. Despite having formed some quite close relationships with people on the ward, they had never before discussed why they were in hospital. He did not volunteer much information about his own experience of hearing voices, but seemed interested in hearing about the experiences of others. He was more comfortable entering into the discussion about the different models of explanation for hearing voices. The facilitator allowed the group quite an unstructured and wide ranging discussion about this, with some members voicing their support for paranormal or spiritual explanations. Ken described what might be described as a metaphysical view, which was at times hard to follow and incorporated theories about quantum physics and string theory. The facilitator asked clarifying questions, summarised, and checked their understanding, without challenging his explanation. In this way, it emerged that his view was that his experiences were part of the natural order and perhaps explicable by future advances in physics, but not currently understandable within a traditional scientific model. It is of note that while Ken's initial explanation had seemed entirely incomprehensible, it was rendered coherent through a little gentle enquiry. The facilitator led the group to reflect on the fact that different people had very different views of hearing voices, and that different perspectives are valid.

In session 2 the group discussed different possible coping strategies. Ken initially started from the perspective that he had no control whatsoever over his voices, and doubted whether he would be able to influence them in any way. However, another group member commented that sometimes when he concentrated on another task, such as playing computer games, his voices diminished. This made Ken consider that when he was concentrating hard on reading the newspaper, he was troubled less by voices. He attributed this to the fact that in reading the newspaper he was obeying the voices and hence they left him alone. However, he was prepared to consider the possibility that it could partly be because he was concentrating on something else. Regardless of the explanation, he concluded that he did have some degree of control over the voices, which seemed highly significant for him. The homework task from this group was to try out one of the coping strategies suggested by another member of the group. Ken opted to try concentrating on other things at times when he was troubled by the voices, specifically, reading the newspaper. All group members wrote down a new strategy on an index card, which they took away with them as a reminder.

Between sessions 2 and 3, Ken experienced some setbacks. He was told that he was not ready to leave the ward, which made him very angry. He was verbally abusive to a member of staff and attempted to kick down the door to the nurses' station, which led to him being physically restrained. This made him feel highly stressed, led to deterioration in his relationship with staff and an exacerbation in symptoms. Nonetheless, he was encouraged to attend session 3, and did agree to come if he did not have to say anything. The group began with feedback about how the members had got on with applying the new strategies. Ken stated that he had forgotten about the strategy he had arranged to try and had lost the card. The facilitator accepted this in a non-blaming way, and supplied

Ken with another card to try the idea again. The group moved on to play the 'self esteem game'. This involves writing each person's name on a card, passing it around, and each group member writes something they like about the person. The person keeps the card and might want to look at it when they are feeling low. This leads to a discussion of whether the person's mood affects their experience of hearing voices. Although Ken had only agreed to attend on the basis that he did not have to say anything, in fact he participated in this discussion quite passionately. He spoke about his anger at not being allowed to leave the ward, and the fact that his voices had subsequently been worse. Together, the group were able to conclude that generally people's voices were better when they were happy and worse when they were unhappy, angry or under stress – a view which Ken endorsed. Using the flipchart, the facilitator attempted to pull together all the things that were said to influence voices, drawing on the discussions from all three sessions. This was framed in terms of the stress-vulnerability model, emphasising the ways in which participants had described having a degree of control over their voices.

In feedback about the group, Ken was most positive about hearing from people who had similar experiences. It came as a revelation to him that other people did experience something similar. He also stated that he had learned coping strategies in the group which he would like to try out, although there was no evidence of him actually having done this. Like many aspects of the group, this element would not be expected to be an immediate success, but merely to sow the seeds of ideas participants might return to later. It was clear that taking part in the group was not, nor was it expected to be, in any sense a 'cure' for Ken's psychosis, nor did it eliminate his voice hearing. The main benefits for him were the opportunity to discuss his experiences with others, practicing appropriate social skills in the group, and developing a sense of control over his voices.

Self esteem group

The stigma associated with mental health problems is widely known (see Hayward and Bright, 1997, for a review). There is also evidence for the negative impact of stigma on people's self-esteem, social functioning and recovery (Knight et al 2003). Many service users report continuing to experience distressing symptoms despite appropriate levels of medication, and this is associated with continued depression and low self-esteem.

As part of the same initiative to improve therapeutic interventions described above, a 'Self-Esteem and Coping with Stigma' group was implemented in several sites in South London. This was based on the model developed by Knight et al (2006), and the protocol can be found in Appendix 2. The intervention is a CBTp approach, and addresses the negative self-evaluations that may be involved in maintaining low self-esteem. The focus is to target the service users' responses to public and self-stigma, challenge the legitimacy of discriminatory and stigmatising attitudes in others, and combine this with self-esteem and empowerment work. The group format is thought to be an advantage here, as it provides additional support to counter the effects of isolation and exclusion experienced by people who are stigmatised. It is intended that the intervention will lead to an increase in levels of self-esteem, empowerment, and a reduction in distress. The intervention does *not* seek to modify service users' faulty beliefs about stigma: it is assumed that stigma, prejudice and discrimination are present in society, and service users are accurate in their perception of this. It would be predicted that there would be no significant change in the perceived level of stigma reported by participants.

This approach has not previously been used with inpatients, and hence we have no data to support its efficacy with this client group. Previous evaluations of the approach with outpatients with psychosis showed a significant increase in self esteem over the course of treatment, and a significant decrease in depression, although these benefits were not maintained at follow-up (see Knight et al., 2006). As with the Hearing Voices group the positive evaluation of participants was considered to be a particularly important outcome. In all responses, participant feedback was positive, and the overall group experience was highly regarded. In particular, service users highlighted listening to other's experiences, discovering that they were not alone in having the experiences discussed, and having the opportunity to express their views, as being the elements of the group they found most helpful. These initially positive findings therefore justify further research to establish whether the benefits of this new approach would generalise to an inpatient setting.

Community Group Meeting

This form of group is less specific in its focus and there have been no formal published evaluations. The rules to guide both the leaders and service users are clear: in this group, personal issues which do not pertain to other individuals (e.g. medication doses or individual leave from the ward) are not discussed, unless of course it relates to a specific general issue (e.g. the difficulty of accessing leave by a number of individuals because of staff availability).

The focus of the group is on encouraging a more active role by service users in how the ward is run. Two broad goals are overt: (i) to increase the responsiveness of the ward to service user goals through the monitoring of key changes in the ward milieu and (ii) to increase feelings of empowerment in service users. Less overt is the way in which the group leaders act as role models and encourage personal problem solving. For instance if patients want unfettered access to the internet group leaders can ask the group to discuss why this may not be beneficial to all. Similarly if there is a suggestion that the TV should be allowed at any time of the night the group can be guided to discuss why this may be disadvantageous in relation to sleep hygiene.

The process for the group leaders is not to intervene except when asked about specific issues of ward or hospital rules but to provide support to guide discussion between all individuals who may also include nursing and medical staff not taking part as leaders.

A Note on the evidence base

As we have seen, CBTp groups can be utilised in an acute inpatient setting, and there is an emerging evidence base for their efficacy in this setting. It is worth noting that pharmacological treatments for psychosis are based on an acute treatment and prevention model, in the same way diabetes or asthma drugs would be evaluated. If a drug reduces symptoms, it would be expected that withdrawal of the drug would lead to the symptoms returning. However, psychological treatment is often evaluated as if it was analogous to an antibiotic, whereby success means the person remains symptom free when the course of treatment is finished. This leads to the conclusion that if symptoms return following psychological treatment then the treatment has failed. This is clearly not the case: a group CBTp intervention will have measurable benefits, although these benefits are not always maintained at follow-up. Our argument suggests an alternative treatment approach, whereby psychological treatment should be provided in maintenance doses every few months. These assumptions about treatment efficacy have seriously hindered the adoption of psychological treatments in health services. Because the maintenance component would increase costs, it is not often adopted, despite the fact that there is likely to be a further benefit in terms of quality of life for service users (Castle et al, 2003).

References

Castle, D., Copolov, D. and Wykes, T. (Eds.) (2003) *Pharmacological and Psychosocial Treatments in Schizophrenia*. London: Martin Dunitz.

Clarke, I. and Wilson, H. (eds.) (2009) *Cognitive Behavioural Therapy for Acute Mental Health Units*. London: Routledge.

Durham, R., Guthrie, M., Morton, R., Reid, D., Treliving, L., Fowler, D. and Macdonald (2003) Tayside-Fife clinical trial of cognitive behavioural therapy for medication-resistant psychotic symptoms: Results to 3-month follow-up. *British Journal of Psychiatry, 182*, 303-311.

Fowler, D., Garrety, P. and Kuipers, E. (1995) *Cognitive Behaviour Therapy for Psychosis*. Chichester: Wiley Blackwell.

Gledhill, A., Lobban, F. and Sellwood, W. (1998) Group CBT for people with schizophrenia: a preliminary investigation. *Behavioural and Cognitive Psychotherapy, 26*, 63-75.

Hayward, P. and Bright, J. (1997) Stigma and mental illness: a review and critique. *Journal of Mental Health, 6*, 345-354.

Hearing Voices Network (2001) *Starting and Supporting Hearing Voices Groups*. Manchester: Hearing Voices Network.

Kingdon, D. and Turkington, D. (eds.) (2002) *The Case Study Guide to Cognitive Behaviour Therapy of Psychosis*. UK: WileyBlackwell.

Kingdon, D. and Turkington, D. (2008) *Cognitive Therapy of Schizophrenia*. London: Guilford Press.

Knight, M., Wykes, T. and Hayward, P. (2003) 'People don't understand': an investigation of stigma in schizophrenia using Interpretive Phenomenological Analysis (IPA). *Journal of Mental Health, 12*, 209-222.

Knight, M., Wykes, T. and Hayward, P. (2006) Group treatment of perceived stigma and self-esteem in Schizophrenia: a waiting-list trial of efficacy. *Behavioural and Cognitive Psychotherapy, 34*, 305-318.

Linehan, M. M. (1993) *Skills Training Manual for the Treatment of Borderline Personality Disorder*. New York: Guilford Press.

Morrison, A. (2002) *A Casebook of Cognitive Therapy of Psychosis*. London: Routledge.

Morrison, N. (2001) Group cognitive therapy: Treatment of choice or sub-optimal option? *Behavioural and Cognitive Psychotherapy, 29*, 311-332.

National Institute for Clinical Excellence – Guideline Development Group (2009) Core interventions in the treatment and management of schizophrenia in adults in primary and secondary care (update). Available at: http://www.nice.org.uk/nicemedia/pdf/CG82FullGuideline.pdf

Newton, E., Landau, S., Smith, P., Monks, P., Shergill, S. and Wykes, **T.** (2005) Early psychological interventions for auditory hallucinations: an exploratory study of young people's voices groups. *Journal of Nervous and Mental Disease, 193*,1, 58-61

Newton, E., Larkin, M., Melhuish, R. and Wykes, T. (2007) More than just a place to talk: Young people's experiences of group psychological therapy as early intervention for auditory hallucinations. *Psychology and Psychotherapy: Theory, Research and Practice, 80,* 127-149.

Romme, M. and Escher, A. Hearing Voices (1989) *Schizophrenia Bulletin, 15(2),* 209-216.

Tarrier, N. and Wykes, T. (2004) Is there evidence that cognitive behaviour therapy is an effective treatment for schizophrenia? A cautious or cautionary tale? *Behaviour Research and Therapy, 42,* 1377-1401.

Turkington, D., Kingdon, D. and Turner, T. (2002) Effectiveness of a brief cognitive behavioural therapy intervention in the treatment of schizophrenia. *British Journal of Psychiatry, 180,* 523-527.

Wykes, T.. Parr, A. and Landau, S. (1998) Group treatment of auditory hallucinations: exploratory study of effectiveness. *British Journal of Psychiatry, 175,* 180-185.

Wykes, T., Hayward, P., Thomas, N., Green, N., Surguladze, S., Fannon, D. and Landau, S. (2005) What are the effects of group cognitive behavioural therapy for voices? A randomised control trial. *Schizophrenia Research, 77,* 201-210.

Wykes, T., Steel, C., Everitt, B. and Tarrier, N. (2008) Cognitive behaviour therapy for schizophrenia: effect size, clinical models, and methodological rigor. *Schizophrenia Bulletin, 34,* 523-537.

Appendix 1 – CBT Hearing Voices Group

Session 1. *Aims:* Sharing information about psychosis

Models of psychosis

1. Set Agenda

2. Introductions
   - Introduce selves and the group's purpose (to talk about voices: the goal is to lower distress and not to eliminate voices completely).
   - Confidentiality (don't talk about what others have said outside of the group).

3. Show first 15 minutes of DVD (Horizon – 'Hearing Voices')

4. Ask what is the same or different about the voices experienced by people in the group compared to the people in the video
The similarities between group members' experience is emphasised.
   - When did you begin to hear voices?
   - How often do you usually hear your voices? How long do they usually last?
   - Are they loud or quiet?
   - What kinds of things do they say?
   - When do they usually happen? (i.e. when alone or with other people, time of day, when busy or bored?)
   - How do the voices make you feel?
   - Do you know anybody else who has similar experiences?

5. Introduce the normalising rationale and continuum of experience model
   - Leaders relate any 'odd' experiences they might have had.
   - Findings suggest that many people hear voices.
   - The wide variety of the experiences of the people in the video is noted.
   - Some people who hear voices come into contact with services (about 40%), but others don't.

6. Different models / views of psychosis
Ask the group to comment on the issues covered in the video (people in the video had different views).
   - Medical Model: chemical imbalance in the brain, illness, needs medication to put it right, although the meds might not always work.
   - Stress-Vulnerability Model: describe the model on the flip-chart using the words used by the group members.

♦ Acknowledge that there are different ways of making sense of hearing voices, and different interpretations are valid.

7. What makes the voices better or worse?
♦ When and where are the voices worse?
♦ What stops the voices or makes them less upsetting?
Discuss whether people feel that they have some degree of control over their voices.
(a) Medication
♦ Is it helpful? If so, how? What are the risks and benefits?
♦ Does it get rid of the voices? Does it make them more bearable?
(b) Other treatments for voices
♦ Does it help to talk about voices?
♦ Does it help to know that others have the same experiences?

8. Summarise the group's discussion.

Session 2. *Aims:*   Models of hallucinations

Effective coping strategies

1. Set agenda

2. Show 15 minutes of the video

3. Models of hallucinations
♦ Where do voices sound as though they are coming from? Inside or outside your head?
♦ If they sound like they are coming from outside your head, why is it that no-one else can hear them?
♦ What do you think the voices are?
♦ What causes the voices? The brain, spirits, God or the Devil, other people's thoughts, your own thoughts?
♦ How should you treat the voices? What happens if you disobey them?
Emphasise this point and ask about behavioural tests of hypotheses.

4. Discussion of stigma and labelling
♦ Do you think that your symptoms are due to mental illness?
♦ Diagnosis: does it help you to think that your voices are due to an illness, or do you prefer other explanations?
♦ Does the fact that you have 'different' experiences make you any worse than others?
♦ Is it hard to tell others that you hear voices? Who would it be safe to tell?

5. Methods of coping

- What do you do to cope with the voices?
- How well do the strategies work?
- Have you tried any of the following strategies?:
- Distraction – listening to music, watching TV, talking to somebody.
- Increased or decreased stimulation.
- Ignoring / disobeying the commands of the voices.
- Telling the voices to go away.
- Postponing the voices until later in the day.
- Focussing on the physical characteristics of the voices: volume, tone, male / female etc.
- Concentrating on a task – reading, playing computer games.
- Thinking about something nice/positive about yourself while you try to ignore voices.
- Humming or singing to yourself. *If the group doesn't suggest this strategy, the facilitator should, as there is evidence for its effectiveness.*

6. The Role of medication

- Does it help? How is it helpful?
  The facilitator should provide some basic information about psychopharmacology. If the group wishes, the facilitator can offer to get further information, e.g. arrange an education session from a pharmacist.

7. The role of recreational drugs

- Do these make the voices better or worse?
- Cannabis is worse than alcohol (it relaxes people but also makes them more paranoid).

8. Homework

- Each person is to try a new strategy for dealing with the voices.
  Each person writes down a new strategy on an index card to take away as a reminder.

9. Summarise the group's discussion and remind about homework.

Session 3. *Aims:* Improving self-esteem

Overall model of coping with voices

1. Set agenda

2. Feedback on the success of new strategies

- Have the new strategies been applied since the last meeting?

+ If so, what did you do and was it helpful?
+ Did the strategies need modifying?
+ Do different members need to use different methods of coping?
+ Are there other coping strategies that you can think of?
+ Encourage the experience of self-efficacy.

3. Self-esteem

+ Play the 'Self-esteem Game' using index cards, but only if group members wish to do so. Everyone writes their name at the top of the card, and then passes it around. Each group member writes something they like about the person whose name is on the card. This continues until the card is passed back to the person, who receives a card with things people like about them written on it. The facilitator takes part too.
+ Does your mood affect the experience of voices, e.g. frequency, severity?
+ Do the voices effect your mood (i.e. is there a circular, maintaining model)?
+ What do other people think about you?
+ Discuss how group members can use cards or think of positive things about themselves, especially when they hear voices. Group members are encouraged to use the cards to improve their mood or remind themselves about their good points.

4. Homework

+ Try to modify coping strategies and encourage 'positive thinking' with the use of the index card from the self esteem game.

5. Sharing coping strategies

+ Identify with group members the different possible ways of helping to reduce distressing experiences, e.g. medication for biological vulnerability, improving coping strategies, improving mood, decreasing stress, etc. Often members want to write this down so ensure that there are enough writing tools available.

6. Discuss members' experiences of the group

+ What do you think you have learned?
+ How many different coping strategies do you know of?

The service users could be asked to write down one or two different strategies which they found most helpful on index cards so they can remember them more easily when they are experiencing voices.

7. Summarise discussion and remind of homework.

Appendix 2 – Self Esteem and Coping with Stigma Group

Session 1: Stigma: The concept and experiences

1. Introductions
+ Introduce selves and the group's purpose (to talk about the stigma of mental health problems, ways of overcoming stigma, and improving self esteem).
+ Confidentiality (don't talk about what others have said outside of the group).

2. Show first ten minutes of video 'Myths about Madness' (Glasgow Media Group)
+ Sections on facts and dangerousness (Blondes).

3. Sharing of information regarding stigma
+ What do the words stigma and discrimination mean to you? (Similar words, examples, definitions).
+ Have you ever felt stigmatised or discriminated against in your life?
+ Have you ever felt stigmatised or discriminated against due to being a hospital patient?
+ Do you feel stigmatised now due to being a hospital inpatient?
· *Being Sectioned (only discuss if group members raise topic). Disseminate facts, acknowledge its distressing nature, discuss methods to avoid sectioning*
+ Do you feel there is a difference between being a patient in a General Hospital and a Psychiatric Hospital? (E.g. breaking a leg, vs. having depression).
+ Who causes you to feel this way? (Family / friends / public / hospital staff).
+ Do you feel you are prejudiced against yourself? Do you stigmatise yourself?
Emphasise the similarities between group members' experiences.

4. The 'normalising rationale'
This theme is returned to in each subsequent group.
+ Leaders relate any experience of stigma.
+ Note different experiences of stigma in the group.
+ Findings suggest that mental health problems are surprisingly widespread in the general population. Around 1 in 3 people will experience mental ill health at some point in their lives.
+ Continuum of normal-abnormal experience, not two distinct categories.

5. Sharing of information of mental health problems
+ How do you see your difficulties (do you see yourself as having difficulties)?
+ Do you have mental health problems / schizophrenia?
+ Is that why you are here (in hospital)?
+ If you do not see yourself as having mental health problems, are you different

from other people?
+ Do people stigmatise / discriminate against you because of this difference?
+ Is schizophrenia a 'label'?

5. Facts and myths about schizophrenia / psychosis
This is an educational component where the facilitator provides some basic information.
+ It is **not** split-personality.
+ The cause is probably a combination of genetic factors and life experiences.
+ This is not your fault / a sign of weakness.
+ Problems are not untreatable / incurable. People can and do make a recovery.

6. Models of mental health problems
+ Medical Model (chemical imbalance in the brain, illness, needs medication to put it right, although the meds might not always work).
+ Stress-Vulnerability Model: describe the model on the flip-chart using the words used by the group members.
+ Acknowledge that there are different ways of making sense of hearing voices, and different interpretations are valid.

Session 2: Myths about dangerousness & methods of coping

1. Sharing of knowledge and experience of dangerousness
+ What does it mean to be dangerous?
+ Which kinds of people are dangerous?
+ Do you think people with mental health problems are dangerous? Have you seen violence / aggression by service users in hospital or a clinic?
+ Have you ever read about / seen on TV, stories of violence by people with mental health problems?
+ Are they fair representations?
+ Do people think of you as dangerous because of having mental health problem / being different from others?

2. Dissemination of facts concerning violence, dangerousness and mental health
+ Facts: the vast majority of people (including those with mental health problems) are not dangerous.
+ Who is most dangerous?
+ Where / how do most acts of violence occur?
+ What is the proportion of those incidents with the general population?

3. Discussion topic
+ If 'men' and 'young people' are the most dangerous / violent section of the population, should we avoid all of them? Should we be scared if they move in

next door? *This can be related to issues of location and housing for people with mental health problems.*

- Violence: the best predictors of violence are factors outlined above (male / age), and history of past violence.

4. Normalising rationale

- Stress-vulnerability approach: a variety of factors, such as age, gender and substance abuse, may increase propensity to violence. The additional element of psychosis *may* alter this vulnerability further, but it is one element among many.

5. Sharing of methods of coping

- The leaders should acknowledge that many if not all group members have been using coping strategies, and have been coping with stigma, stigmatisation and discrimination, prior to the group.
- What do you do to cope with stigma / discrimination?
- Which strategies work well and which do not work? *(N.B: some strategies may be counterproductive, and the facilitator should encourage discussion of the pros and cons)*
- Public may have negative reactions, due to a lack of understanding of mental health problems. This is their ignorance, not your inferiority.

6. Hidden stigmas

- If a person makes a derogatory comment regarding people with mental health problems, without knowing you have (or have had) similar difficulties, what do you say? Ask the group to generate possible options, e.g. ignore comment, express your concern without revealing own illness, express your concern while also revealing own illness.
- Discuss the advantages and disadvantages of these strategies.
  Acknowledge that coping strategies require considerable effort, and that different coping strategies may be appropriate for different occasions. They may not work every time.

Session 3: Self-esteem

1. How stigma affects us

- Does your mood affect your feelings of stigma, being stigmatised?
- Does feeling stigmatised affect your mood? How?
- What do you think that other people think about you?

2. Play the self-esteem game.

- Discuss how group members can think of positive things about themselves, particularly if feeling stigmatised.

3. Discussion Topic: Responses to overt stigma, discrimination, or abuse by others

+ Are people stigmatising you due to your mental health problems / being different, or are they simply rude? Use racial and gender commonalities, is the offensive person racist or sexist, or is their rudeness irrespective of that?
+ You may stigmatise me, but you don't know me.

4. Practical skills: How to complain

+ Making a formal complaint if one is the target of abuse or discrimination (e.g. in a shop).
+ Speaking with one's key-worker, preparing a formal letter.

5. Discussion of methods to increase assertiveness and feelings of empowerment

+ Use of empowerment to choose which coping strategy is most suited to specific circumstances.
+ Role-Play (As basis: Christine Padesky - Social Anxiety - Signing Cheques).

7. Discussion of how members experienced the group

+ What do you think you have learned?
+ How do you want to deal with feelings of stigmatisation in the future? (*Additional role-play could be used if desired*).

8. Advocacy: Taking my empowerment further.

+ The facilitator should disseminate information about local advocacy services.
+ Discussion of how this may impact on one's life, and others' lives, in a positive way.

13
Applying the Kanas Model on an Acute Psychiatric Unit

Ronan J McIvor and Wil Pennycook

Purpose and Structure

In this chapter we describe the development of a group therapy programme in an acute inner city setting. The programme is based on the model developed by Professor Nick Kanas at the University of California at San Francisco, using an integrative approach for treating patients with psychosis and severe mental illness. We explore the social context in which the group takes place, as well as practical aspects of setting and running it on a busy acute psychiatric ward. We discuss some of the challenges of running the group in such a setting. Case vignettes are used to illustrate themes and interactions.

The Social context

In many parts of the United Kingdom, acute inpatient psychiatric units struggle to maintain a therapeutic environment for their patients in the face of staff shortages, unsafe environments, poor ward design and overcrowding (Holloway, this volume; McGeorge & Rae, 2007). As a result, wards can be frightening places in which to be admitted and may not provide the sanctuary envisaged by many service users. Periods of intense activity and arousal, with anger directed towards staff and patients alike, alternate with long periods of inactivity and boredom (Chaplin et al, 2006). In such an environment it is difficult to develop and maintain structured therapeutic activities.

Radcliffe and Smith (2007) noted that at any time during the day 84% of inpatients were socially disengaged and mainly inactive.

This situation is more marked within an inner city environment, the setting for the group under discussion. The London borough of Lambeth is an ethnically diverse, socially deprived inner-city area with high levels of unemployment, criminal activity and drug abuse. The borough has above average rates of psychiatric morbidity, characterized by high levels of psychosis and psychiatric illness.

Aubrey Lewis 3 Ward (AL3) at the Maudsley Hospital is an 18 bedded acute inpatient unit for male patients living within Lambeth. The majority of patients suffer from acute exacerbations of severe mental illness, such as schizophrenia or bipolar disorder. They are frequently admitted compulsorily under Mental Health legislation, because of associated risks of self-harm or harm to others. Dual diagnosis and personality issues frequently complicate their clinical presentation. Average duration of admission is twenty eight days.

Despite this background, staff have endeavoured to develop initiatives for improving the therapeutic environment for patients, through the provision of daily organisational meetings, art and music therapy and an extensive occupational therapy programme. In addition, the authors wanted to introduce a therapeutic group onto the ward for those patients suffering from acute psychosis, in an attempt to provide a specific psychological intervention for symptom management and maintenance of interpersonal connections with the outside world. Given the high acuity, rapid turnover and clinical profile of patients, the integrative model developed by Kanas provided a useful framework to develop the group (Kanas, 1996).

Theoretical aspects

The approach taken by Professor Kanas evolved over more than 20 years of clinical and research activities. As the model was refined with clinical experience and important components clarified, outcome and process studies were performed. Between 1975–77, Kanas conducted a controlled study of inpatient group therapy in San Antonio, Texas and began some research in San Francisco in 1978, initially on acute, inpatient settings. Patients were randomly assigned, for example, to one of three experimental conditions: group therapy; activities-orientated task group and a control group, where patients were not involved with small group activities. His aim was to create a model based on research - his own and others - which could be replicated and taught. He wanted 'to acquaint mental health practitioners with a safe, helpful, and cost-effective method of treating schizophrenic patients using the integrative model of group therapy' (Kanas, 1996).

Why groups?

Schizophrenia and other significant, enduring mental illnesses are complex disorders comprising biological, psychological and social causes and effects. In developing a treatment programme for patients with such disorders, psychosocial as well as biological approaches need to be considered. An effective way of addressing the psychosocial nature of this illness is through working in groups. This allows the social elements associated with these conditions to be addressed in an environment of direct observation and learning from others. Review articles completed by Kanas supported this assumption, demonstrating 67% of inpatient studies found group therapy being significantly better than the non-group controls. There was a non-significant trend in favour of longer-term groups (ibid Pg 22-28).

The integrative approach

In his research, Kanas found that three main theoretical approaches for conducting group therapy for inpatients were highlighted in the literature. These were the educative, the psychodynamic and the interpersonal. In the educative approach, the orientation was towards biological aspects of schizophrenia, including the disease model of illness and the role of medication. The main goals were to enable patients to learn strategies in order to cope with their symptoms and everyday issues surrounding their illness. In this approach, therapists gave advice, created question and answer sessions, used problem-solving and techniques such as role play.

The psychodynamic approach focused on early psychological difficulties and unconscious conflicts rooted in early developmental experience which impacted on subsequent relationships. The treatment goal was to improve ego functioning, through gaining understanding of how long-standing problems created maladaptive behaviours. This was achieved through discussion and interpretation of transference reactions. This approach is well illustrated by Kernberg, although his work was mainly within the outpatient setting (ibid pg. 36). The psychodynamic approach is explored in greater depth in this volume (Radcliffe & Diamond).

The interpersonal approach views patients as socially isolated, with its goal to improve their ability to relate to others. The interpersonal approach relies on using structured techniques exemplified by Yalom (Hayek, this volume; Jefford et al, this volume; Yalom 1995), with emphasis on reality-based, structured approaches over those that are insight oriented and unstructured.

Kanas thought that all three approaches lacked something on their own. He felt the educative approach did not pay enough attention to the psychosocial needs of patients, while the psychodynamic approach was too intensive and risked exacerbating patients' symptoms by increasing anxiety. Finally, he thought the interpersonal approach did not pay sufficient attention to psychotic symptomatology.

Kanas' Integrative Model

The integrative model incorporates elements of all three approaches, but rejects or de-emphasises others. Like the educative approach, an important goal is to help patients manage their symptoms from a position of knowledge, but the integrative model does not use a didactic format. For example, psychosocial strategies are given more emphasis than medication strategies. Like the psychodynamic approach, there is an emphasis on open-ended discussions, with patients being able to generate topics from session to session, as long as the topic is congruent with the goals of the group. Transference issues and an exploration of the unconscious are not developed, for fear of provoking anxiety or worsening psychosis. The focus is generally on the present rather than the past, with an emphasis on ego strengthening through reality testing or reality sense. Long term maladaptive problems are examined with reference to current problems.

Like the interpersonal approach, a major goal of the integrative model is to help patients become less isolative and improve relationships with others through the group process. There is an emphasis on coping with symptoms and strengthening functioning. The model focuses on working in the 'here and now' of what is going on in the session, to reality test and identify maladaptive behaviours and psychotic beliefs which could be challenged.

There are two aims of this integrative approach; firstly to help group members cope with their symptoms through reality testing and sharing of ideas, and secondly to improve their interpersonal skills and relationships. Patients can discuss their isolation and relationship difficulties in the group and together consider possible solutions. In the process of discussion, they practice and improve their interpersonal skills. Healthy interactions can be reinforced by the therapists and eventually by patients themselves.

Kanas also points out that, when psychotic symptoms are perceived to be unpleasant and foreign, patients are motivated to discuss alternative coping strategies. However, if they are perceived to be positive there develops a motivational problem that needs to be challenged and resolved. In the case of psychotic symptoms that are perceived to be comforting and useful, such as auditory hallucinations which are reassuring, Kanas argues that the focus of treatment should be on helping patients understand how such experiences interfere with their lives, such as voices that give unrealistic advice or encourage avoidance of social contact.

Kanas suggests co-therapy in groups, as two therapists are better able to manage the sometimes chaotic feel of the group. They can model non-psychotic interactions with one another, such as test reality and play off each other to assist the group in challenging distorted beliefs. Co-therapy helps to protect against burn-out and stress, assuming they form a good working alliance.

In the integrative approach, therapists need to be active and directive in sessions in order to keep patients focused on the topic under discussion. Interventions need to be clear, consistent and concrete. Therapists can give advice and personal opinions if this helps advance reality testing. Therapists can support one another in the group by reinforcing what the other is saying. In addition, co-therapy can facilitate the creation of a safe environment. Patients need to feel safe when discussing problems in a group setting in order to minimise anxiety and conflict.

Practical aspects

Setting up the group

We considered it essential for the group to be viewed by staff as being part of the ward milieu and a recognised component of the range of therapeutic interventions available. We were anxious for staff to be supportive of the group and take ownership of it. We discussed our proposals with the ward manager to ensure her support and encouraged interested staff to attend two seminars chaired by ourselves, each lasting about an hour and a half. Prior to the first seminar, a number of relevant papers were distributed to staff, which outlined some of the practical aspects of Kanas' model, as well as concepts relating to transference and group dynamics (Stock Whitaker, 1985; Edelson & Berg, 1999). In the first seminar, attended mainly by nursing staff, we discussed the papers and group processes. We talked about bringing together patients and staff, and acknowledged that patients in general wanted more contact with staff, contact that was not focused only on medication or perceived or actual coercion. We discussed the importance of allowing patients to talk openly about their experiences and providing a resource for each other.

We discussed the model that we wanted to adopt for the group, stressing the importance of maintaining relationships and connectedness. Staff expressed some apprehension that the group would have an interpretative element, which they felt unskilled in managing. We clarified that the group would not be a psychodynamic group, in the sense that we would also not be making interpretations, nor allow the group to become too anxious, which we felt would be intolerable. We emphasised the focus would be on the 'here-and-now', and reinforced that the group was about fundamental and basic needs, such as recovery from the 'acute' phase of illness and relationships. We encouraged staff to have a sense of owning the group. The goals of the group were summarised, with the focus on improving interpersonal communication, coping with symptoms and managing feelings as a result of admission.

In the second session, we discussed practical aspects, such as frequency (weekly), duration (40 minutes), numbers (minimum 4, maximum 9) and location (meeting room on the ward). Given the turnover of patients on an acute ward we decided that the group would not have a fixed membership but would be open to new members each week. It was agreed patients could not join the session late, after it had commenced. Ground rules were devised, focusing on confidentiality and safety. It was agreed that we would not restrict attendance to those with a diagnosis of schizophrenia, but would include patients with any psychosis, including mania. This was a deviation from the Kanas Model (which is homogeneous for schizophrenic diagnosis), but we felt it was justified given local pressures and for reasons of inclusiveness, as we felt it would benefit this wider group of patients. Patients were excluded if they did not have a psychotic illness or their behaviour was deemed too aroused or disruptive. The group was to be facilitated by two people, initially the two authors. We were keen for ward staff to be part of the process and for one to attend on a rotating basis for one month at a time. It was agreed that a debriefing session would take place after each meeting. To emphasize the importance of maintaining relationships both within and outside the hospital the group was named the Connexions Group. It was appropriately advertised on the ward prior to commencement.

We had one additional advantage in the planning process. One of the authors (RM) organised a day long seminar focusing on inpatient group therapy and delivered by Professor Kanas. This provided first hand experience of his expertise in the theoretical and practical aspects of his model.

Typical structure of each session

On average, six patients attended the group each week, the range being from four to nine. Ground rules were described at the beginning of each session. These included listening to others, not interrupting when another person was speaking and refraining from inappropriate behaviour or violence. We stressed confidentiality within the service setting rather than the group setting, so that patients understood that we could share important clinical or risk information with the wider team. We also explained that the group was not the forum to discuss individual leave arrangements or changes in medication, as these topics could be more appropriately discussed at ward rounds. If such subjects did arise, we reframed them to trigger general discussions on, for example, the impact of hospitalization on outside relationships or what it was like taking medication when patients did not feel they needed it.

At the beginning of each group everyone introduced themselves. After the introductions, and following what was usually more general discussion, a theme emerged. The group ended by both therapists summarising what had been discussed.

Themes and interactions

Although patients regularly requested talking therapies, it was a struggle to persuade them to attend. Part of this was that staff did not always remember that the group was due to take place, and had to be reminded regularly. This indicated to us that we were not fully successful in achieving the shared ownership to which we aspired. This resistance was, perhaps, a complex interaction between staff ambivalence and patients' anxiety about being together. In addition the ward environment can create a culture of dependence and passivity. Prior to the meeting, it was not unusual for us to 'round up' patients, encouraging them to attend. RM also 'prescribed' the group at ward rounds, to patients he and the team felt were appropriate to attend. In addition, one or two of the higher functioning and verbal patients helped with recruitment.

The group lasted for one year, and stopped due to a major reorganisation of the service, which included a change in job for RM and a change in physical location for the ward. Over the year, a number of themes regularly emerged during the sessions, including issues of safety, powerlessness, personal and professional care and isolation. In general it could be said that the themes focused on the nature of this temporary, ever-changing community and the task of being a member of it. The issue of safety, encompassing personal well-being as well as worries about theft of personal possessions and fear of fire came up in almost every session. Occasionally, there would be specific concerns about feeling intimidated by other patients and even staff, and issues relating to trust. Such concerns were expressed in terms of the fabric of the ward: what would happen if there was a fire, for example, or how could safety be maintained? Linked to this was the issue of hygiene. This was a frequent topic and of great concern. This seemed to be linked to the wish for privacy, to be able to use the bathroom without interruption and, more importantly, to find it clean. There was considerable distress expressed about the general lack of cleanliness on the unit, which was justified to some extent. It was sometimes hard to grasp whether these were complaints about fellow patients or directed towards staff, for not looking after them or taking care of their basic needs and comforts.

As an all male group, the conversation often focused on powerlessness, the feeling of emasculation and the pain over the loss of relationships. The absence of female patients may have allowed for the expression of such vulnerable feelings, aided by the presence of a female therapist. Reflecting the name of the group (Connexions), members often talked about their sense of isolation and difficulty in maintaining contact with family and friends whilst in hospital. Many believed they had been forgotten and felt cut-off from the outside world. Sometimes this was expressed in physical terms, such as worries about lack of control over bodily functions. At other times, the men would talk of their sorrow over not being able to maintain relationships, not only because they were separated through hospitalization, but because of the nature of their illness. We sensed this loss was seen as more acute on an all-male ward, and many patients expressed regret at the lack of contact with female patients. We wondered if female nursing staff or the female therapist were seen as having a parenting or nurturing role in this regard. Patients spoke of long standing difficulties in developing relationships, including intimate relationships:

Example: Steven

Steven, who had a diagnosis of schizophrenia, mentioned that, as a child, he never had friends and indeed paid other children to play with him or accompany him to the cinema. As an adult, he said he tended to 'hunt' for women in the form of one-night stands. He said he fell in love immediately and asked them to move in with him. Some of the other patients offered Steven advice about this, saying that he was like an open book. They advised him to hold back in terms of expressing his emotions too quickly when he met women. Other patients said they had been in long-term relationships, although they tended to talk about their failure in relationships rather than any successes. The group often touched on the impact of inpatient confinement and repeated admissions to hospital on relationships, including intimate relationships. One patient spoke of his difficulty in maintaining his relationship with his girlfriend. He said she wanted to have baby, but he did not feel he was ready to become a father. He subsequently learnt that his girlfriend became pregnant by another man, which caused him some regret.

Group therapy, by its very nature, is a social exercise and discussions such as these were encouraged, particularly as patients became less psychotic over time. We gained the impression that patients got to know each other better on the ward as a result of group attendance, and this helped to make the atmosphere friendlier. Contact with group members, both in and outside the group, began to alleviate the fear and mistrust often experienced by patients. We were at times surprised by the amount of personal information patients revealed to the group and heartened by the support they got from fellow patients.

Linked to a sense of powerlessness on the ward was the challenge of how to influence others in order to change things. The sense of hierarchy amongst patients was keenly felt, both with their peers and with staff, as was the importance of securing one's place in the pecking order. Some felt that in order to get through their admission they had to be obedient and conform, which lead to a discussion about control or the lack of it. Other patients challenged the stance of obedience and admitted they pushed boundaries in order to achieve some sense of control, although the reality was that these usually lead to less control, as care plans became more restrictive. Rules seemed to be both craved and loathed. Many seemed genuinely despondent about this and feelings of apathy and depression could quickly descend.

The issue of exercising control is illustrated in the following example, which took place only weeks after the group had commenced on the ward:

Example

The group was interrupted by a nurse who wondered if another patient called John could join the session. RM said it was not possible, in accordance with the ground rules. However several minutes later, the patient was brought into the meeting by another member of staff and sat down. The discussion underway was interrupted and the group was asked what we should do about John's presence. Some members of the group believed John should be allowed to stay for the duration of the session, while others felt that, as he arrived late for the group, he should be told to leave. There was some discussion as to how a decision could be arrived at, but it was eventually agreed that there should be a vote on the matter. The group discussed who was eligible to vote, with some members suggesting that staff should not. It was eventually agreed that staff could be part of the voting process. Interestingly, John then decided to leave the group of his own accord. However the issue of late attendance had still to be resolved and the group again voted to exclude patients who arrived late for sessions.

The example illustrated the ability of patients, even when acutely psychiatrically unwell, to negotiate a complicated range of processes and decisions, leading to a clear outcome. It was hoped that such processes would be remembered and used in other settings. For us as therapists, the incident reflected the evolving nature of the group and its rules. It reminded us that the ground rules of the group had not been clarified, and it was our responsibility to clearly state them and avoid boundary infringements. As it turned out, the group resolved the issue itself, although the decision may have appeared punitive to John, who was not at fault for being brought into the session. The example also illustrated how difficult it was to manage boundaries and perhaps it could be argued that, with such patients, we should have been more relaxed and inclusive. We felt that having clear boundaries would enable the group to feel safe and contained. There was subsequently very little movement in and out of the group once a session had started. The mechanism of the resolution, by voting, was not specific to the Kanas model, but the general theme was, that of socialisation and negotiation.

In a number of sessions the subject of managing symptoms arose, either from direct patient questioning of the therapists or from general discussion. Many patients were confused about why they were in hospital and were unable to comprehend that they were ill, as the following examples illustrate:

Example

Mohammed asked about the definition of delusions, which opened a discussion on recognizing and dealing with them more effectively. Mohammed noted that trust and paranoia did not go together. We asked the group what effect their delusions had on them, and how they made them feel. A number of people mentioned that they enjoyed some of their delusional beliefs, particularly the grandiose ones. When the delusions disappeared, they felt it was sometimes difficult to adapt to being an ordinary person. We reflected that there may a desire to maintain their delusional beliefs or impulsive behaviour so patients did not have to think of the consequences to their daily lives. The group went on to discuss coping strategies.

During another session, the group talked about auditory hallucinations. Most had experienced these. Some found them distressing because of their content or meaning, while others found them comforting and supportive. Most recognized them as being part of their illness and outside themselves. We asked how patients coped with the distressing symptoms. One listened to music, while another used other activities and distraction techniques.

From one session to the next, a number of regular group members reflected that patients' behaviour and presentation had improved from the previous week. This positive feedback was reinforced by the therapists, reflecting our role in encouraging and supporting patients in their recovery.

Delusions present a good opportunity for the group process, because their unreality may be challenged by other group members and coping strategies put in place for those which are distressing. One could speculate that patients develop delusions because they find it difficult to adapt to being an ordinary person. This example is from a patient with acute mania:

Example

Peter started the group by saying he didn't know why he was in hospital as he was the right-hand man of a famous British entrepreneur. He added that he was rich and had a yacht. Group members looked at him warily. They began to question him – why were his clothes so dirty if he was so important, why did he live in a bed-sit if he was so rich and why did the entrepreneur not visit him in hospital. The therapists took a back seat for a time, except to ensure that the group was not ganging up on Peter and the questions remained good humoured.

The challenge for the group in this example was not to collude. The persistent challenging of delusional beliefs can be counterproductive without the support of the group. In addition, the patient's version of reality should be acknowledged, with a reflection on how the belief might interfere with the patient's life. Dealing with patients with mania in a group setting presents particular problems. One session was dominated by a manic patient, who was intrusive and rambling in speech, and difficult to interrupt. Some members of the group reflected this back to him, but he did not take it onboard at the time. About half way through the meeting, the patient appeared to feel persecuted and left the group. This issue is explored further in the discussion section.

The use of illicit drugs, both on the ward and in the community, was frequently discussed. The following is a typical illustration of the issues that arose:

Example

At one meeting, Derek began to talk about his use of cannabis prior to admission to hospital. He said he used it because it helped him relax and he didn't see why he had to stop it. He added that all his friends used cannabis and it was normal. He did not think it had any negative impact on his mental health. Another patient acknowledged cannabis made his paranoia worse, if used continuously. Some patients expressed how difficult it was to stop illicit drugs on admission to hospital, particularly when they had no leave. Another patient acknowledged the difficulty of remaining off cannabis on discharge, because his friends used it.

As therapists, we took a directive stance in the discussion, noting recent research highlighting the risks of cannabis on mental health. Some patients took this on board; others dismissed it, citing their own experience. For the therapists' standpoint, the issue illustrated the directive nature of our position at times and the psycho-educational component to our role. We were unambiguous in our position, while at the same time being supportive and encouraging.

Discussion

The challenge of developing inpatient groups for those who are acutely psychiatrically unwell is considerable, both in terms of support and commitment from staff and bringing together patients with a variety of diagnoses. The group took place in a ward that had already made progress developing a therapeutic milieu, with art and music groups established as part of the weekly practice. Yet initially, we found it difficult to encourage staff to take ownership of the group and embed it in the therapeutic ethos of the unit. For example, it was difficult to get the same nurse to attend the group over even a relatively short number of weeks, as envisaged in the planning group. Was there some kind of mystique that surrounded the group, even though both psychotherapists clearly stated these were not psychodynamic groups and not about 'fiddling with people's heads?' Was there a more prosaic issue, related to the amount and intensity of work on an acute psychiatric unit, with a sense that the group was simply just another thing to do or a victim of the rigid shift system?

How do treatment groups become embedded within the ward and what are the pre-requisites for this to happen? We considered several strategies of importance. One of the therapists was the consultant psychiatrist for the ward, while the other worked as a group psychotherapist in the hospital. The group therefore had a local connection that minimised the perception that it was somehow imposed on the unit. Our group did survive with good patient attendance and we wondered whether some of the coherence of the group owed much to the fact that both therapists were senior in their fields. In our case, RM was the ward consultant with many years experience and WP was a Consultant Psychotherapist and trained Group Analyst. Her experience included not only theoretical aspects of group processes, but hands on experience of being in groups, of managing herself in groups and in leading them.

We also attempted to prepare staff adequately for the group, through seminars, informal meetings and encouragement. The issue of how staff are rostered is key to the well-functioning of any group, as we found to our cost. In our specific case, an added complication was considerable uncertainty amongst staff over the long-term viability of the ward because of service re-provision. In addition, the permanent ward manager, who was supportive of the group, was on long term leave during the planning and early stages of the group. This impacted, we believe, on the staff's capacity to commit to the project. We also noted that it was not unusual for those running groups to encounter staff resistance or, at the very least, staff apathy. However, the difficulties we encountered with nursing participation could reflect the downside of having two experienced clinicians running the group. The main problem may have been one of envy at being unable to offer something good to patients which other staff could.

One answer may be that on-going education and training on therapeutic engagement of nursing and other staff needs to be established, perhaps through the group process itself. A staff group may reduce anxiety levels about groups in general and what happens to people in them. This inevitably involves leadership and the demonstration that such groups are supported from those in charge. This, in turn, is demonstrated by practical support for the groups.

Linked to this, we set time aside to have a discussion about the group following each session. Whilst this was not formal supervision, in that we did not have a supervisor, we were rigorous in both talking about the group and our experience of it and each other on a weekly basis. We think that this was very important in our management of the group process.

For the most part, Kanas developed his model with homogenous out-patient groups and one of the difficulties that he identified was working with patients who were experiencing different symptoms. He recognised, however, that homogeneity was almost impossible to achieve within the inpatient setting and this was certainly the case with our group. We decided, for practical reasons, to include patients with a range of psychotic diagnoses and to have an open group whose members changed from week to week. This largely worked, despite the risk that the manic or acutely aroused patient might interfere with the group to some extent. In such a setting, useful work can still be achieved, helping patients relate to one another in the 'here-and-now' and finding ways to manage symptoms and develop interpersonal skills. Keeping in mind Kanas' description of the two main treatment goals – management of symptoms and improvement in interpersonal relationships – enabled us to have a clear sense of what we were trying to achieve in each session. We firmly believed that patients can challenge other patients more powerfully than therapists.

Working in such a way with inpatients, therapists have to behave differently than they would if they were working with higher functioning patients (in outpatient settings). Kanas suggests that therapists need to be:

'active and directive in keeping group members focused on the topic: clear, consistent and concrete with interventions; supportive and diplomatic with comments; open and willing to give opinions and advice that are appropriate to the discussion; here and now (rather than

there and then) focused; encouraging of patient to patient (rather that patient to therapist) interaction'. (Kanas, 1996, p. 70)

Finally, the issue of our gender was one that we thought was relevant to our work on this ward. RM is a man and WP is a woman and at no point did we consider that WP's gender should bar her from co-leading the male group. Indeed we saw it as an advantage. We also encouraged female nurses to participate. We believed the group was contained in the way that it was because we were a working couple, modelling positive and helpful interactions. We also believed that the presence of a woman in this all male group was an influence on the content of the work of the group. Whilst on one occasion, a patient became overly sexualised towards WP, this was challenged and contained by both therapists. Although the behaviour did not diminish much in that session it improved in the next. Given that we were trying to promote more positive interpersonal engagement and relationships, we felt our own relationship was a helpful role model for patients. To that end, it was important we took time to talk about the group and our feelings within the supervision process.

Summary

The Integrative Model proposed by Kanas provides a useful framework for group therapy on an acute inpatient setting, specifically aimed at patients with psychosis. With its emphasis on maintaining connectedness, managing symptoms, advice giving and interpersonal sharing, it provides a practical and implementable therapy for use in an environment which can be, at times, aroused and unstable. Careful planning and constant encouragement of both staff and patients is essential to maintain ownership by the ward and embed the group into its therapeutic programme. For the group to be a success, it requires the support of senior staff. Training for staff may be necessary. If the group is to develop its own momentum and be self-maintaining, ward staff have to assume the role of co-therapists over time, maybe with the ongoing involvement of a trained group therapist.

References

Chaplin, R., McGeorge, M. and Lelliott, P. (2006) The National Audit of Violence: inpatient care for adults of working age. *Psychiatric Bulletin*, 30, 444-446.

Edelson, M. and Berg, D. (1999) *Rediscovering Groups*. London: Jessica Kingsley.

Kanas, N. (1996) *Group Therapy for Schizophrenic Patients*. Washington DC: American Psychiatric Press.

McGeorge M. and Rae M. (2007) Acute inpatient psychiatry: service improvement - the time is now. *Psychiatric Bulletin*, 31, 259-261.

Radcliffe, J. and Smith, R. (2007) Acute in-patient psychiatry: how patients spend their time on acute psychiatric wards. *Psychiatric Bulletin*, 31, 167-170.

Stock Whitaker, D (1985) Using Groups to Help People. International Library of Group Psychotherapy and Group Process. London: Routledge & Kegan Paul.

Yalom, I. (1995) *The Theory and Practice of Group Psychotherapy*. New York: Basic Books.

14
Kibel groups and their dynamic perspective

Torben Heinskou

Introduction

Patients admitted to acute wards face major psychological challenges. To begin with, many do not fully comprehend the reasons for admission. Their ability to understand and orientate themselves is often reduced as a result of their breakdown. The structure of the ward and of the treatment can be difficult to grasp, and during their stay the patients are likely to continue to feel disoriented at times and to struggle to emotionally process what is happening. Patients commonly find it difficult distinguishing whether their emotional reactions are the result of their altered emotional state or represent a normal response to a highly abnormal situation. Other patients' behaviour, for instance, is sometimes irrational and hard to make sense of. One of the key roles of staff is to reduce the negative impact of these difficulties and to help the patients gain a realistic perspective on what is going on. This is not straightforward as the staff themselves do not know everything about everything that is happening on the ward, for example relationships between patients, how patients are experiencing the ward and whether particular issues need to be talked through. What patients make of their experiences are often not revealed when talking to them individually but this often emerges when groups of patients get together. This makes groupwork especially valuable. Helping patients put their experiences into words in groups helps them understand the structure and interplay of everyday ward life, combat anti-therapeutic factors and create the conditions for a 'living-learning milieu' (Kennard, 2004).

Therapeutic factors in the therapy group

Certain inherent forces are brought into play when therapeutic groups meet. Foulkes (1964) outlined some key therapeutic factors in his description of group analysis, including socialisation, mirroring and exchange. *Socialisation* refers to the opportunity that the group provides participants to understand and reach out to each other, giving a sense of belonging. Sharing experiences of difficulties previously experienced individually helps participants break out from their isolation. Conflicts and anxieties can be viewed alongside those of others. As one Patient A. put it, 'Having talked about it now I realise that I was probably not the only one to be scared in the night when I was woken up by all that noise'. Secondly, individuals can also see aspects of themselves *mirrored* in the way other people describe similar experiences. They can then reflect on reactions they may have previously neglected, and understand them in a new light, for example, Patient B. said 'I was afraid of being a nuisance last night if I went and asked what was causing all the commotion.' Patient A. answers 'Yes, fear of being rejected and being misunderstood probably held me back too. That often happens to me.' Thirdly, patients can share information with each other and the therapist. What is *exchanged* on an equal footing between the patients is often easier to accept than from a professional, for example hearing another patient recommend a medication can be far more powerful than hearing a doctor recommend it.

Kibel groups

Howard Kibel, an American psychiatrist, developed a specific form of group therapy for psychiatric inpatients (Kibel 1981, 1987a, 1993). In the beginning of the '90s, Kibel was invited to Denmark by a group of psychiatrists interested in psychotherapy in order to conduct a psychotherapeutic seminar and lecture on the principles of inpatient group psychotherapy. His visit created considerable professional interest. He has since visited Denmark several times and has conducted numerous courses. At one stage, junior Danish psychiatrists were taught a qualifying course on the principles of group psychotherapy mapped out by Kibel. Supervised participation as a co-therapist in such a group will also be accredited as part of the psychotherapeutic qualification of psychiatric training. Kibel's approach has been adopted in a number of Danish acute psychiatric wards, where the therapy groups are referred to as 'Kibel groups' (Heinskou & Kristensen, 2002; Heinskou, 2007). At present there are Kibel groups on all the unlocked, acute psychiatric wards in the northern part of the Copenhagen Metropolitan Psychiatry (Nordsjælland, population 350,000) as well on several wards elsewhere in Denmark. Kibel's approach rests on the general principles of group psychotherapy with a number of additional characteristics. Kibel describes the impact on patients of joining the ward social structure. They are exposed to both helpful influences, and harmful or incomprehensible influences. These result from fellow patients, from the treatment milieu and from the wider hospital system. The Kibel group forms the place in the ward social structure where these anti-therapeutic experiences can be identified and dealt with. The group becomes an interface between the ward milieu and the intra-psychic experience of each patient.

The key features of the Kibel approach are:

1. An object relations and open systems theory approach.
2. A focus on parallels between what is taking place in the group and what is happening on the ward and wider hospital systems.
3. Nearly all patients are encouraged to attend.
4. The aims are to reduce maladaptive defence mechanisms and to strengthen the therapeutic alliance.
5. Staff learn how patients are responding to the ward milieu and this aids planning and treatment.

Theoretical foundations

The first theoretical basis of Kibel's approach is *object relations theory*. This refers to internal representations and images of other people ('objects') who are important and significant to us, built up in our minds during our childhood together with internal representations of ourselves. Significant people from our external worlds are represented as objects in our internal world, and we develop our own inner image of ourselves or self-representation (Kernberg, 1976). Early intra-psychic objects are initially poorly differentiated but as we grow and develop, self and object representations become more distinctive. An object relations perspective supplements the medical model by providing psychological explanations and a language to describe mental breakdowns. Patients' object relations and how these are related to their difficulties can be explored in the group with an emphasis on supporting and validating their experiences.

Kibel (1981) describes how the core of the ego is made up of self and object representations, and how prior to psychotic breakdowns, patients with schizophrenia hold tenuous distinctions between the two. Like Kernberg, Kibel describes how a good constellation of self-objects functions as a secure base from which the individual can engage with the social world. When a patient starts to break down, in order to protect the constellation of good objects, aggressive parts of the self and its objects are split-off and denied. A psychotic breakdown can be understood as the dissolution of the connection between the self and its objects leading to a fragmented sense of self. To defend himself or herself against internal conflict, the person with psychosis projects the aggressive feelings onto the outside world. These projected aggressive objects are then experienced as paranoid and persecutory elements which exist in the environment. For instance, patients can experience other patients or staff as harbouring ill intent towards them and so may misinterpret what is being said as negative and persecutory. In the group we try to help patients disclose their perceptions of others, understand what leads to these paranoid states of mind, and attempt to contain these in order to calm the paranoid thinking.

With regard to borderline patients, Kernberg again describes a defect in the integrative capacity of the ego. As with the schizophrenic patients described above, there is a splitting of good and aggressive experiences in order to protect the ego. When the splitting between the good and the aggressive parts starts to break down, the ego is threatened by aggression, leading the individual to feel threatened and become extremely anxious. These considerations are in accordance with Melanie Klein's object relations theory and her description of the paranoid schizoid position (Klein, 1946). A split in the perception of the outside world accompanies the internal division between good and bad, with some aspects becoming idealised and others being denigrated. For instance, a patient complained about the lack of empathy from his key nurse and contrasted her with the kind and generous group therapists. Another patient devalued the ward whilst idealising a ward that she had stayed on previously. In the group we try to help patients achieve a more balanced and realistic view, whilst acknowledging that splitting is an important defence against instability, chaos, anxiety or paranoia. Being able to divide experiences into good and bad at least affords the borderline patient some sense of control.

Hospital treatment, including medication, may be understood as a means of reducing the destructive effects of patients' pathological reactions to external stress. The task in the group is to help patients regain their normal coping mechanisms. We do this by focussing on the stresses of life on the ward. This includes any perceived threats and anything that creates a sense of chaos. The primary therapeutic means are not trying to give patients insight into the psychological mechanisms of splitting and projection, but rather gaining a sense of belonging and support. The therapists use empathic understanding to contain and moderate patients' destructive and aggressive experiences. The group acts to detoxify these and help patients develop greater tolerance and understanding for internally and externally derived aggression, and to increase their self-esteem and self-respect in the face of their experiences. This will increase ego strength, particularly in the area of the observing ego, and it will improve reality testing.

The second theoretical basis of Kibel's approach is *open systems theory*. According to this, the hospital is a system containing hierarchically organised sub-systems. Sub-systems include the administration and clinical departments, individual wards and ward round meetings. Interfaces operate between sub-systems and between the system and the outside world. Resources and information move back and forth and up and down across interfaces or boundaries. The boundaries are permeable in the sense that the wider organisation affects patients on the wards and information and knowledge pass upwards as well. Knowledge about the patients, for instance, may be passed elsewhere in the wider system. The movement of information and impact of events are like rings on the surface of water. Because of this, events in the psychotherapeutic group often reflect dynamics in other parts of the hospital system. Carrying this further, each individual patient's mind is also a sub-system of the wider system. There is thus a dynamic interaction between individual patient's 'systems' and the group, the ward and organisation systems. For example, one patient's divided inner world of black-and-white understandings may cause a split in the staff group, which may in turn create splits elsewhere in the system.

Cultural influences operating in the system show themselves in language, the manner that people speak to and about each other, and the degree of tolerance and containment in relation to the pain and powerlessness caused by the patients' paranoid withdrawal, devaluation, aggression and splitting. Patients' intra-psychic worlds are affected by decisions made in the external system, and hence parallel processes are at work, whereby patterns of conflict are repeated in different sub-systems. The aim of group therapy is to bring together these fields of experience and to make them more comprehensible, so that the ward milieu becomes less mystifying and more meaningful, thereby reducing frustration and anger at what takes place.

As can be seen, the ward is a complex social system for patients to understand and adapt to at a time when they are already in difficulty. Not understanding how the system operates can lead patients to have unfulfilled expectations and experience staff as controlling or punitive and this can feed into existing tendencies. A common reaction is for many patients to withdraw, which can perpetuate their distorted perceptions. It can then become difficult to motivate patients to attend group therapy.

Example

A patient reports to the group that she has been told that she is soon to be discharged. She says that she wants to go home but does not feel well enough. She has told the doctor who has reassured her that the medication will soon clear up her symptoms but she does not know whether staff are competent enough to assess her properly. She did not want to come to the group today and did not have the energy to participate. Two other patients continue the theme of criticism towards treatment. The session is taking place after some regular staff members have been away for two days on training and have been replaced by substitutes. Unsurprisingly it emerges in the group that these absences have created insecurity and anger in many patients. With the help of the therapist, the patients voice their frustration, powerlessness, and sense of lack of control created by the changes. The group becomes calmer and the conversation turns to the difficulties making oneself understood when feeling low. One patient says that when she feels let down by the people who are important to her this makes her feel insecure and doubt everything and everyone.

This example shows how the group session is like a biopsy of the ward, reflecting events, the prevailing feelings and the atmosphere.

The group therapists often become the target of projections. They represent the institution, regardless of whether they carry out any other aspects of treatment and will at times represent both biological and psychological frames. It is therefore important that the group therapists point out such projections when they occur and thereby strengthen both relations with the ward and provides a realistic perspective of others plus a clearer understanding of the therapeutic boundaries, which may enhance the therapeutic alliance with the individual patients. Focusing on the significance of external factors underscores the weight that this approach places on both the patient's intra-psychic world and the organisation and culture of the institution.

Participants

Kibel recommends eight to twelve participants in the group sessions (Kibel, 1987b). If fewer than eight, then patients may find the group too demanding. Larger groups run the risk of individuality disappearing. Irrational large group processes also increase if there are more than about twelve (Turquet, 1974). In principle, as many patients from the ward as possible should participate and the group should form part of every individual's treatment plan. It is recommended that patients do not participate in the first 24 hours of their admission, to give them a chance to acclimatise to the ward and for the staff to assess any counter-indications for joining the group. Patients are also excluded if they would be unable to understand what goes on or stop the group operating as a therapeutic group. This applies to patients with cognitive disturbances such as severe dementia and those suffering from the after-effects of ECT, and patients behaving bizarrely who create severe anxiety in others. Patients who could be dangerous and patients who are severely self-mutilating would also be excluded. For most patients, however, participation is viewed as an integral part of treatment. In collaboration with the patient, the participation in the Kibel group is included with other elements of treatment in the treatment plan. The patient's key worker on the ward may also remind the patient to attend. Experience shows that most patients, often about three quarters of those admitted, are motivated to participate in the Kibel groups. This high rate of participation is dependent on the ward staff supporting this element of treatment, including refraining from scheduling other activities during the group sessions. Patients with severely psychotic thinking can participate and their inclusion facilitates greater understanding of their behaviour on the ward. If a patient is unsuited to the group, that patient's key worker is asked to talk to the patient during the group session to combat feelings of exclusion and neglect.

The therapist's tasks and knowledge about occurrences at the ward

One therapist usually leads the session, working with one or two co-therapists. The lead therapist should ideally be a regular staff member on the ward with psychotherapeutic group training, typically a senior psychologist. A doctor in psychiatric training can be a co-therapist, but usually the co-therapists should be members of the ward staff. This combination signifies to the patients that the group emphasises both psychotherapeutic qualities and the importance of the everyday therapeutic environment. The therapists take responsibility to ensure that the therapy room is ready with chairs placed in a circle around a small table. Start and end times are kept to. Groups are 45 or 60 minutes, at a designated time, held in the same room. The reliability of the frames helps contain anxiety. Originally Kibel recommended that this kind of group meet two to five times weekly. The greater the patient turnover, the more frequent the group meetings should occur, since many new and acute patients may contribute to creating an unstable atmosphere. In fact, the frequency of group meetings on Danish acute wards is twice weekly at the most, as the average admission is about 15-20 days. Due to lack of resources, several wards have reduced the group activity to once a week, making it difficult to ensure continuity and possibly carry on with topics from the previous group session.

The therapists find out about important events on the ward at the ward handover meeting before the group so they can be alert to the impact of events which may be mirrored in the group's behaviour and material.

Example

A patient says she is angry about having no say about what activities are provided on the ward. She gives the timing of meals as an example, and recounts that she raised this at the morning community meeting without getting a satisfying answer. The therapist says perhaps the important feeling is the wish to be able to have some sense of control over the environment. Another patient maintains that it would be better for everyone if the patients took over running the ward. There is laughter, and the therapist comments that it is probably difficult to be taken seriously with such radical calls for change. One patient says that she feels safe with the staff taking care of the planning and organisation of ward routines. Another says everything is at a standstill for him and he is pleased for other people to take responsibility as he has trouble enough taking charge of himself. The first patient says that she when she was hospitalised previously the staff were far less rigid with the rules and routines. The therapist asks the other patients who been hospitalised before whether they shared this view. None reply directly but one person says that he believes that it is important not to become to too dependent on the staff or to constantly fight against the rules and routines if you are to become more independent yourself. He said he was always overly dependent on his parents.

This example shows how the group allows patients to express their shared experiences in different ways. Individuals' thoughts are gathered into a whole, promoting a sense of security and a chance for reflection. After each session the therapists meet to debrief and discuss the group process and its themes. They convey significant themes to the wider staff group, ensuring the group remains integrated in the milieu. After this particular session the therapists fed back that the patients had discussed the wards rules at the staff meeting. Several staff members reflected that staff were thinking about guidelines, systems and rules being developed in connection with a planned hospital accreditation. The staff discussed how this could be affecting the patients and agreed that it should not impinge unnecessarily. They reflected that the patients' preoccupation with the rules could reflect a parallel process, which in this case could represent an unhelpful displacement from one situation to another.

Conducting the group

The therapists often sit next to anxious patients if they feel this would be reassuring (although some anxious patients prefer to sit away from the therapists). Special attention is paid to the importance of providing a calming, physical presence towards particularly uneasy, severely psychotic and anxious patients. The main therapist often starts the group by recalling the group task, which is to discuss experiences of the ward, of being admitted and of the treatment. Patients are reminded of the time-frame and are asked not to disclose any information with patients who are not present. The therapists explain that they will share relevant information and themes with other staff members. There follows a round of introductions, but without the patients being expected to give a detailed description of their problems. The therapists aim for a sense of security. Problems may be taken up, but an emotionally charged atmosphere is avoided and communications should not be critical or persecutory. The atmosphere should be friendly and accommodating, with the therapists helping give a sense of coherence to what the patients bring and show interest in each contribution. Patients can talk about others who are not present in the group, but the therapists focus the discussion on what participants felt in relation to these others. Any acting-out of aggression in the group should be dealt with firmly so that the group remains safe. It is the therapists' responsibility to provide containment. Conflicts and contradictions can be voiced but the therapists use their authority to interrupt verbal attacks and arguments when necessary.

The therapists need to be up-to-date on what has been happening on the ward that could be influencing the group, but first and foremost they listen closely to what the patients bring. Where possible they link this to occurrences on the ward. If the patients are reticent, the therapists may raise a topic or a significant event for discussion. Prolonged silences are unconstructive and tend to provoke anxiety which can aggravate symptoms. At times, the mere fact of the therapist commenting on a silence can reduce the tension. The therapists help patients start talking and may make links to topics raised earlier in the session or previous sessions. They try to help the talk flow freely and provide a safe environment for problems and dysfunctional aspects to be raised. The therapist must, as far as possible, facilitate a containing atmosphere within the group. This allows problem-solving without destructive aggravation from patients' projections. It is important to comment positively on mutual support between patients whilst at other times acknowledging differences of views.

Kibel (2003) refers to 'clarifying interpretations' directed towards topics in the sessions that unconsciously or pre-consciously are reflecting dynamics of the milieu. The therapist helps patients create meaning out of what seems incomprehensible. Patients gain an increased tolerance of frustration, greater capacity for self-observation, and are able to carry out a communal reality-testing of what may be happening on the ward. Most therapeutic interventions are directed at the group as opposed to individuals, which promotes group cohesion.

Example

Several patients in a group on a locked ward talked about the noise and commotion which had kept them awake the previous night. They said that a patient not present had tried to barricade several ward exits. He had been gesticulating wildly and crying loudly that everyone should defend themselves as something terrible would happen because it was September 11th (anniversary of the New York twin towers attack). The therapist said he wondered whether others had also been afraid of something happening. Several patients said that they had indeed felt frightened and angry. One said that those who create terror should be smashed, as should 'biker types' he knew. The therapist said that it can be difficult to know what to do when you feel under attack, but that hostile feelings can come from inside, particularly if you are feeling bad. Another patient said that there is a big difference between feeling angry and aggressive and actually acting it out; 'If you first let go – then there is insecurity all the way through. And by the way, I feel more secure now about what happened last night, although I can understand his reactions'.

This shows how with the help of the therapist patients can work on distinguishing between what is coming from outside (terror, bikers, and other patients' reactions) and emotions originating in themselves. This theme was repeated for a long time in the group and as a result the ward atmosphere became gradually less tense. The distinction between 'me' and 'others' made it easier for patients to take responsibility for what they could increasingly recognise as their own feelings.

Group supervision

Therapists running groups with acute inpatients are under considerable pressures. Containing patients' fragmented communications and communicating these back to the patients in a thoughtful, benign manner requires flexibility and personal resources. At the same time, the therapists have to hold in mind what is happening in the staff group. They can provide other staff with insight into how the patients' psychopathology is playing out on the ward, and this allows other staff to think about the unhelpful aspects of their interactions with patients as revealed in the group. If patients, for instance, believe that some members of staff are uncaring, and the therapists believe this has some basis in reality and is the result of staff fatigue, they must think carefully about how to convey this to the staff group. For these reasons, on-going supervision is essential. The therapists are under pressure from both the patients and the surrounding system and supervision enables influences from each on the other to be considered. Patients' criticism may represent the projection of their inner conflicts onto the ward (eg splitting) but may also have a reality base. Supervision is concerned with finding meaning and coherence between themes raised in the group and the situation on the ward. Supervision is a vehicle for identifying unhelpful dynamics operating on the ward. Most patients experience a loss of personal competency as a result of their breakdown. This and the associated feelings of loss will be projected onto the staff and the therapists. Devaluing is therefore common and will at times create despondency and demoralisation in the group. This can be unpicked in supervision. An experienced group supervisor can supervise several group therapists in a monthly or preferably weekly supervision group. Weekly supervision makes the group therapy more prominent within the curative work of the ward.

Milieu reflection

The therapists attempt to bring the experiential spheres of the ward together to create a coherent, meaningful whole and counter the forces of fragmentation, frustration and aggression. The knowledge obtained in the Kibel groups can be used as a focus for the monthly staff meetings. All treatment staff join these 'milieu reflections' and it is a chance for everyone speak their minds. Staff consider the extent to which themes from the Kibel groups mirror issues in the staff group and milieu, as the following example illustrates:

Example

Several patients in the group said that they were mainly staying in their bedrooms because the nurses were stressed all the time. At the milieu reflection meeting several people said that their workload had become unusually heavy. Individuals were trying to cope with this in their own way but generally people had not realised the impact on patients. This led to a discussion about best how to deal with the increased work demands without passing the pressure on to the patients.

In another Kibel group several patients said that their admission was a waste of time with little opportunity to do anything remotely inspiring. In the milieu reflection staff commented on how difficult it was to initiate anything new because of the bureaucratic demands for everything to be approved by the hospital management. The staff group went on to consider whether decision-making processes could be improved.

Conclusion

Kibel groups can be at the heart of a ward's social structure. First and foremost they are a tool for investigating and helping patients express their experiences and conflicts. During group sessions important themes and psychological problems emerge, and to the extent that these reflect individual versus systemic issues can be clarified. Patients' reflective capacity is increased. Kibel groups form a meeting place where psychological influences from the different parts of the systems can be considered. Through a group dialogue and by reflections in the ward system, unhealthy patterns of relating can be discussed and thereby reduced within the therapeutic milieu.

References

Foulkes, S.H. (1964) *Therapeutic Group Analysis*. London: Allen & Unwin.

Heinskou, T. and Kristensen, J. (2002) Gruppeterapi med Døgnindlagte Patienter ad Modum Kibel. *Matrix, Nordisk Tidsskrift for Psykoterapi*, 19,2, 131-148.

Heinskou, T. (2007) Den miljøterapeutiske samtalegruppe. In : Schjødt, T. and Heinskou T. (eds.). *Miljøterapi – På Dynamisk Grundlag*. København: Reitzel, 108 -121.

Kernberg, O. (1976) *Toward an Integrative Theory of Hospital Treatment in Object Relations Theory and Clinical Psychoanalysis*. New York: Jason Aronson, 241-275.

Kennard, D. (2004) The therapeutic community as an adaptable treatment modality across different settings. *Psychiatric Quarterly*, 75, 3, 295-307

Kibel, H.D. (1981) A conceptual model for short-term inpatient group psychotherapy. *American Journal of Psychiatry* 138, 1, 74-80.

Kibel, H.D. (1987a) Contributions of the group psychotherapist to education on the psychiatric unit: teaching through group dynamics. *International Journal of Group Psychotherapy*, 37, 1, 3-28.

Kibel, H.D. (1987b) Inpatient group psychotherapy - where treatment philosophies converge. In R. Langs (ed). *Yearbook of Psychoanalysis and Psychotherapy*, 2, 94-116.

Kibel, H.D. (1993) Group psychotherapy. In E.Leibenluft, A. Taman and S.A. Green (Eds.),

Less Time to do More - Psychotherapy on the Short-Term Inpatient Unit. New York: American Psychiatric Press: 89-109.

Kibel, H.D. (2003) Interpretive work in milieu groups. *International Journal of Group Psychotherapy*, 53, 303-330.

Klein, M. (1946) Notes on some schizoid mechanisms. In: Riviere J. (ed.). *Developments in Psycho- Analysis*. London: Hogarth Press,1952 : 292-320

Turquet, P. (1974) Leadership: the individual and the group. In: Colman A.D and Geller M.H. (Eds.). *Group Relations Reader 2*. Washington: AK Rice Institute: 71-87.

15

A psychodynamic inpatient group

Jonathan Radcliffe and Debora Diamond

Introduction

This chapter describes a weekly one-hour psychodynamically informed therapy group on an acute ward, based on work at Lewisham Hospital, London. We describe the aims and principles, the group structure, different levels operating in the group, and some psychodynamic formulations of patients' problems. We give examples and there is a transcript of a session in the appendix following the chapter.

Outpatient psychodynamic group therapy is time-limited or slow-open but the membership is continuous. The acute inpatient group is based on psychodynamic principles and techniques but group membership is rarely the same from one week to the next. Many patients attend only once whilst others come for several weeks or even months. In common with other forms of dynamic therapy (Gabbard, 2004), the aims are to help patients express their feelings within a supportive space and to increase their insight through interpretations. Support of expression is always present in our group and we aim to offer some interpretation though this varies. Some writers suggest that acutely disturbed patients are suited to supportive expression only and should not be encouraged to experience feelings that are too upsetting. Our view is that the disturbing feelings pushed out of mind are the very thing causing the problems.

The unconscious consists of ideas, wishes, memories pushed out of mind, and those that may have never been conscious, for example pre-verbal childhood experiences. Many of the choices we make are affected by our unconscious. This can be seen in problems at work, choice of partners, tendencies to get into the same kind of relationship difficulties; all areas of life in fact. People bring their experiences into the group, where their unconscious feelings can be understood from their behaviour and what they say. Patients can benefit from interpretations of their unconscious feelings if these are carried out skilfully in a supportive environment. When unconscious feelings are given expression and helped to enter conscious awareness this can provide some relief. The psychodynamic view is that tackling the symptoms, for example with medication, without examining the underlying causes of the distress will lead the problems to come out in some other way.

At a conscious level patients do not fully understand why they have broken down. They may have partial awareness of the impact of precipitating factors and ongoing stresses or there may be little or no awareness. Because of extremes of distress, they have pushed from their mind the painful or anxiety provoking feelings. These unconscious feelings find expression in the symptoms, which have become so severe that they prevent independent functioning. Many patients pass through hospital without anyone understanding fully what has gone wrong and why. In the group we aim to discover the link between symptoms, and the unconscious feelings and conflicts that are causing them. Together with one-to-one assessments and therapy, and supportive relationships with staff and other patients, psychodynamic groups are an opportunity to explore problems and this can increase the team's understanding of the patient.

Reasons for breakdown vary widely. An interaction between each patient's psychopathology and their predicament has pushed them over the edge. The aim is to help patients to reconnect with the disturbing feelings by engaging with other patients and staff in a safe, containing space. Expressing hitherto unexpressed feelings may make patients feel worse in the short-term. However, if the feelings can be sustained and some understanding gained, this may reduce symptoms, lead to greater integration and aid the re-establishment of more adaptive defences. This can be seen in the group when patients who are thought-disordered or largely mute are able to engage and communicate far more than they have been doing on the ward, often to the surprise of staff who know them.

In order to allow unconscious conflicts to emerge, the therapists do not determine the content of discussion. Instead patients are encouraged to talk about whatever comes into their minds and respond freely to each other, which is the equivalent of free association, one of the hallmarks of psychodynamic therapy. Spontaneous content and interactions reflect both conscious and unconscious processes, which can be reflected upon. Working in this way can itself create anxiety especially in new patients who may feel exposed. The therapists need to create and maintain a space that is safe whilst at the same time not structuring the time so much that spontaneous material and interactions cannot take place. The approach requires therapists to tolerate uncertainty and their own anxieties. It can help to remember that simply getting people talking and engaging together for an hour is an achievement and anything more is a bonus. The success of the group depends on the patients as well as the therapists.

The group is open to all patients willing to come, apart from the most acutely disturbed or those who are very likely to abscond whilst off the ward. Running a mixed group can help patients tolerate each others' chaos and can foster a sense of community between those who come.

Structure

Membership

We occasionally hold the group with one patient and have had as many as 12, but the norm is 3-6. There are usually two therapists. The nurse attending the group provides an invaluable bridge between group and ward, communicating information between one and the other. Junior doctors are also a great asset in working as co-worker or observer if they have an interest in this kind of work as they have useful background information and are in touch with all aspects of patients' care.

Preparation

The group needs to become established in the minds of staff and patients. A working alliance with ward nurses is especially important. One of the therapists goes to the ward twenty minutes before the session to identify the nurse co-worker. Nurses and doctors are often familiar with patients' histories and backgrounds, which are of great help to those running the group.

Recruitment

Nurses who patients like are best placed to encourage them to attend. They need to find the right tone of expectation and encouragement. The therapist provides back up. We work hard to keep to the start-time as far as possible. Patients can come up to 10 minutes late if they are not ready but no later.

The room

The room should be quiet and interruption-free. There are pros and cons for holding the group off the ward. The advantage is a more protected space and calmer atmosphere and is our preference. Working on the ward makes the group more visible and contiguous with the ward, but because it is easier for patients to walk out and return it can be less contained and containing.

Observers

We are fortunate in having a family therapy room so one or two observers can watch from behind the one-way screen if the patients are happy with this. Observers come out to say hello at the start of the group and often return for the feedback at the end. Otherwise an observer sits-in on the group. Three patients is our minimum for three non-patients present in the room (therapist, nurse, and co-therapist). Watching a session and working as co-therapist are good learning experiences and observers contribute to the sense of a therapeutic team.

The session

The therapists explain that the group happens every week at the same time and it is a chance for patients to talk about their experiences and think about them together. They are asked not to share each others' personal information with others outside the group. We have found that patients respect this. People introduce themselves. A spontaneous discussion may then start, but in any case the therapist makes sure that each patient finds their voice, for example saying what is on their mind or how they have been finding the ward. This typically takes 15 -20 minutes. There follows a freer period when the therapists encourage discussion. Groups will vary as to how much patients are able to interact with each other as opposed to listening to each in turn engaging with the therapists. The therapists draw out themes, clarify, comment and make interpretations. It is a fine line between offering helpful insights and trying to have all the answers, which can reinforce dependency, however an active stance is needed. Nurses are encouraged to contribute and not worry about saying the wrong thing. Faith in the process is needed. It is also not unusual for a patient to ask to leave; we encourage them to stay and say what is bothering them. At the end the therapists invite each person to say something on the session before summing up, giving positive feedback and encouraging participants to come back the following week.

Debrief

Therapists and observers discuss the group and decide what can be shared with other ward staff. The nurse co-worker then writes the names of attendees in the ward diary to attend the following week. One of the group therapists writes a brief paragraph on each patient in their notes omitting any personal information that we judge that they would not wish to be shared more widely. If a patient has had a difficult group for example walking out, we discuss how this can be followed up after – for example the nurse will speak to them individually about what happened, how they felt about it, give them positive feedback and encourage them to try again the next week.

Continuity

The group includes patients who attend once only, patients who come every week, and patients who come back to the group after attending on previous admissions. Each session should be of value to one-off attenders, but it will be of more value to those who come more often. The therapists learn more about patients over time, the therapeutic alliance deepens, and patients carry forward their memory of earlier groups and the group culture. A proportion of patients also return to the group on successive admissions in some cases over periods of several years and are held in mind by the therapist.

Levels of focus

The content of discussion and the interactions within a ward group can be complex and confusing. A number of therapists (e.g. Rice & Rutan, 1987) have written about different levels operating:

- the individual patient: personality, experiences and psychopathology
- the interactions that occur between patients and between patients and therapists
- whole group processes
- the ward and hospital
- wider society

The emphasis on different levels of focus will vary according to the type of group therapy. In our group there is an element of conducting individual therapy with patients in turn: (1), in order to engage and help patients share something of themselves and their circumstances. This alternates with interactions between patients with the therapist as group conductor (2), facilitating, clarifying, and making intrapsychic and interpersonal interpretations and occasionally group-level interpretations. There is an equal emphasis on patients engaging with each other, and voicing anxieties relating to their situation and why they are in hospital. Flexibility of style is needed. A therapist may comment on whole group process (3), for example commenting on themes at the end of the group. Patients sometimes discuss what has happened on the ward such as thefts or upsetting incidents (4). Patients occasionally express concerns about social stigma of mental illness (5), and naturally their lives outside hospital. Further reading on object relations and systemic thinking of this type can be found in Brabender and Fallon (1993).

Psychodynamics

Data used to make hypotheses about unconscious processes are gathered from observing patients in the group as well as from nurses, doctors, electronic patient files, ward-rounds and in some cases from individual work with patients. Malan's triangles are a classic way of conceptualising psychodynamic defences, unconscious feelings, and the anxiety associated with allowing the unconscious feelings expression (Malan, 1995). The examples used in this chapter are retrospective summaries of group sessions that show how the group can be used to bring hitherto unexpressed feelings to the fore.

Example

Samantha was suffering from anxiety but otherwise was totally passive and devoid of discernable feeling. When asked why she was in hospital she said that her son was repeatedly becoming violent and intimidating when drunk and she could do nothing about it. When pressed how she felt about this Samantha said that she was angry. However, instead of expressing her anger she started weeping. In the same session, Frank, a manic patient, raised the death of his father and that of an older sibling before he was born. He spoke about this in a non-stop, matter-of-fact way, later becoming angry, swearing and describing violent feelings towards his step-son. It was pointed out that Samantha was unable to experience anger whilst Frank was unable to let himself become sad.

Each of these two patients became anxious when the normally repressed feelings were fleetingly experienced. Davanloo very clearly describes the way repressed feelings are defended against. Some techniques from his intensive short-term dynamic therapy can be used in the group, for example asking patients how they are feeling and pointing out how they evade the difficult feelings, although not as intensely as in Davanloo's method (Davanloo, 2000; Coughlin Della Selva, 1996). Malan and Davanloo describe exploring hidden feelings in relation to the here-and-now of what is going on in the room, relationships in the patient's life, and early formative relationships. Sadness and anger are often evaded because of early childhood experiences. Unconscious feelings are also expressed behaviourally outside the group and in the group.

Example

Rosa absconded from the ward twice and rang the police who brought her back. She frequently had to be called back on the way to the group, and in the session often started walking out. She always responded to being asked to stay. The therapists felt this expressed both her conscious feeling that she should be at home looking after her children as well as her unconscious wish to be wanted. The therapist commented that Rosa had mixed feelings about being in hospital; on the one hand she wants to go home and look after her children; on the other hand she knows that she is unwell and wants to stay here with people who care about her. This conflict was also expressed in Rosa's preoccupation with her house and garden. After putting two and two together, the therapist suggested that the real anxieties were not the hole in her roof and the grass growing too long, but whether the hole that was her psychosis could be mended and her concern that her children were growing up without her. Her response was non-committal. However at the end of the session she said uncharacteristically that her husband was doing a good job with the children. Having previously attacked and criticised him this represented a shift in the direction of a more realistic perception of reality.

Rosa's hidden feelings were of wanting to remain in hospital, which clashed with her strong wish to be with her children and the associated guilt about abandoning them. Her anxiety about whether she would be able to manage as a single mother with schizophrenia was expressed in her preoccupation with the hole in the roof. Her mixed feelings about wanting to be in hospital and wanting to be at home were divided between herself and staff – she ostensibly wanted to go, whilst the staff wanted her to stay, and this was constantly acted out behaviourally. Putting some of these dynamics into words helped reduce Rosa's need to enact them. Being committed to the group and forming a therapeutic alliance was an excellent indicator for individual work for which she was referred on to and which she used well.

Another patient in these sessions had also had a psychotic episode, which she also blamed on her husband. During Rosa's description of her hatred of her husband this patient listened intently. She felt similarly furious with her husband but was resistant to talking about any difficult feelings, and often stood up and went to stand near to the wall. Both women were able to express anger and hatred, but found it more difficult expressing sadness and loss. In the case of the second patient this included a recent bereavement, her daughter leaving home, hitting age 60 and the prospect of retiring from her much loved job and spending more time with her demanding husband. She was offered follow-up couple therapy as a result of the group.

Early experiences, containment and projective identification

The psychodynamic approach emphasises the continuity of human experience from infancy through childhood and adolescence to adulthood. Later problems are seen as reflecting developmental difficulties, which have created vulnerability to later problems, which especially occur when there are difficult developmental tasks and transitions, or in the context of losses or conflicts. Psychotic patients are seen as having experienced significant early developmental problems that have left them especially vulnerable. Bion (1959; 1962) describes the immature mind of the baby lacking the capacity to process fear, neediness, pain, hatred, hunger and so on, and the baby projecting these experiences into the mother's mind, for example by crying. The mother allows herself to experience the disturbance, processes it and then offers containment, thereby transforming the experience into something that can be borne or understood. This is one of the functions of the group leader and the group for the distressed members attending. Bion (1961) also describes how certain types of groups have tendencies to become highly dependent and impose pressures on group leaders to provide all the answers. Bion emphasises the importance of not doing this; by being open to the projected feelings and sustaining uncomfortable states of uncertainty, thinking becomes possible.

Institutional and individual defences may make staff less receptive to disturbing projections (Menzies-Lyth, 1979). The therapist must sustain interest and curiosity in patients but must also be able to be disturbed by their projections and those of nursing staff and process some of these projections and the feelings they stir up. If a reflective stance can be maintained it may be possible for patients to think about hard-to-bear experiences and to adopt interest in the contents of their own minds instead of trying to get rid of them. The group offers a starting point for processing of unconscious emotions when projections are accepted and fed back to the patient in digestible form.

Example

Melissa, in her second group session, started crying as she revealed that her fiancé had told her last night that he wanted to end their relationship. Ade said 'Do not cry, be cheerful!' Stephen said 'look to the future, you are a beautiful girl, you will easily get a new boyfriend.'

The therapist said 'It's good to be able to cry when there is a loss' (losing his reflective stance and becoming directive). The other therapist asked Melissa how she was feeling and said 'that must be very painful'. At that point Melissa was able to access painful feelings of loss and seek support.

The first therapist, regaining a more therapeutic stance, asked Ade whether he has ever felt like crying. Ade said 'Christ told me, do not cry'. He explained that he came to this country after his wife died. After her death he cried for two days but Christ told him to stop because he is a man. He had continued to cry, but inside his head.

It seems that Melissa touched a raw nerve in Ade, putting him in touch with feelings that he would rather not experience. Ade went on to explain that he left his two children in Africa and came to the UK to earn money to send home, but he could not manage to get a job, which made him feel very bad. Ade too has been able to expressing painful feelings that had so disturbed him instead of suppressing them.

At this point, Stephen berated Ade for letting his children down. The therapist, remembering a previous session, asked Stephen about his own parents. He said that his parents did not deserve to be called 'parents'. When he was five his mother broke many sticks beating him. His grandmother took over raising him and did a good job. The second therapist suggested that perhaps Stephen's comments to Melissa to leave the past behind and look to the future reflected his way of dealing with his painful experiences from childhood and this was perhaps why he felt annoyed with Ade for letting his own children down. Stephen was clearly in touch with anger towards his parents. However, given his recent violent behaviour in hospital it seemed likely that he was not in touch with the associated violent rage, which had to be acted out towards innocent nurses. Beneath the displaced violent feelings were unconscious feelings of sadness and vulnerability at the damage he had sustained.

The discussion returned to Melissa, who said that she often felt mistreated. The therapist asked: 'Did you feel betrayed or let down by your boyfriend - did you feel angry with him?' Melissa did not respond, leading the therapists to believe that she was defending herself against feeling angry with her boyfriend and was directing it elsewhere, perhaps using the defence of attacking herself (described by Freud, 1917). Later, Melissa talked about her experiences of her grandmother's death and her mother's manic-depressive breakdown. She did not mention the experience of her rock like father becoming depressed which emerged in a different context. In a subsequent group Melissa became so angry with the therapist that she managed to undermine his ability to conduct the group.

This group shows the interplay that can take place between patients if they engage with the group process. Stephen and Ade could not cope with the discomfort of hearing Melissa talk of her sadness and despair, because each had been warding such feelings off themselves. These patients each contributed different feelings; Melissa and Ade had each lost a partner; Ade had also in effect abandoned his bereaved children. Stephen had been abused and rejected by his parents. The group became a container for feelings of sadness, loss, betrayal and victimisation that were present in patients' conscious and unconscious minds. The intermingling of different tasks can be conceptualised in terms of patients projecting different parts of themselves into each other, such as the sad helpless parts (projected by Alan into Melissa), or the useless neglectful part (projected by Stephen into Ade), or the resourceful capableness (projected by Alan into the therapist). There is no space to go into this in more detail, but the reader may be interested to read Hinshelwood (1987) for a further description of this phenomenon in groups.

Psychodynamic formulations of common psychiatric presentations

Psychoanalytic theories of unconscious feelings and defences against them can be used to explain different types of mental health problems. There follows a description of four commonly found presentations to illustrate psychodynamic formulations.

Psychotic delusions

The gap between reality and delusion reflects an especially unmanageable conflict causing the sacrifice of an element of reality. The approach here is to examine the content of the delusional beliefs and relate them to the patient's life experiences. Delusional beliefs can represent the fantasied fulfilment of a wish that becomes a substitute for a reality that is too painful to bear. This can be clearly seen in the case of grandiose fantasies that are a substitute for feelings of low self esteem, powerlessness and often anger.

Example

Alice was a Caribbean woman in her 60s who said she was Jewish, Scottish, had a special relationship with Cliff Richard and was due to have tea with the Queen. She came to several sessions and at the beginning mainly listened. When she did speak, her strong accent made her difficult to understand and her relentless delivery led group members to stop listening. The therapists eventually noticed how little Alice had said about herself and invited her to say more. She then described a history of early deprivation and trauma including the murder of her father. She was now living on her own after decades working to support her family as a cleaner. Her husband had left her and her daughters were busy with their own families. A stark contrast was apparent between Alice's delusions of what she perceived as being high-status races and mixing with admired celebrities, and an internal reality of feeling unwanted after years of hard work. This point was gently made over several sessions. This, together with the value placed on her contributions in the group led to an improvement in her interactions in the group.

Alice's earlier relentless delivery caused people to disregard and sideline her, repeating the very experiences that were disturbing her (Freud, 1914). Rather than feeling annoyed when her symptoms were interpreted, Alice made an emotional connection to the underlying feelings. Patients do not always respond so well. Such interpretations work when patients are well enough to access internal resources and form a therapeutic alliance.

Paranoia

Cognitive approaches treat paranoia as distorted perceptions based on faulty schemas and misattributions of internal emotional states onto external phenomenon. In contrast, the psychoanalytic view is that the forces of persecution originate in aggressive parts of the personality. This aggression causes excessive anxiety and guilt and so is split-off and projected onto others who are experienced as the aggressive ones (Freud, 1896, pp 174-185). The patient usually cannot tolerate their aggressive impulses because of excessive guilt. By getting rid of the feelings the person becomes guilt-free but they are then at the mercy of the imagined persecutors. Helping the patient reality-test can be used at times, for example other patients reassuring them that they mean them no harm. However, exploring the internal source of the projected angry feelings is potentially more useful. The patient is encouraged to describe current relationships and may be asked for historical information. Detective work and intuition are needed to track down disowned feelings. If the therapists and other patients can successfully encourage the patient to express and experience the anger they have been avoiding then the paranoia will often reduce.

Example

Michael was passive and compliant. He had been admitted after climbing onto the roof and throwing tiles at people. He believed people were spreading rumours that he was a paedophile, which made him angry and anxious. The therapists were aware from ward nurses that Michael's wife was divorcing him and planning to make him leave, and asked Michael about his relationship with his wife. Michael denied any anger towards her. Instead, his anger was directed towards the vindictive, threatening people who were out to get him. In this case, our formulation was that Michael was denying his angry attacking feelings towards his wife, and projecting an attacking aggressive part of himself onto the environment, creating sinister forces that then frightened him. We asked Michael to tell us about his background. Michael described an unhappy childhood during which he was brutally beaten by his stepfather whilst his passive and depressed mother looked on.

Michael took to walking out of hospital and going home. His wife would phone the hospital or police to take him back, repeating the painful rejection. He learned from the nurses that she wanted him to leave. Michael's feelings of wanting to be with his family and feeling unwanted and rejected were repeated each time he went home, resulting in him remaining under section and not facing up to the reality that his marriage was over. Being ill was preferable to the pain of rejection by his wife and his consequent homelessness. Michael attended several groups and was able to see links between his early experiences of violence in his family and his paranoia that others wanted to kill him. Over the course of time, he came to acknowledge that he was angry with his wife although he never acknowledged the extent of his despair about the ending of his marriage in the group.

Melancholic depression

According to Freud (1917, p244), mourning and melancholia share some important common features, including a profoundly painful dejection, cessation of interest in the outside world, loss of the capacity to love and inhibition of activity. The feature that sets melancholia apart from mourning is extremely low self-regard connected with attacks on the self. This takes the form of self-reproach and self-reviling, and culminates in a delusional expectation of punishment. In extremis this can cause suicidality or psychotic voices criticising and attacking the self. Freud explains this type of depression as being caused by a significant loss of a loved person or ambition. The depressed person identifies with the lost person or ideal self and then attacks the part of this identified self. Although this attack is directed at the self, the hidden aspect is an attack on the lost object, which is identified with, as a way holding onto it. Unconscious hostility toward the lost object prevents the person from carrying out mourning which is the essential work of dealing with loss. In the group, as a step in the direction of dealing with the loss we attempt to establish the source of the loss, and encourage the expression of the full range of feelings including sadness and anger or rage.

Example

Stephanie was a 52-year-old woman whose husband had died a few months before her admission to the ward. He had been an alcoholic for all of the 18 years they were together and he had attacked Stephanie several times resulting in hospitalisation. Despite this, Stephanie chose to stay in the relationship even though this meant that her three children refused to speak to her. They had tried for many years to get her to leave her husband, who was not their father, but each time she went back. Finally, they refused to have anything to do with her. Stephanie came onto the ward following a suicide attempt. In the group she presented as low in mood and self-effacing.

Stephanie: (head bowed, speaking in a whisper) If people knew what I'm really like they wouldn't want anything to do with me. Even my own children won't talk to me.

John: I think you're a really nice person Stephanie. You've always got time for me when I need someone to talk to.

Malcolm: You're a good person Stephanie but I think you've been through a lot. Your husband (hesitates)…what sort of man beats up a woman?

Stephanie: He couldn't help it, alcoholism is an illness, he couldn't stop drinking. What would he have had if I'd left him?

Therapist: Stephanie, it sounds like other people are angry at your husband on your behalf. Do you think maybe you should be the angry one?

John, Malcolm and Katrina: Yeah, that's right (nodding their heads in agreement).

Stephanie attended the group for eight consecutive weeks and she eventually did express her anger towards her husband. It had been difficult for Stephanie to mourn the loss of her husband because of the rage she felt towards him when he was alive and her wish that he would die. In the group, Stephanie also spoke about her childhood when she was beaten by her father and ignored by her mother. The group members helped Stephanie to see a link with her adult life and to challenge her perception that she was worthless. On discharge from the ward, Stephanie resolved to try to make amends with her children.

Mania

Mania is seen as a defence against sadness and loss (Abraham, 1911; Freud, 1917). Manic patients are especially challenging in the group as if not handled firmly they can dominate with a non-stop flow of talk and emotion designed to prevent them from becoming depressed.

Example

Deirdre, now in her 40s, had regular admissions since her late teens and worked on the unit in a service-user role when she was well. She knew the therapist in this capacity. Upon speaking to him early in her admission, she erroneously informed the ward manager and deputy that his wife was expecting another baby, and she would organise a card for him. In the first group, as though anticipating problems, Deirdre went to sleep and remained asleep until the last five minutes when she exploded into life, storming out when she was not allowed to take over. In two subsequent sessions she unleashed a stream of talk about herself and her life, then attempting to act as co-therapist by instructing the other patients how to solve their problems. On both occasions she left after furious outbursts when the therapist did not let her dominate. She managed with some difficulty to remain throughout the fourth session after being told three times that if she did not stop talking she would have to leave.

The therapist and nurse had powerful counter-transference reactions towards Deirdre but despite their reservations invited her to successive sessions. Her body language showed she wanted to come but knew that she might not be wanted. She would often apologise after sessions. In the fifth session the therapist tackled some of these dynamics near the start of the session, commenting on how angry Deirdre became towards him in previous sessions and asking her what she thought the triggers were, which she found hard to a answer. The nurse present also gave some helpful direct feedback, namely that Deirdre wanted to express her feelings but that if others wanted to talk they had to speak over her and push in. The therapist had pointed out that Deirdre wanted to help others but found it hard accepting help herself. She accepted this, and she was encouraged to focus on these aspects in the session. Deirdre wanted to complain about the behaviour of others outside the group (staff) and medication, and blame them for her problems, but was redirected back to the group. On this occasion Deirdre became more integrated and was able to make helpful contributions towards others. She was especially stirred up by a woman who expressed no feelings about the death of her boyfriend. Deirdre became suddenly tearful saying 'how can you sit there and claim to love someone you've lost and not be upset or sad about it in any way? You must be a hard woman; I could never do that, never'. Deirdre later spoke about her former boyfriend who she still loves, but who now lives with another woman. She herself lives quietly in a flat, guarded by an elderly white couple who live downstairs. She also spoke of being raped, a vivid instance of people 'pushing in' to her, as happened in the group when she did not allow people a gap to speak.

Deirdre appears in the transcribed session in the appendix following this chapter.

Conclusions

This type of group can help patients by giving them a better understanding of their own state of mind and thus have therapeutic value. It also helps staff present understand better what is going on. Anecdotal evidence suggests that once-weekly groups run by psychologists, psychiatrists or nurses are the most common type of psychodynamic group on UK adult acute wards but these have become less common in recent years (Robertson & Davison, 1997; Radcliffe & Smith, 2007). Groups run more often than once a week are rarer still. The psychodynamic approach is less at the forefront of individual psychological therapy in the NHS at the present where cognitive approaches have become the dominant and look set to become more so. However, psychodynamic psychotherapy and its insights have much to offer to the acute inpatient setting and need not be in competition with other approaches (Martindale, 2007). It is believed that the group described in this chapter can operate as a stand-alone group operating separately from the rest of the ward. However, it works best when integrated into the ward discussion of patients with ward staff and in ward rounds. In this sense it becomes part of the ward milieu. It can provide a valuable clinical collaboration between professionals of different disciplines as well as a good training experience for other interested staff members. Working with patients in the group enables the group leader to contribute more to the ward round discussion, and to use this to promote psychological explanations and formulations. The group gives access to the patients who want psychological therapy when insufficient individual time is available. It can be used to identify suitable patients for individual follow-up, and we have found that although this needs handling sensitively, can complement individual work running in parallel. The group does not provide a cure, but can form an important part of the service to inpatients and can make a significant difference for some.

References

Abraham, K. (1911) Notes on the Psycho-analytical Investigation and Treatment of Manic-depressive Insanity and Allied Conditions. In K. Abraham (1927) *Selected Papers on Psychoanalysis*. London: Hogarth.

Bion, W.R. (1959) Attacks on Linking. *International Journal of Psycho-Analysis*, 40:308-315.

Bion, W.R. (1961) *Experiences in Groups and other papers*. London: Tavistock.

Bion, W.R. (1962). *Learning from Experience*. London: Tavistock.

Brabender, V. and Fallon, A. (1993) The Object Relations/ Systems Model (chapter five).

In *Models of Inpatient Group Psychotherapy*. Washington DC: American Psychological Association.

Coughlin Della Selva, P. (1996) *Intensive Short-term Dynamic Psychotherapy: Theory and Technique*. New York: John Wiley

Davanloo, H. (2000) *Intensive Short-term Dynamic Psychotherapy: Selected Papers of Habib Davanloo*. Chichester: Wiley Blackwell.

Freud, S. (1896). Further Remarks on the Neuro-Psychoses of Defence. In *The Standard Edition of the Complete Psychological Works of Sigmund Freud, Volume III (1893-1899): Early Psycho-Analytic Publications*, 157-185, London: Hogarth.

Freud, S. (1914). Remembering, Repeating and Working-Through (Further Recommendations on the Technique of Psycho-Analysis II). In *The Standard Edition of the Complete Psychological Works of Sigmund Freud, Volume XII (1911-1913): The Case of Schreber, Papers on Technique and Other Works*, 145-156, London: Hogarth.

Freud, S. (1917). Mourning and Melancholia. In *The Standard Edition of the Complete Psychological Works of Sigmund Freud, Volume XIV (1914-1916): On the History of the Psycho-Analytic Movement, Papers on Metapsychology and Other Works*, 237-258, London: Hogarth.

Gabbard, G.O. (2004) *Long-term psychodynamic psychotherapy: A basic text*. Washington DC: American Psychiatric Publishing.

Hinshelwood, R.D. (1987) *What Happens in Groups: Psychoanalysis, the Individual and the Community*. London: Free Association

Malan, D.H. (1995) *Individual Psychotherapy and the Science of Psychodynamics*. Oxford: Butterworth-Heinemann.

Martindale, B.V. (2007) Psychodynamic contributions to early intervention in psychosis. *Advances in Psychiatric Treatment*, 13, 34-42.

Menzies Lyth, I. (1960) *The functioning of social systems as a defence against anxiety*. London: Tavistock Institute of Human Relations.

Radcliffe, J. and Smith, S. (2007) How do patients spend their time on acute psychiatric wards? An observational study of social interaction and audit of attendance at organised group activities. *Psychiatric Bulletin*, 31, 167-170.

Rice, C. and Rutan, J (1987) *Inpatient Group Psychotherapy: A Psychodynamic Perspective*. New York: MacMillan.

Robertson, S. and Davison, S. (1997) A survey of groups within a psychiatric hospital. *Psychoanalytic Psychotherapy*, 11, 2, 119-134.

Appendix: verbatim notes of a session

Present: therapist, observer, nurse, Deirdre, (46), Samantha (43), and Helen (55)

Helen has schizophrenia. Little is known about her on the ward, other than that she had been living on her own. When she became ill she moved into an empty flat, which she insisted was her own. Samantha has a diagnosis of personality disorder and suffers from acute panic attacks when out, when she believes she will have a heart attack. Deirdre's diagnosis is bipolar affective disorder. Each has attended the group two or three times.

Therapist	How are you Helen?
Helen	Getting better, it's good here. First class treatment and very good food. I'm really enjoying my stay. But I'm not being discharged yet.
Therapist	Why's that?
Helen	Well, the doctors think I still need treatment, but I don't.
Therapist	Have you appealed against their decision?
Helen	Yes – I want more time off the ward you see. I'm not complaining.
Therapist	And how do you feel about that?
Helen	Disappointed
Nurse	You do have some leave though.
Helen	Yes, I'm happy about that.
Therapist	And Deirdre – How are you?
Deirdre	I'm back on section. I put in a complaint against staff, but then we all have bad days.
Therapist	So you were brought into hospital on a section?
Deirdre	No, they promised I wouldn't be on a section but they lied and I was put straight on one.
Therapist	How do you feel about that?
Deirdre	I knew they would. It wasn't a surprise.
Therapist	Was it a blow?
Deirdre	No, I'm always on a section. I couldn't go home because of the lock situation. And I didn't try to kill myself, I had three hours of leave but I had too much to do, there were so many letters from all the voluntary organisations I do work for that I had to reply to.

Therapist	Why did they think you'd tried to kill yourself?
Deirdre	The police did, not the nurses. They broke into my house because I wasn't answering the door.

...

Therapist	I know Deirdre that sometimes you become very angry here and it often comes as a surprise when you do. What do you think the triggers are for your anger?
Deirdre	When I know my facts are not fiction. The tablets don't make the memories go away. Last week (in the group) brought them out [memories].
Therapist	What do I do that makes you angry?
Deirdre	You're a man Jonathan, you remind me of my husband. You're a mouse, not a man. Men make me angry because I was raped. Women didn't rape me, men did, so I only get angry with men.
Therapist	So it sometimes feels as if I am forcing myself upon you?
Deirdre	Yes. He [husband] controls my daughter which makes her angry, and that makes me angry too.
Therapist	Do any of the others in the group see anything that triggers Deirdre's anger? Can you look out for them today as well Deirdre?
Helen	She only gets a little bit angry.
Therapist	And why do you think that might be?
Helen	Well she's on the ward twenty-four seven.
Therapist	(nurse's name) - any thoughts on Deirdre's triggers?
Nurse	Sometimes when she feels that she hasn't had her say, or that she's not been listened to properly she can become angry.
Therapist	When people don't listen or hear her properly?
Nurse	Yes, when she speaks she needs to leave a pause so that people can respond to her, but she just wants to talk and express her feelings and when others want to talk they have to speak over her and push in.
Deirdre	People think it's because of my illness, they think that I don't talk the truth; I do, they just don't want to hear it because they think 'oh you're mentally ill, you must be lying' and they just won't believe us.
Therapist	Often, Deirdre, you want to give help to other people here in the group, but you find it hard to accept help.
Deirdre	I've always been like that.
Therapist	Perhaps that's one of your problems?
Deirdre	My 13-year old grandson says to me 'Nan, you need to put yourself first,

before other people'.

Therapist	And what does that mean in the group? Can you accept people gently challenging you and pointing things out to you that perhaps you've not thought of before? Maybe today you could focus on what it is that triggers you?
Deirdre	I'm angered by the mannerisms of the bank staff. They don't listen to you; they just slam doors and don't help.
Therapist	Yes, but let's try to keep it in the group. What is it in the group that triggers you?
Deirdre	The side-effects of my medication means...
Therapist	Maybe there are things you don't know are happening and we can try to focus on those today. Samantha – how are you?
Samantha	OK. I went home for the weekend. It was very bad. I was really anxious on Saturday. They increased my meds.
Therapist	What happened on Saturday?
Samantha	I felt like I was going mad, I had no control and it just got worse until Monday.
Therapist	This is the second time you've been home for the weekend?
Samantha	My son came home and when I got back to the ward I just lost it. I was pinned to the floor because I threw chairs around and they injected me with meds.
Nurse	They offered you some lorazepam but you declined it. You got very upset with a nurse who was offering you a cup of tea I think and you got really angry.
Samantha	I was angry because I was back there.
Therapist	Why did you get angry when the nurse made you a cup of tea?
Samantha	She was offering to make me some food and I can't eat at the moment because I'm so anxious and I just exploded.
Therapist	At the weekend, did something build up inside you and came out when you came back here? (She nods). What do you think was inside that exploded on the ward?
Samantha	I don't know.
Deirdre	With the illness it's twice as hard to be normal. Society doesn't accept us, and our kids don't accept us either.
Therapist	Would you like to put that to Samantha?
Deirdre	Our kids want a normal mum, but we are normal. Having a diagnosis that says I'm mad makes me really angry.

286

Samantha	My kids aren't like that, they don't talk to me like that. They worry about me [couldn't hear] … I got the cord from my dressing gown and I was measuring it up against the banisters but I stopped myself because I don't want my son to see me like that.
Therapist	Helen, what do you think about what Samantha's just been saying?
Helen	She's going through some sad times, but she's a nice person. She'll get better.
Therapist	Why did you think of hanging yourself?
Samantha	Because I can't take any more.
Deirdre	Your kids love you, Samantha, you need to live for your kids.
Samantha	They don't feel like my kids anymore. They seem like impostors.
Therapist	Why do they seem like impostors?
Samantha	I love them, but it doesn't feel real.
Therapist	Do you normally feel like this towards them?
Samantha	No, and I don't want them to see me like this
Therapist	It's awful for you to have them see you like this – what is 'this'?
Samantha	My diagnosis… the feelings just flooded through me in the morning
Therapist	The last time you went home you found out about your son's behaviour. Could you let the group know about that?
Samantha	It doesn't bother me any more, He got drunk and argued with people and threw a bin through a window and got arrested.
Therapist	And how did that make you feel?
Samantha	Angry, but now they're talking about sending him to prison
Therapist	Do you think they should?
Samantha	Yes.
Therapist	And why do you want that to happen?
Samantha	It's not that I want it to happen.
Therapist	But you think it should happen, why's that?
Samantha	For help. He needs help.
Therapist	He'd be forced to face up to the consequences of his actions – including the actions against you.
Deirdre	He might go into prison and come out worse.
Therapist	What do you think about Samantha wanting her son to go to prison?
Helen	Well, I think she's a fool. He's not been accused. I always believe people are innocent.

Deirdre	How old is he?
Samantha	Twenty-two.
Deirdre	Oh well then, he's big enough and ugly enough to look after himself. Don't you worry about him.
Therapist	Do you feel responsible in some way, Samantha?
Samantha	Yes, of course I do, I brought him up.
Therapist	And so you decided to punish yourself for this by hanging yourself. What is the link there? You punish yourself as a punishment for him?
Samantha	No, I just think I'm going mad.
Therapist	What is the link though?

[Deirdre interrupts. Can't hear what is said clearly]

Therapist	Helen?
Helen	Yes, well, I'm on the ward 24/7 and I just feel like people should mind their own business and leave me alone.
Therapist	You feel that others are wrong to pry and you don't want them to pry into your business, like we've just done with Samantha?
Helen	Yes, people I don't know should just stick to their own affairs.
Deirdre	They don't try to pry, they try to support you.
Helen	Well they shouldn't.
Observer	You don't want support?
Helen	No, it's not that, it just makes me all confused. It goes in the end. This hospital is very nice though.
Therapist	Helen, I see you looking at the clock a lot – why is that?
Helen	I just like to know the time.
Therapist	Are you looking to see how long is left in the group?
Helen	No, no I just like to know the time.
Therapist	What is striking about you Helen is how hard it is to get to know you. What is it about that?
Helen	It's just in my nature.
Therapist	It's hard to let people know you?
Helen	I did know a man once and had a relationship with him for four and a half years but he died in 2006
Deirdre	How did he die?
Helen	Natural causes.
Therapist	How old was he?

Helen	He was in his early 50's at the time.
Therapist	It's very rare for someone of that age to die of natural causes. What was his name?
Helen	I don't want to say.
Deirdre	How can you sit there and claim to love someone that you've lost and not be upset or sad about it in any way – how can you not be sad?! You must be a hard woman, I could never do that, never (crying).
Helen	Well, I'm not sure if he's dead. We sort of lost contact a bit before he died. He was of no fixed address. But you know, it just sort of goes quiet when someone dies, so I think he has.
Therapist	Do you go quiet when people die?
Helen	No, no it's not that. I don't want to say really.
Therapist	There seems to be a parallel with Samantha in how you deal with things. You both go quiet and try to get on as normal but find it hard to let yourself feel things.
Samantha	hmm.
Therapist	Samantha, what do you think of what Helen was saying?
Samantha	I think she's strange – she doesn't even know if he's dead. She needs to know if he's dead or just disappeared.
Therapist	I notice that you don't look at Helen when you're speaking about her, why is that?
Samantha	It's hard to, I've tried before and she doesn't respond.
Therapist	What would you like to say to her?
Samantha	Helen, you seem to be a loner, you don't have many friends.
Therapist	Helen, what Samantha said was that when she talks to you, you think you're being kind and friendly but she thinks you're blanking her, so there seems to be a gap between your perceptions. (Observer's name), can you cast any light on this?
Observer	Well it's quite common for people to have differing perceptions on things, which is why we have groups like this really, so that people can talk about how these are different and get feedback, whereas in normal life there are polite rules which stop this from being able to happen.
Therapist	Helen, do you feel upset by what Samantha said?
Helen	Yes.
Observer	It can be very hard to hear something like that.
Deirdre	But your body language is saying something very different.

Therapist	When you're upset, you can't tell because you keep it so under wraps, do you agree?
Helen	Yes.
Therapist	But you've chosen to come to the group again and to tell us about yourself. You've been very brave and done well. When people leave us we feel sad, but we can feel angry too. I don't get the feeling that you're very angry.
Observer	But he's dead, he hasn't left.
Therapist	But is he?
Observer	Perhaps she's killed him off in her mind.
Therapist	Helen, do you think you might have killed him off in your mind, perhaps because he committed a crime against you and so it's easier for you to kill him off than to accept that he's left you?
Helen	Yes.

Therapist rounds off group and each person says something about how they've found the group today (not transcribed).

Later we discover that the person Helen 'lost' was in fact a fantasied relationship with a newsreader she watched on TV.

16
Making connections:

Thoughts on the nature of thinking and relating with reference to people with severe psychotic difficulties

Jack Nathan

Introduction

This chapter aims to elaborate ideas developed over a number of years at the Maudsley Hospital, England. These ideas originally began through co-therapy in a mixed outpatient group with Wil Pennycook, a group analyst, and an inpatient group on an all-male acute ward with consultant psychiatrist, Dele Olajide. It is in these groups that I developed two interlinking theoretical perspectives as a way of thinking about this particularly demanding patient group. Each theoretical idea will be elaborated and woven into clinical vignettes from both groups. The first concept, 'the mentalisation hierarchy', is a development of the work by Fonagy and others on mentalisation (see Fonagy et. al. 2002). The second, I call 'psychic states of engagement' (PSE), a model for locating the levels at which patients with psychosis are able to emotionally engage with other people. These two constructs are profoundly interconnected since the mentalisation hierarchy addresses the patient's internal *intra-psychic experience*, whilst the PSE model focuses on interpersonal communication, *the inter-psychic ways of being with the other*. Through the use of these ideas I hope to demonstrate the part inpatient group therapy can play in working with patients who have the severest of psychotic illnesses. This is particularly timely as a Healthcare Commission Report (Department of Health, 2008) on inpatient care services recommends improving access to psychological therapy. As a reviewer of the report made clear, 'the best performing trusts were those that provided a therapeutic environment and engaged people in meaningful activities' (Wooster, 2008)

Attuning to the psychotic wavelength

From the start, we found the work of Michael Sinason (1993) particularly helpful, especially his notion of 'internal co-habitation'. This concept emphasises the immutability and ever-presence of 'the other mind' (the psychotic self) alongside the healthy self. Internal co-habitation is a mind-disturbing concept to conjure with as it takes seriously the idea of 'the co-habitation of two minds in one body'. Conceptually this is a key to our understanding of work with profoundly ill psychotic individuals. No philosophy of despair, where no change is possible, is involved. Indeed it will be shown that the opposite is the case since, like Sinason (1993), we work from the assumption that even when in its most acute and florid form, people with psychoses have what Dele Olajide refers to as, 'an oasis of sanity'. As Freud (1938) understood a long time ago when talking to patients after a psychotic breakdown: 'in some corner of their mind, there was a sane person hidden, who, like a detached spectator, watched the hubbub of illness go past him'. It was Bion (1967) who first distinguished between psychotic and non-psychotic parts of the personality. The psychotic part is so intolerant of frustration that it attempts to eliminate reality through pathological projections that result in hallucinations and persecutory delusions. Yet, Bion (1977) later went onto to suggest that there is a sane person within the self that the practitioner can address. Jackson (2008) understands this possibility by suggesting that the 'mind can operate at different levels at the same time or may regress so that earlier and less differentiated states of mental function predominate for shorter or longer periods'. In order to detail the way in which these 'different levels' of intra-psychic activity operate, I shall now present what I call, 'the mentalisation hierarchy', a development coming out of contemporary thinking on mentalisation.

The mentalisation hierarchy

Although mentalisation was originally described in the psychoanalytic literature in the late 1960s, the term has more recently been associated with the research on borderline personality disorders by Bateman and Fonagy (2004). It refers to a capacity to understand and think about both one's own and other people's mental states (thoughts, feelings and so on). It is essential for healthy adult functioning and provides a basis for affect regulation, impulse control and empathy. The mentalisation hierarchy (Nathan, 2008) is a development of this work, refining the concept into a hierarchy of three levels of mentalisation; rudimentary, simple and complex (see Box 1 for summary). These are the different levels at which patients with psychosis can reflect on their own as well as other people's experience. This hierarchy assumes a sane, differentiated self, the Adult Self, every individual carries within (Nathan, 2007). These ideas emerged from a group in which one member, Leone, had talked of hallucinating on a bus that people were being stabbed. We interpreted these experiences as symbolically meaningful, reflecting Leone's unconscious rage about the summer break. We suggested that she was angry, and was finding it too scary to let us know because she loves the group (and us), and instead had experienced these violent images of people 'out there' being stabbed. They reflected an expression of an emotional experience she could not allow herself. Leone nodded politely, apparently agreeing, but with encouragement acknowledged that she found this idea difficult to accept. Alongside our interpretations the group came up with helpful practical solutions, including one which 'simply' required her to get off the bus. In subsequent weeks Leone was able to do this.

Some months later in the group, Leone once more brought up the fact that she was having visual hallucinations, except on this occasion these took the form of her *being stabbed*. After asking for further clarification about what was happening and what she thought about these terrifying experiences, Leone spontaneously came up with the following, 'I don't know if it's got anything to do with the fact that I was not able to go to my mum's at the weekend'. Leone had mentioned the previous week that her mother was not allowing her to visit that weekend. I suggested that perhaps this related to her feeling that her mother had stabbed her by not allowing her to visit. Once more, Leone smiled in a bemused manner but this time was able to say that this was going too far and her thinking had not taken her to that conclusion. The co-therapist in the group added that perhaps this was another reflection of Leone's own anger attributed to her mother and turned inwards, against herself. It seemed that instead of getting angry with her mother, an affect she found too disturbing, she experienced her mother as attacking her. Once more this was 'accepted' with a view to avoiding any possible conflict with us. However, we were able to think, aided by Leone's comment, that in not being allowed to see her mother at the weekend,

Leone's experience of rejection took the concrete form of a visual hallucination through seeing herself being stabbed. For Leone, what her mother did by not meeting her, was experienced as nothing less than *an act of violence*. It was highly significant that there was no 'as if' in the construction of this experience. It marked out a key distinguishing feature of the way in which a psychotic patient could experience the full physical force of an emotional exchange at a 'hallucino-somatic' level; i.e. as an hallucination experienced in the body. It is what Lucas (2008) thinks of as operating at 'a psychotic wavelength'.

Does this mean Leone is unable to mentalise; i.e. reflect on her own and other people's experience? Perhaps the best way to approach this question is by looking at the nature of non-psychotic forms of mentalisation. For the 'normal-neurotic' - having an intense paranoid experience of being hated on a bus, does not produce concrete hallucinations or paranoid delusions. We can describe such a person as functioning in what Melanie Klein (1946) has called the paranoid-schizoid position; i.e. seeing the world in black and white terms, involving projection of their own, often hostile, emotions. This, of course, means that the projecting person is prone to experience other people as equally hostile, and is thereby ready to feel tormented and attacked, invoking the feeling of being hated.

Clearly here the person is demonstrating, even if wrongly, a capacity to think about the meaning of the other person's mind and their experience. This level of paranoid-schizoid functioning is reactive rather than reflective, invoking persecutory anxiety and even hostility. The key point however, is that it does not result in visual hallucinations or paranoid delusions. Because the reactions are non-psychotic in nature, I term this level of functioning *'simple mentalisation'*.

Such a level of mentalisation should be distinguished from the healthiest state of mental functioning, and one all of us veer from occasionally. In this most sophisticated form of mental functioning, the person is able to reflect on the possibility that the person looking at them on the bus may be angry, but may be thinking about something entirely different and/or that it is *they* who are in a bad mood. This capacity for reflection I term, *'complex mentalisation'*, and I most closely associate it with what Klein calls the depressive position (Klein, 1935).

Clearly, Leone is not operating at either of these levels. Unlike the non-psychotic form of paranoid-schizoid functioning, her form of projections, termed 'pathological projective identification' (Bion, 1967), are on an entirely different 'psychotic wavelength'. These projections result in what Bion (1967) calls, 'bizarre objects' producing the kind of visual hallucinations, like her or people being stabbed, that Leone experiences. And yet I want to argue that through the work in the group, she is capable of exhibiting a form of mentalisation, which I call *'rudimentary mentalisation'*. Firstly, being able to get off the bus demonstrates that she is able to 'take in', 'hold' and use what the group advised. This implies a space in her mind to take an action that counters the psychotic experience, since she can now listen and take the group's suggestion. Without that capacity she would not have been able to do even this. Secondly, Leone is now able to connect not going to her mother's and being stabbed. In other words, there is a space for a healthy, Adult Self that can *think and make links between two separate phenomena* - her visual hallucination (the symptom) and her previously denied feelings (the 'cause'). Now Leone's visual hallucination has meaning. Moreover, this experience can be observed and commented on. The experience demonstrates that Leone has a healthy mind which has an *observing self*, however primitive. Such an exchange goes beyond the 'concrete' and demonstrates that she is able to think symbolically (by which I mean something representing something else). In Leone's example, being stabbed represented being rejected by her mother. This connection highlights how the healthy mind can make links between apparently disparate phenomena. It shows that *meaning* can be derived even in the severest psychotic patient. However, this meaning remains a rudimentary form of mentalisation because of the concretised (e.g. getting off the bus) and less conscious nature of Leone's capacity to make links in her mind. Nonetheless, the most important point is that despite its rudimentary nature, people with psychosis, like Leone, clearly manifest a fragile, (even if almost overwhelmed), healthy self. It is this Adult Self that we as therapists align with and encourage the group to support.

Interestingly, subsequent to this period of work, the hallucinations decreased and perhaps just as importantly, Leone began to talk more openly about the way she more generally experiences herself as someone who can be easily overlooked. Since then, Leone has been able to talk about her relationship with a particularly significant male friend and how emotionally upset this makes her.

Talking about two types of self is not meant to imply that this is a non-complex dialectic. Sinason (1993) makes clear that for those with the severest psychotic illness, the psychotic and healthy selves 'will co-habit, 'til death do they part'. From this vantage point, two assumptions arise. First, for many in this patient group, there is no notion that the therapeutic task leads to these patients becoming free of their psychosis. This assumption can pose particular counter-transference problems for staff that have unrealistic expectations about their patients being cured. As Main points out, 'the sufferer who frustrates a keen therapist, by failing to improve is always in danger of meeting primitive human behaviour disguised as treatment' (Main, 1957 p.129). For practitioners this means having to carefully attune to their counter-transference responses, which include forgoing the narcissistic gratification of working with patients who, in some cases, will *never* get better. Secondly, and as profoundly important, practitioners need to hold to the notion of a healthy self that is invested in living as positive a life as possible, even within the limitations caused by the illness.

A patient once rebuked me in a group when I insensitively referred to him as 'schizophrenic', correcting me by suggesting that he was 'a person with a schizophrenic illness'. The patient was in effect demonstrating something about the ways the healthy self developed in the context of psychosis. This development is the subject of the next section.

Box 1: Summary of mentalisation hierarchy

Rudimentary Mentalisation
* The patient has little capacity to reflect on their own or other people's mental states.
* There is almost no mental space. The mind is dominated by the psychotic wavelength, where no other version of reality exists.
* Even black-and-white thinking is thoroughly undermined.
* There is almost no capacity for thought: alternative explanations for a particular experience cannot be tolerated.
* It is an interior world taken over by delusions and hallucinations.
* The Adult Self is a virtual spectator. It is this Self that is mobilised in therapy.
* Rudimentary mentalisation is most closely associated with the psychotic form of Klein's (1946) paranoid-schizoid position.

Simple mentalisation:
* The patient maintains a capacity to reflect on their own and other people's mental states.
* Thinking is much more black-and-white. The capacity to think in shades of grey is severely compromised: *either/or thinking* rather than *both/and thinking* dominates.
* There is much less mental space available for complexity.
* There is a rigidity of thought: alternative explanations for a particular experience cannot be easily considered.
* Conflict internally, or directly with other people, is a key characteristic.
* It does not include paranoid delusions or hallucinations.
* Simple mentalisation is most closely associated with the non-psychotic form of Klein's (1946) paranoid-schizoid position.

Complex mentalisation:
* The patient can reflect on their own and other people's mental states.
* There is a capacity to think in shades of grey, not just in black-and white terms: allowing for *both/and thinking* rather than just *either/or thinking*
* There is therefore the mental space for complexity
* There is flexibility of thought allowing for a range of responses to a particular experience, including reconsideration of a previously-held view
* Complex mentalisation is most closely associated with Klein's (1935) depressive position

The relational as core of human experience

We begin from an understanding that the development of the healthy self comes about from the experience of life lived in relationship, an idea articulated by Winnicott (1971), and more recently corroborated by infant research (Boston Change Process Study Group (BCPSG), 2007). In a similar vein, our work borrows heavily from the ideas developed by the innovative thinking of group therapists such as Kanas (see chapter by McIvor and Pennycook in this volume) who developed his integrative model of group therapy with people with schizophrenia, and Yalom's interpersonal model of inpatient group therapy (Yalom, 1983). Hajek (see 2007 and her chapter in this volume) provides a useful summary of Yalom's model. She describes how because we are formed in a social context, our mental health is 'influenced by, and dependent on interpersonal relationships' (Hajek, 2007). Kanas and Yalom each privilege social engagement as a key human activity in the promotion of psychological well-being. As will have already become clear, our way of working more specifically emphasises the psychodynamic as well as the interpersonal dimension.

It is worth noting that this form of therapeutic work is the 'other side of the coin' of the extensively researched work on 'expressed emotion' (EE) (Vaughn & Leff, 1976). Through psychoeducation, this approach has focused on helping carers and patients to *reduce* their levels of engagement with their psychotically ill loved ones; encouraging them to avoid getting over-involved, critical or hostile. In fact, relatives with a high degree of EE are urged to have less than 35 hours face-to-face contact per week with their ill family member (Vaughn & Leff, 1981). Research has demonstrated that in combination with medication, these patients have a much lower chance of further psychotic episodes by a factor of 5 (see Bebbington & Kuipers, 1994). This work is clearly important in families where relationships have become critical, hostile or over-involved, but it does not address the key issues raised by Kanas and Yalom; namely, the profound *loneliness and isolation* these patients experience precisely because of their alienating illness. Nor does it explore the nature of any longing for emotional engagement.

The group therapy experience for patients with psychosis attempts to address these issues by helping them develop more enriching relationships outside the group. The question arises: how can these relationships be developed in an inpatient therapy group where as many as half the members are there against their will? Indeed, discussion in the group is often couched in penal language – 'Doctor, when am I going to be *released*?' We are left in no doubt that for some patients the nomenclature 'patient' is clearly understood to be a veil masking the status of 'inmate'. Whatever comfort we may garner from our working assumption of a healthy self, inpatients often have little sense of this, and some are instead consumed by delusions and hallucinations. We have to manage these massively contradictory paradigms. We think them 'mad' because they deny reality. Many patients' experience is of being denied freedom. The patient knows enough about the nature of reality to recognise that we are agents of social control, that they are being incarcerated and we are their gaolers. On this particular ward up to 50% of patients are detained under the Mental Health Act 2007 (section17) which requires the approval of the ward consultant and Home Secretary before any kind of leave can be granted. Such legal restrictions reinforce the view of the psychiatric ward as a prison. 'Out in the community, I have my own front door whereas here, I don't. And I need the permission of staff to do most things'.

In response to these issues and challenges we, as therapists, make much greater efforts to actively engage with patients in the group as we attempt to create what Lucas (2003) calls the 'exoskeleton'. Lucas defines this as 'a supportive environment that can think and care' for the patients. We would add, an environment that also facilitates their own capacities to think and care for themselves and each other. This is a much harder task than this adroit concept implies. Again, in our all-male group, massive and regular attacks on the nature, purpose and function of the group are repeatedly expressed: 'what is the point of this so-called therapy group?' John contemptuously roars. 'All I want to talk about are women – their tits and arses', he mockingly adds. The exoskeleton (in effect the therapeutic couple), is instantly and thoroughly undermined by a determination to bring about its collapse, perhaps mirroring the state of their own internally collapsed skeletal structure. At this point in the proceedings our primary task is set no higher than simple survival. Bion's enjoinder to 'think under fire', seems impossible at this moment for in these groups it is often our capacity to think that is under profound attack. Any enlightening interpretations that might address this patient's sense of collapse (and enhance our sense that we are functioning as therapists), is way beyond our reach, as we struggle to survive the projection of extremely disturbing emotions of anxiety, guilt, rage and psychic collapse.

Before too long another patient is determined to have his voice heard: 'I am Anton, I am Anton', repeated over and over with one of us literally having to put our hand out to him, telling him to 'wait a minute' whilst the other sets out the ground rules. It is often a moment of great irony as the ground rules have already been thoroughly trashed.

We press on clear at least about the need to create a space for a reality that can stand firm against the psychotic process already so manifest in the group. We begin by stating our commonality - that we are all men in a group that is open to all ward patients, with no set agenda, where they are invited to talk about issues that brought them to hospital, their experiences on the ward and concerns relating to their discharge. We explain that it is not an alternative ward round with the consultant psychiatrist being pressed to discuss specific care plans.

In an attempt to empower and, as importantly, to communicate that they too have a functioning sane self, we make clear that if group members feel a patient is being too disruptive, then they can ask him to leave. We add that, as staff, if we feel this needs to happen, then we will ask the disruptive person to leave ourselves. Strikingly, in the five years of the group's life, these measures have not been invoked by the patients or us.

What we are attempting to do above all is provide a therapeutic environment where the level and quality of engagement between patients as well as us, is enhanced. Recent psychoanalytic research (BCPSG, 2007) lays particular importance on the primacy of lived experience, essentially from birth. This work powerfully argues that it is no exaggeration to suggest that interactive relational processes are at the very core of human experience. They suggest that the interactive process itself is primary and generates the raw material from which we draw the generalised abstractions that we term conflicts, defences and phantasy...and that relational is the level of deep experience' (BCPSG, 2007 p.856).

In its most mature form a number of expectable relational variables are present. These include secure attachment, acceptance, warmth, security and trust, as well as tolerance of challenge, ambivalence and even hatred; in other words, everyday experiences of human engagement. There are of course other, less benign, levels of such engagement. *The psychic states of engagement model* (PSE) will now be presented as a schematic way of understanding the different levels at which human engagement, or what I call inter-psychic ways of being with the other, takes place.

The Psychic States of Engagement (PSE) Model

Various levels of the Psychic State of Engagement can be identified. The following is a review of these possibilities.

Psychic State of Engagement 1 (PSE1): Withdrawal and disengagement

For the therapist, group or individual, this level of engagement is perhaps the most frustrating experience of being-with the psychotic patient. This level of functioning comes closest to what Sinason (1993) refers to as 'the other mind', invested in maintaining that which is to remain beyond words; nameless and incomprehensible. This state is associated with the individual almost totally taken over by the seduction of psychosis, divested of any apparent need for relational engagement, leaving the patient in an almost entirely withdrawn state. In the group, this state takes the form of a blank, staring grimace, punctuated from time to time with conversation that is a response to an *internal* engagement, psychiatrically understood as auditory hallucinations. Whilst patients in such a state are virtually unable to participate, they are invited to sit in the group, introduce themselves and be part of the experience.

When asked their thoughts about a particular topic under discussion, they will have no idea what has been discussed or simply reply with a nod of the head, a shrug of the shoulders, a stony discomforting silence or, at best, a whispered, 'I don't know'.

With one less acute patient in an outpatient group; Alan, this state took a physical form. Alan would literally be staring out of the window and be seemingly entirely taken over by a fixed delusion, which took some year and a half for him to disclose. The delusion included the idea that whenever he heard police sirens, this was a signal that the police were after him. This delusion was accompanied by a rescue fantasy in which God would one day let the police authorities know that Alan was innocent of all charges, though the charges themselves were never disclosed. The impact of this delusional system was that Alan hardly participated in the group at all.

Alan's scenario powerfully demonstrates the workings of the other mind. We see that there is a profound and preoccupying relational but *intra-psychic* engagement, with little or no socio-emotional engagement with the group.

Similarly, one man in the inpatient group spent the first session outwardly silent, dishevelled and broken, in pyjamas exposing his genitals, eyes empty of content, staring blankly into the middle distance, with little or no engagement. When expressions of anger began to emerge in the group the patient began talking to his 'intra-psychic group' to bolster his defences against what he correctly understood to be the increasing tension in the group. The other mind was then indeed a place of comparative refuge.

The dominant feature of this form of PSE1 functioning is, *hallucinatory*. It is characterised by withdrawal and disengagement at an interpersonal level, but *not* at the intra-psychic level, where the other mind is pre-eminent. In this world interactive processes continue to thrive, but articulated, significantly, in the form of *auditory* hallucination; a state of engagement continues to exist, but essentially at an intra-psychic level.

Psychic State of Engagement 2 (PSE2): Engagement by violent impact

If PSE1 is characterised by hallucination, then the feature that marks out PSE2 level of functioning is *denial and delusion*. To maintain this psychic state the patient will use violence, mostly through massive projection, but can also resort to physical violence if necessary. The projective form is clearly demonstrated in the example where John, referred to earlier, wants to sabotage the group. In this patient we see his psychotic self in full flight protesting about the idea that not only is he an inpatient for no good reason and against his will, but also that we have the temerity to suggest he may need therapy. Lucas (2008) puts it like this:

'The psychotic part of the personality hates to be confronted with the fact that he is going about things in a mad way (i.e. that he is mentally ill)' (p.59).

This reality has to be projected as soon as we try to begin the group. There must not be a nanosecond of space that might allow this possibility to enter his consciousness. We are meant to carry this burden. To not do so can arouse such rage that there is always the potential for violence. In one group a patient, Tony, was causing manic hilarity when he described his grandiose delusion that he was an all-powerful man, a billionaire who employed all NHS staff, including us. We were meant to understand that *we* (as his employees) were the powerless, impotent ones. When we challenged this, the patient exploded with rage, stood up and came close to hitting one of the therapists. As with many acutely psychotic patients, Tony was reacting in two interconnected ways. *Cognitively*, he reacted viscerally, with murderous rage, at his version of reality being questioned. *Psychodynamically*, he will have unconsciously experienced our intervention as pushing the projections of our being the powerless impotent ones, back into him. This frightening outburst led to a discussion in which group members were able to acknowledge how vulnerable they felt. Tony then apologised; not because he no longer believed his psychotic narrative, but rather because of group member feedback about the terror he had invoked in them. Perhaps this once more highlights the oasis of sanity available even to someone consumed by the other mind bent on promoting only delusion and denial.

Psychic State of Engagement 3 (PSE3): Engagement without risk

This state is most clearly associated with the individual's capacity to interact with greater complexity in their environment. It is a form of relating that I call '*engaging without risk*'. Engagement without risk is a development from the previous forms of psychic engagement, as the patient engages with people in a superficial, discrete way. It is often followed by a cavernous, empty silence as the patient carefully ensures that 'nothing personal' or 'intrusive' is touched on. It is, however, the first move to a more interpersonal and reality-based engagement. This manifests itself in the group through factual discussions about what kind of medication group members are on, how many milligrams and for how long, what the most recent junior doctor is like, have they seen their consultant recently, and so on. Interestingly, it is a state of engagement more often associated with outpatient therapy groups and but also features in the life of inpatients through the exchange of cigarettes, for instance.

Psychic State of Engagement 4 (PSE4): Engagement with risk

Engagement with risk is a further development from the previous forms of psychic engagement, as it means the patient is able to engage with people in a way that allows for risk taking that is more interpersonal and reality-based. However, because of the pre-eminence of PSE1 and PSE2 forms of engagement, *'engagement with risk'* (PSE4) remains highly problematic for two reasons. Firstly, the use of denial and delusion - the key pathological response in PSE2 (engagement by violent impact), ensures that the patient can evade the hated reality of their situation. Secondly, such engagement would mean challenging the code of silence that operates, based on an implicit hierarchy of intimidation. Where 'risk' is taken, it is often against staff. This normally takes the form of a patient complaining, justifiably, about conditions on the ward; e.g. staff not spending time talking about his care plan.

Nonetheless, this is not always the case; sometimes the risk involves challenging a patient. On one occasion a patient, Daniel, expressed his rage that a fellow patient, Frank, was making homosexual advances, baldly stating: 'come to my room, I will fuck you up the arse'. Frank tried to suggest that it had been 'just a joke'. Daniel did not accept this. A row ensued, which, though ferocious and loud, did not threaten to become violent; each protagonist remained seated. Our task was to operate as referees, facilitating the conversation. This meant using communication techniques that required our intervening to ensure they spoke to each other in turn, listened to the other's viewpoint, etc. it is worth adding that as well as actively conducting the group process, we also interpreted Frank's behaviour as dangerously provocative. Although contemptuously dismissed, Frank returned to this theme in a subsequent group, suggesting he had been thinking about the issue.

Just as importantly, Edward, another patient, who had been known to the ward consultant over many previous admissions, suddenly and bravely, acknowledged having had homosexual experiences. Edward was thereby also challenging the group to face this highly unconscious dynamic in the group. One actively psychotic patient, who has been talking to himself through much of the group 'awoke' to what was being discussed. He emphatically stated his wish to leave because he was so appalled. Another member also expressed disgust. The sense of horror and tension was palpable, highlighting the ferocious hatred some of this patient group feel toward what to them was 'perverse' sexuality. This may reflect their own self-disgust, as if their madness, one form of 'perversion' from the 'norm', lays them vulnerable to another 'perversion' - homosexuality. This is a particularly sensitive subject as it touches on a number of painful dynamics: the nature of their own sexuality, being in an all-male ward with all its sexual connotations and their vulnerability as 'men' to exploitation. As men on the ward, for many against their will, this violent intercourse expresses in sexual terms, their sense of 'being fucked' passively; and 'raped' of their dignity and freedom. It is perhaps no wonder that when an issue like homosexuality arises, some patients resort to PSE2 level of engaging by violent impact.

Psychic State of Engagement 5 (PSE5): Engagement with ambivalence

For all of us, engaging with ambivalence; for example, managing both affectionate and hostile feelings towards the same person, is by definition the most difficult of psychic states to reach or sustain. I most closely associate this state with Klein's depressive position as well as complex mentalisation. This state of engagement requires an ability to manage powerfully divergent feelings that may include warmth and admiration mixed with angry, even destructive feelings. It is not surprising, therefore, that an inpatient group rarely achieves this level of engagement between members. At an individual level, Edward was demonstrating a more developed capacity to tolerate uncertainty, where his sexual world did not have to be rigidly organised. He could tolerate thinking about possibilities outside the range of many of his fellow patients, who determinedly and violently (by expressing disgust and walking out) wished to assert their *heterosexuality* as the defining characteristic of their maleness. Interpersonally, the key point about successfully negotiating ambivalence is that engagement at this level of functioning does not lead to violent disruption (PSE2 functioning), but a toleration of even intensely conflictual emotions. More often than not, such experiences are intolerable for both parties. In one group a patient quietly and unwaveringly 'chants' over and over again that his fellow patient has 'a black heart'. Another patient, Thomas, retorts with impotent rage that he is 'stupid, stupid, stupid', and becomes increasingly aroused. The first patient continues his chant. By now Thomas, unable to take any more, is screaming and beginning to get up from his seat, resulting in him having to be restrained from becoming physically violent.

It is clear that in this form of engagement what is being fought over is nothing less than the *survival of self*. What is now being defended against, violently if necessary, is ending up with the other's violent projection. Put the other way round, each patient is trying, as Freud (1925) put it, 'to spit out the bad' (and this means *all* that is bad, or mad or dangerous, etc. and locate it in the other. Engaging with ambivalence would require each of these patients to do what they *cannot do*; i.e. own intolerable and unwanted parts of themselves. Indeed, the psychotic process, articulated through the 'voice' of the other mind, is geared to maintaining the precise opposite: *to spit out, eliminate and deny any such knowledge.*

Box 2: Summary of Psychic States of Engagement (PSE) Model

Psychic States of Engagement 1 (PSE1):
- State of almost total withdrawal and disengagement
- Most closely approximates to Sinason's notion of being taken over by 'the other mind', where hallucinations dominate.
- Where there is engagement it is with this other mind and includes auditory hallucinations ('the voices') with whom the patient does engage.

Psychic States of Engagement 2 (PSE2):
- Engagement by violent impact, psychological or physical.
- Denial and delusion dominate e.g. the billionaire patient, Tony.
- Hatred of reality most apparent and will be defended against by physical violence, if necessary.

Psychic States of Engagement 3 (PSE3):
- State of engagement where no risk is taken. Engagement usually revolves around facts e.g. patients sharing the name of their psychiatrist.
- A development from PSEs 1 and 2, where reality is accepted to a greater extent e.g. the patient acknowledges their 'illness'.
- Interaction is superficial, discrete and 'thin' – a quality of it 'going nowhere', most often followed by an empty, cavernous silence.

Psychic States of Engagement 4 (PSE4):
- State of engagement where risk is taken
- Risk taking is generally reality-based, with less use of denial.
- It allows for personal disclosure and/or greater inrpersonal exchange of authentic issues in the patient's life.

Psychic States of Engagement 5 (PSE5):
- State of engagement where ambivalence is accepted or even openly acknowledged.
- It is reality-based and includes a capacity to think, as in complex mentalisation.
- There is the mental space for complexity as in depressive position functioning .

Conclusions: What lessons can be learnt?

These psychic states have important implications for how therapists need to work in groups. Firstly, the difficulty of engagement requires therapists to engage with each other as well as other group members in a way that is playful, supportive, even risk taking, but above all survivable. The nature of the emotional engagement, therefore, is real and of the moment. Research lends support to this view. In a review of the literature, Lambert and Barley (2001) conclude that 30% of treatment outcome is attributable to the therapeutic relationship and, tellingly, this was found to be twice as important as therapeutic technique. In another review, Orlinsky, Grave, and Parks (1994) identified key therapist variables shown to have a positive impact on treatment outcome. They pinpoint a range of factors such as empathic understanding, affirmation of the patient and *the ability to engage the patient*. The PSE model adds to this finding by drawing attention to the fact that such engagement includes not only the therapist's capacity to engage, but also the patient's own, usually hidden, capacity to do so. The great advantage in group therapy is that an additional resource is brought to bear; namely, the feedback available from other patients.

This is not to deny that running an inpatient psychosis group is different from an outpatient group. The most obvious difference between the two groups is of course the acute severity of illness. Inpatients are extremely ill but do not always believe that they are ill, and therefore resent being in-patients and perceive interventions as imposed. We have learned that each session should be run as if it is a 'one-off' or 'single frame' group. This is based on the observation that no group ever comprises the same members due to patient movement. These issues, as Hajek (2007 and her chapter in this volume) recently pointed out, are compounded by the fact that running inpatient psychotherapy groups is, by definition, highly problematic as patient turnover is high, especially these days as they are always extremely ill and usually heavily medicated.

Each session is thus a discrete experiential moment with the therapist directing individuals within the group to two fundamental tasks. The first supports patients to go beyond their current psychic states of engagement (PSEs 1-3) by encouraging greater levels of interpersonal collaboration (PSEs 4-5). Secondly, through promoting these higher levels of psychic engagement, group members have the potential to go beyond rudimentary mentalisation. This shift involves a movement, however small, from a previously rigidly-held position where no reflective thought is available, to one where the patient begins to evolve a mental space where such mentalisation can emerge. This was demonstrated by the 'billionaire' patient; Tony, who - after getting feedback about his frightening outburst in the group, was able to express regret for his behaviour. Strikingly, Tony continued to hold onto his delusional narrative about his status. However, through his emotional engagement with group members, he was able to move from a state of rudimentary mentalisation, where no reflection was possible, to a form of simple mentalisation where he could take in other people's emotional experience. He could recognise that he had been 'bad' and for this he wanted to apologise.

It is through these types of emotional engagements that we have come to understand that for the group to be meaningful, the most helpful therapeutic work takes place when the session focuses on patients' 'here and now' preoccupations. This is why the group has no set agenda. A deliberate attempt is made by us to explore each issue raised and strive to achieve a resolution, or at least reach a point when the fears – the sense of 'nameless dread', have been named and contained before the end of the session. This approach places a lot of pressure on us as therapists to make the group work in the present rather than defer any serious problem to the following week. There is, of course, the possibility that patients continue to discuss the issues raised outside the group. Resolution, in this sense, means that the toxic dynamics that sometimes grip the ward have been sufficiently detoxified, to allow further exploration amongst themselves. To that end, the chronic interpersonal relationship difficulties and poor communication skills are both directly worked on in the group. In the best of circumstances, a safer space has been created to continue their own therapeutic work. This might mean that patients are then able to socialise more on the ward.

Perhaps the most important lesson we have learned is that through encouraging greater therapeutic input on wards, the group symbolically and literally represents a recognition of the oasis of sanity that each patient carries. Although not always pretty - from this base, the work of therapy can begin.

References

Boston Change Process Study Group (BCPSG) (2007) The foundational level of psychodynamic meaning: Implicit process in relation to conflict, defence and the dynamic unconscious. *International Journal of Psychoanalysis*, 88, p.843-60.

Bateman, A. and Fonagy, P. (2004) *Psychotherapy for Borderline Personality Disorder: Mentalisation based treatment.* Oxford: Oxford University Press.

Bebbington, P.E. and Kuipers, L. (1994) The predictive utility of expressed emotion in schizophrenia: A aggregate analysis. *Psychological Medicine*, 24, p.707-718.

Bion, W.R. (1967) *Second Thoughts.* New York: Jason Aronson.

Bion, W.R. (1977) *Seven Servants: Four works by W.R. Bion.* New York: Jason Aronson.

Department of Health (2008) The pathway to recovery: A review of NHS acute inpatient mental health services. London: Healthcare Commission.

Fonagy, P., Gergely, G., Jurist, E. and Target, M. (2002). Affect regulation, mentalisation, and the development of the self. New York: Other Press.

Freud, S. (1925) Negation. The Standard Edition of the Complete Psychological Works of Sigmund Freud, Volume XIX (1923-1925): The Ego and the Id and Other Works, p.233-240. London: Hogarth.

Freud, S. (1938) An Outline of Psycho-Analysis. In *The Standard Edition of the Complete Psychological Works of Sigmund Freud, Volume XXIII (1937-1939): Moses and Monotheism: An Outline of Psycho-Analysis and Other Works*. p.139-208. London: Hogarth.

Hajek, K. (2007) Interpersonal group therapy on acute inpatients wards. *Groupwork* 17, 1, 7-19.

Jackson, M. (1985) A psychoanalytic approach to the assessment of a psychotic patient. *Psychoanalytic Psychotherapy*. 1, p.31-42.

Klein, M. (1935) A contribution to the psycho-genesis of manic-depressive states. *The Writings of Melanie Klein*, vol. 3, 1-24. London: Hogart.

Klein, M. (1946) Notes on some schizoid mechanisms. *The Writings of Melanie Klein*, vol. 1, 306-343. London: Hogarth.

Lambert, M.J. and Barley, D.E. (2001) Research summary on the therapeutic relationship and psychotherapy outcome. *Psychotherapy*, 38, p.357-361.

Lucas, R. (2003) Psychoanalytic Controversies: The relationship between psychoanalysis and schizophrenia. *International Journal of Psychoanalysis*, 84, p.3-15.

Lucas, R. (2008) The psychotic wavelength. *Psychoanalytic Psychotherapy*. 22, p.54-63.

Main, T. F. (1957) The Ailment. *British Journal of Medical Psychology*. 30, p.129-145.

Nathan, J. (2007) Self-harm: a strategy for survival and nodal point of change. *Advances in Psychiatric Treatment*. 12, p.329-337.

Nathan, J. (2008) Rudimentary mentalisation in a psychotic patient. (Unpublished paper – available from author).

Orlinsky, D.E., Grawe, K. and Parks, B.K. (1994) Process and outcome in psychotherapy. In A.E. Bergin and S.L.Garfield (Eds.) *Handbook of Psychotherapy and Behavior Change*. New York: John Wiley.

Sinason, M. (1993) Who is the mad voice inside? *Psychoanalytic Psychotherapy*. 7, p.207-221.

Vaughn, C.E. and Leff, J.P. (1976) The influence of family and social factors on the course of psychiatric illness: a comparison of schizophrenic and depressed neurotic patients. *British Journal of Psychiatry*. 129, p.125-137.

Vaughn, C.E. and Leff, J.P. (1981) Patterns of emotional response in relatives of schizophrenic patients. *Schizophrenic Bulletin*. 7, p.43-44.

Winnicott, D. W. (1971) *Playing and Reality*. Middlesex: Penguin.

Wooster, E. (2008) Some mental health trusts provide poor care. *Openmind* (MIND magazine) 153 p.4.

Yalom, I.D. (1983) *Inpatient Group Therapy*. New York: Basic Books

17
Structure and containment in an adolescent inpatient acute unit and its groups

Dylan Griffiths

Introduction

I want to describe in detail how we use three particular groups on our adolescent unit. The thinking around these groups informs a view of the overall structure necessary to ensure that troubled and vulnerable adolescents can be helped restart and continue their arrested development. The goal of treatment is the achievement of as much reasonable autonomy as possible in this population, although this may eventually be limited by factors broadly called 'illness'. The groups encourage communication and reciprocity between adolescents and staff.

Groups on adolescent units and the provision of a 'therapeutic milieu' with practical activities based around residential life have their origins in the principles of therapeutic communities, a movement begun around the second world war to treat and rehabilitate soldiers. Its principles stressed the development of personal autonomy and the strengths of patients as core values. The structure of most adolescent units owes much to these principles.

Adolescent units in the UK exist primarily to assess and treat severely psychiatrically or psychologically disturbed adolescents, the age range being from about 13 years to 18 years. Younger patients needing specialised help may be treated in Children's Units, most over 18s find themselves in the adult psychiatric setting. Acuteness and severity of the presenting problem will be seen to be part of the need for admission but the deciding factor is often whether or not structures in the community are robust and safe enough to deal with the problem. The level of unpredictability and risk presented by an acutely psychotic or suicidal young person can challenge the best of community arrangements. Anxiety needs containment in both the referred patients and their referrers.

At any one time the make up of a typical unit of 12 to 14 young people might consist of up to a third of young people with psychosis (schizophrenic and mood disorder presentations), usually one to two will have been sectioned. The rest are made up mostly of acutely or chronically suicidal and depressed young people often with varying degrees of deliberate self-harm. These and other presentations may include aspects of Conduct Disorder, Developing Personality Disorder, OCD, Tourette's syndrome, Asperger's Syndrome, Abnormal Illness Behaviour, ADHD, drug problems or post abuse or trauma issues with PTSD. Eating disorders are increasingly being admitted to more specialised units. The normal development of all the young people is severely compromised at the point of presentation.

Adolescent units can be difficult and challenging places for both patients and staff. Although there is some movement towards specialised units, the average unit has to fulfil a large number of functions and there is always an uncomfortable tension between its acute admission function and its assessment and treatment functions. Central to its continued functioning is the ability to maintain a consistent, clear and flexible structure in terms of staff and treatment availability, day to day timetabling and unit 'rules' and expectations. The successful unit works hard to support staff and provide containment for their anxiety also. The rules provide a background level of expectation and statement of staff intent and values against which the troubled adolescent can begin to measure the reality of the limits set and commitment of the unit and staff. This is often done by direct challenge and testing usually involving some form of behavioural acting out. The unit strives to be able to contain these physical excesses but the emotional tension generated is equally important to contain. Hopefully the physical activity and high emotional charge of the communication inherent in the acting out can eventually be transformed into verbal form. This allows acceptance and negotiation of needs on a more advanced developmental level.

Psychoanalytic concepts can inform the work on the unit. They can clarify the 'basic task' of staff and the unit by providing a structure for thinking about unit events and a rationale for support of staff members with an understanding of significance of a particular conflict and action. Briefly put, I see the function of an adolescent unit is to act as a 'good enough' (Winnicott, 1960) 'container' (Bion, 1967) to allow the adolescents time and space in a suitable environment which helps them to restart and appropriately continue their development. Challenge by the adolescent and the appropriate adult response to it, neither too authoritarian nor too liberal (Winnicott, 1971) is an essential part of the process. According to Bion the properties of a container, include its availability and consistency. This allows the transformation of early communication in the form of primitive emotional gamma elements into usable, more potentially verbal, alpha elements, heralding the beginning of the capacity of a mind for thought. The atmosphere on a unit consists, at times, of high levels of 'paranoid schizoid' thought process characterised by splitting, projection and projective identification (see Segal, 1973, for a summary of Melanie Klein's ideas on this). There is a high level of anxiety, with various protagonists apparently clearly in either the right or wrong. Thought and compromise are difficult. There are calls for immediate action with the hope of an instant solution for all, usually by expulsion of a designated 'bad' object. This is also replicated in the tenacity with which the young people hold onto symptoms, and certain unhelpful behaviours, with the prospect of change being feared. Individual therapy provides a setting for examination of the latter, though it can also be recognised and challenged in the wider group. For the institutional issues, regular or special groups, including supervision and meetings for the staff can provide a containing function giving opportunity for more realistic reflection on anxiety and process. Hopefully this leads to a change to more 'depressive position' functioning marked by concern, discussion of meaning, reflective ability, a spirit of compromise and sometimes sadness. As in normality and normal development, unit life consists of endless oscillation between these two states of mind.

Example

A young man with a grievous history of childhood abuse and a chequered attachment history regularly attacked the nursing staff. He was contained on two to one nursing and exploration of his mental state over subsequent time revealed extreme anxiety over his fantasies of the staff's intentions with him. He was able to recognise this and eventually volunteered he had never talked of his previous abuse, it was just too overwhelming for him. This linking of his behaviour and the past and clarification of the projective nature of his attacks, where the fear was to be felt by staff, leaving him feeling in control of his aggression, was the start of a more reflective process and a more positive engagement between him and the staff.

Floridly psychotic young people often need to be actively managed and treated to keep themselves and others safe and to begin to challenge the attack on reality of the psychosis. Hopefully more reasonable communication can resume, though the psychosis may also contain some meaning.

Example

A young man admitted with depressive delusions and hallucinations of having special powers that he was misusing, eventually revealed his long standing pre morbid preoccupation about his development and its presumed effect on his family. When his psychosis had settled with medication and an extended period of one to one nursing, this important issue could then be explored in individual and family sessions.

Troubled behavioural presentations, which almost invariably continue within the unit, are very often a transference reworking of basic intra-familial conflicts. These revolve around responses to authority and perceived, or real, deprivation and trauma. The unit staff, having assumed a parental role, are very much in the firing line. The parents are very often relieved to also find the 'so-called' experts to be struggling with these difficult and disturbed adolescent behaviours. These points of identification can make a good transference based starting point in family work.

Example

A young girl with a long standing history of self harm continued to threaten suicide and react aggressively to staff. Family sessions threw light on family conflict and difficulty in communication, with this often resulting in chronic emptiness and low self esteem for the girl for which she had been 'treating' with the deliberate self-harm. Communication and behavioural improvement with parents and staff went hand in hand.

Groups in the Adolescent Unit

Groups are an integral part of Adolescent Unit life. Most of the adolescents have access to an individual therapist and/or clinical psychologist and all have their own key nurse, consultant, ward doctor and other named support workers. However the majority of their time, perhaps unsurprisingly for an institution, is spent in one form of group or other. Patients have individual rooms but access is limited during the day because of the logistics of supervision of 14 individuals. Morning is spent in School or Skills Centre (for those who have left school or are too unwell to attend formal lessons). Afternoons and early evenings are spent in timetabled group activities such as discussion group, CBT group, DBT (dialectical behaviour therapy) group, anger management group, same sex group, cooking group and a range of occupational therapy activities. Strenuous efforts are made to engage the young people in worthwhile activity and though not changed every day the content of the groups is kept under constant review, and sometimes adapted to a particular unit population. Leisure time, vital to all adolescents, is spent largely within the peer group. Unfortunately for staff anxiety, but developmentally appropriately for the adolescents, staff have limited access to this last group but it is highly important in the life of the unit and the individual. This overall structure forms the basis of the therapeutic milieu, as mentioned above, the basic elements would be common to most adolescent units.

I want to describe in detail a series of three weekly groups which involve representatives of the clinical team meeting with all the young people, very much community meetings. These are :

1.   The Community Meeting, held midweek on Wednesday afternoon.
2.   The Start the Week Meeting, held on Monday morning
3.   The End of the Week Meeting, held on Friday morning.

The Community Meeting

The Community Meeting is an integral part of most adolescent units, bringing with it the opportunity for all to see and be seen and to make the most of 'here and now' communication. When I took over as consultant on an adolescent unit over twelve years ago I decreased the frequency of the unit's community meetings and staff groups from daily to weekly. I did so because the meetings had become ritualised and I judged them, in consultation with unit staff, to be anti-therapeutic and an enormous drain on staff time and effort. This alteration of established structure caused much consternation and anxiety in some staff members, but others felt a sense of change and growth. The timetable was further modified to include a daily half hour staff clinical meeting at the start of the day, a weekly community meeting and a weekly staff support group.

In the spirit of reform, the format of the community and staff groups became less prescriptive and hopefully more spontaneous. This benefited the staff support group immensely, and encouragement of free comment by all on whatever matter seemed relevant, as a starting point for reflection, became well established and valued. However in the community meeting attempts at freer comment with reflective interpretation on the experience of life on the unit did not feel so successful. Long periods of silence seemed to inflict unnecessary discomfort on staff and young people. The adolescents were not an active part of a process that appeared derived mainly from staff ideals; basically it was failing as a community experience. We, as staff, felt we should provide a more positive and useful experience for the adolescents with active modelling of communication skills with the patients. This is a challenging task with troubled and psychotic adolescents. The format we developed provided a didactic framework for communication, based on committee structure, utilising both verbal and writing skills. Adolescent participation was supported and modelled by staff, but there was also space for free comment. It is best described with reference to its unit guidelines at the time.

General rationale of groups

· Reciprocal communication of young people's and staff issues
· Promote verbal communication
· Promote social skills
· Reinforce unit expectations
· Good assessment opportunity

The Community Meeting

Purpose General

Promote social skills, committee skills, verbal, recording and writing skills, leadership opportunity.

Staff opportunity for support and/or challenging unit issues

Staff announcements

Attendance All young people fit

All staff able to, important all disciplines represented

Staff Input Ensure the young persons' Pre Community Group meets

Ensure it produces a written agenda – Business and Feelings

Young people must record who's commented

Young people to nominate Chair and Minute Taker

Bring this to staff Pre Community Group

Decide there on strategy and announcements to add to the agenda

Provide the Young Persons (YP) Chair with written order of meeting and tasks

Provide book and pen to record meeting minutes

Choose Staff Chair – rotating, and support for Minute taker

All staff to support

Format   45 minute group

Started and finished by YP Chair with help of Staff Chair

YP Chair to announce start of meeting, check Minute Taker, consider if introductions necessary, ask if there are any first announcements

YP Chair to ask for minutes of last meeting to be read out

YP Chair to check accuracy, check on progress and matters arising

YP Chair to read through YPs' agenda and staff agenda

YP Chair to go through agenda asking relevant people to comment, allowing discussion – may need help with timekeeping etc.

Meeting finishes at specified time, if applicable ask Minute Taker to carry over items to next week

Staff member checks minutes

YP Chair to congratulate self on chairing meeting

Although the list of guidelines appears daunting they are an attempt to be ready for most eventualities. It will be noted that the community meeting demands two extra meetings – Pre Community Group meetings for both the adolescents and the staff.

Characteristically the Pre Community Group meets with a variable amount of resistance from the adolescents dependent on the unit population and urgency of issues. Though attempts can be made to leave the group entirely in the hands of the young people, these are not always successful. This usefully becomes a live ongoing issue with the adolescents over the amount of reminding and help needed. There is a range of responses. Some groups of adolescents will ask for privacy to prepare an agenda, whilst other less able or motivated will need more active supervision. The group does need to be held in the staff's mind – a reminder in the ward diary the day before and delegation to a member of staff to supervise. The time allotted to this group can vary between ten minutes to a half hour. Most groups produce a page of agenda items. This can range from a barely intelligible scribble of a few points on a piece of scrappy paper to an elaborately and symbolically decorated list on a piece of drawing paper. The decoration may be positive e.g. faces, flowers and comments; or more sinister, daggers, bleeding cuts, nooses and gravestones. This can be commented on in the actual meeting. Splitting the agenda into 'Business' and 'Feelings,' is a response to the agenda and time being filled up with 'Business' items such as complaints, typically about showers, rooms, food and other inanimate objects. These do need to be acknowledged on a practical level and sometimes commented on as a broader emotional communication. We provide a book for entering these housekeeping issues. More pressing unit issues are hopefully broached by providing the 'Feelings' category.

This means any unit event that has led to particular strong feelings of any sort over the proceeding week. These are conflict with staff members, intra group conflict and rivalry amongst the adolescents, episodes of acting out and very often concern about one another and staff members. Sometimes more positive feelings (though with a certain sadness) are discussed e.g. around a young person's imminent discharge or the leaving of a staff member.

The staff's Pre Community Group meeting may not take longer than five to ten minutes. The staff chair, who supports the YP Chair and a member of staff to help the minute taker are chosen. This is done by rotation of disciplines and seniority to prevent too obvious a hierarchy and to give all staff members a chance to take as active a role as possible. The young people's agenda is scrutinised and decisions taken on the need for, and style of response. Significant omissions in the young people's agenda may be addressed via the staff agenda and separate items of importance may be tabled. A decision may be taken to be particularly challenging over some pressing issue like bullying or aggression to staff but alternate strategies may also be considered.

Example

Following two days of relentless but not wholly successful challenge of certain antisocial elements among the young people it was decided not to continue in a potentially bad-tempered and repetitive discussion of events familiar to all, but rather attempt to provide a more light hearted interlude where possibly relationships could be rebuilt. A quiz was organised and teams chosen from young people and staff together. A pleasant time was passed which everyone thought was much needed.

Following the 9/11 disaster, the community group was given over to an exploration of feelings brought up by the tragedy and its' reporting.

When the meeting proper starts it is treated as an extremely important weekly event. This is reinforced by the compulsory attendance of the young people and available staff, including the consultant and doctors. Acutely psychotic or seriously unsettled patients are not expected to attend but if any adolescent wilfully refuses to attend this will be taken up with them later in terms of a lack of motivation to engage. This action (but not any clinical details) is made plain to the rest of the group. Leaving the group for any reason is discouraged, re-entry is discussed with the group.

When it is established by the staff chair who is to be to be YP Chair and minute taker they are handed the written pro forma for the meeting and the minute book and pen respectively. If the young persons' group has not managed to choose a Chair or minute taker, then the staff attempt to resolve this, reminding the adolescents of their responsibilities and the expectation of mature participation. Care must be taken with this last minute 'volunteering', that a young person does not monopolise either function out of convenience for the rest of the group or personal preference. The YP Chair is then invited to declare the meeting open and proceed via the written proforma or with staff prompts. In practice the adolescents appear to value the community group and the thinking behind it. By the time a young person is asked to be the Chair or minute taker they will already have participated in a number of these meetings and will have a good idea of what is expected and the usual conduct of the meeting. Thus the YP Chair will lead the group in a round of introductions. They also find it easy to also give a succinct definition of the meeting at this point for newcomers.

> *'It's a meeting where we make a list of what we want and what's happening on the unit and talk it over with the staff....'*

'First announcements' are invited; these may be points of information about new admissions or members of staff, imminent discharges or staff absences or any other items of relevant information. These items may hold significance in terms of later agenda items and are often better left to be linked with these.

Linking unrest and acting out on the unit with staff absence is a potent reminder of the emotional life of the unit.

The YP Chair then asks for the minutes of the last meeting to be read out. Most of the time, these are surprisingly accurate. The agenda points lend themselves to easy recording as do the responses to straightforward requests, but the minutes often convey the emotional temperature of the last meeting by dint of direct quotation of dialogue and comments. The minute takers take the task seriously without much prompting from staff. 'Matters Arising' is next; there is a real satisfaction in being able to report on a point which has been followed up but a very flat feel to things when the staff have not done so.

When this is complete the YP Chair reads through all agenda items and then takes each item in turn asking the person who added the item to speak to it. The adolescent's agenda might include displeasure or anxiety over a piece of behaviour of another group member or staff member or some perceived or actual slight by the same. Intra group rivalries usually benefit from an airing. Often the adolescent who has made an agenda point has to be supported in changing the proffered 'something an adolescent said/did upset me' into a more definite statement, thus allowing a more real discussion. Conflicting parties are reminded that its everyones privilege to state how they feel, and there may be no immediate solution for their disagreement. Young people are able to appreciate that their behaviour towards each other can be the result of social anxiety or related to their own emotional struggles. However the adolescents can also be intolerant of other's needs and have to be reminded that they too may have had their difficult moments. When members of staff are challenged we try and take specific complaints seriously and the young people know an official complaints procedure exists. More usually the complaints are more general like 'not enough staff' or 'no-one is ever available'. This is sometimes true because staff may be busy elsewhere, especially dealing with distress or acting out, and this is duly discussed. Limited resources and the need to tolerate less than perfect attention within an institution are constant issues and often are at the forefront of discussions. For some troubled adolescents, demanding perfection from staff when their own lives are markedly imperfect, can sometimes be the start of an interesting dialogue. For others it may represent an insurmountable obstruction to engagement.

Example

A young boy with a long-standing behavioural problem, from a deprived and abusive background caused havoc on the unit with his repeated aggressive and destructive behaviour. He put other vulnerable young people at risk and injured staff. He was challenged about this in the group and maintained it was the staff's responsibility, as they were insufficiently skilled to deal with his 'problems'. This view was continued in his family meetings and he was supported in his opinion by his mother. She wondered when we would start 'the treatment' of her son. Although mother conceded that family issues were relevant, in her view we were obviously not treating her son correctly. The boy did not see why he should change and there was a failure to engage in a meaningful discussion. He was eventually discharged.

Unfortunately deprivation and abuse form a conscious and unconscious context for many young people's experience of the unit. One has to be aware of the potent interaction of this and the frustrations of unit life. The group is not often used for 'deep' interpretations. However comments that many people have had unhappy and unpleasant experiences which have affected their lives and made it difficult to manage ordinary things, thus necessitating admission to an adolescent unit to try to work things out, are often repeated and always accepted.

The YP Chair obviously needs help in timekeeping, maintaining order and generally managing what sometimes comes up, though for some not as much as you would think. Sometimes the agenda is rushed through, or items don't seem to stir much comment and then the group is left apparently high and dry for the final ten minutes. Invariably there is an issue that is being avoided.

Example

A recent group coming the day after the unit's move downstairs to new premises came to an abrupt hiatus after twenty minutes. The patients had been very active and helpful in the move, which everyone was congratulatory about. It was a move to brand new surroundings away from a rather tired unit that had seen better days. The comment that young people and staff might be sad at leaving the familiar old unit, and were finding themselves unsettled in unfamiliar territory, at first sparked incredulity. An adolescent said that he had moved many times and it was nothing to get concerned with. However one of the girls stated that she had found moving from her mother's to her father's incredibly hard and this sparked an active discussion about feelings around moving. In the group the staff realised that there had been no goodbyes taken of the old unit and this was duly organised, with full support of the whole group, for the next day.

Finally the meeting is brought to an end by the YP Chair, this part is enjoyed immensely! The minutes are checked through and both the minute taker and the YP Chair are congratulated on their considerable achievement. The staff then meet for a very brief post group to comment on and perhaps discuss aspects of the group before unit life moves on to the next activity.

The Start of the Week Meeting

The Start and End of the Week Meetings were developed to compliment the Community Meeting. The intention was to involve the young people as much as possible in unit life and its groups. We wanted to facilitate something active happening in each of these groups as an antidote to some of the formless, daily meetings that preceded them. We felt that just having a meeting almost for the sake of it provided a safe hiding place for patients and staff. This detracted from people's ability to focus on the hard work of making the most of what is (given the current climate) precious time on the unit. We wanted groups that would mark the beginning and end of the week. The preceding and forthcoming weekends were obvious candidates for review. We would start by asking the young people in turn about their weekends. In keeping with the focus on a work ethic we also decided to set them the task of defining a task or goal for the week. This could then be reviewed at the End of the Week Meeting along with a general review of progress both on the unit and at school. It is useful for all to know in general how things are going, though it is not always appropriate to discuss personal detail. The unit teachers strongly wished to be part of these meetings both because of their work focus but also as it afforded them a different but complementary view of their pupils. The unit guidelines describe the format.

Purpose	General
	Discuss weekend issues
	Plan the week
	Staff announcements
Attendance	All young people fit
	All staff able to, including teachers
Staff Input	One member of staff to lead
	All to support
Format	45-minute group
	Roughly 3 minutes per young person to explore weekend events and forthcoming week's goals
	Rest of time for discussion and staff announcements
	Recording of aims for young people

The group is a very prescriptive group. The adolescents take it in turn to share information on their respective weekends and state or develop a goal for the week. Replies to the weekend query can be monosyllabic, ranging from 'OK' to 'shit'. The adolescent is encouraged to expand on both, and reminded that 'shit' is not a particularly polite form of speech. Adolescents can find open discussion of the details difficult and they are reminded the purpose of the meeting is a general and not a specific enquiry. Details can be discussed later with a member of staff.

The goals too can present a difficulty. Some patients will claim to have no goals and this is actively challenged. If a goal is not forthcoming after some exploration and prompting, the staff can choose one. If an adolescent continues to be resistant, we can call a halt to this particular turn, as often the conflict serves as a secondary reinforcement of unhelpful behaviour. The issue of non-compliance will be dealt with separately.

The young person is usually reminded that the week contains a family meeting or a review/CPA meeting and is invited to plan for this with a member of staff. Group leaders may also diplomatically remind young people of pressing issues.

The goal can sometimes be vague, such as 'to keep myself safe', 'to self harm less', 'to stay out of trouble', 'to get off one to one' (close observation) or 'to be allowed unescorted walks'. The staff encourage the patient both to expand on the meaning of the goal and also to define specific behavioural plans. Thus the prospective self harmer can undertake to actively seek out staff support either at moments of stress or electively at an agreed number of times a day. These arrangements can be finalised with the key nurse as part of a developing care plan. 'Staying out of trouble' is restated as an active undertaking to behave in a positive manner and the young person encouraged to look at this in detail with a staff member. 'Getting off one to one' or being 'allowed unescorted walks' is translated into the young person's responsibility in behaving reasonably. What is it that they should do to increase the chances of aspects of their care being changed? It can be explored as above. Other goals have been to get up or get to school or groups on time. This can be measured daily and for some patients, especially those recovering from psychotic illnesses, this can be a major step on the path to rehabilitation. As adolescents stay longer on the unit the goals set tend to be become more sophisticated. These involve areas of therapeutic work agreed in advance with their therapist and offered to the group as a prospective piece of work.

Recording of the goals is essential though sometimes problematic. Goals recorded on the white board are vulnerable to being rubbed off. Goals recorded on a piece of paper given to a young person can also disappear, a process assisted by that person's ambivalence. The current method is to record the goals together on a suitable piece of paper that can be kept safely until the end of the week meeting, but this means the patients and staff have no direct access to a reminder of the goals.

There can be a tendency for the meeting to appear a dialogue between the staff Chair and the adolescents, but the goal setting discussion usually involves the active participation of the other staff. The meeting is finished on time.

The End of the Week Meeting

The format closely follows the Start of the Week Meeting, the task of the group is to appraise the week for each adolescent and to explore plans for their weekend.

Purpose	General
	Staff announcements
	Appraisal of week
	Exploration of forthcoming weekend issues
Attendance	All young people fit
	All staff able to

Staff Input	One member of staff to lead, preferably member of teaching staff
	All to support/comment
Format	45-minute group
	Roughly 3 minutes per young person to appraise week and explore weekend
	Rest of time for discussion and staff announcements

A senior member of the school staff chairs the meeting because it is useful to amalgamate the review of the week at school with the review of the week on the unit. Most adolescents react positively to the school or skill centre setting. This is due to a relatively high (one to four) teacher to pupil ratio, and a school attitude that is prepared to tailor 'work' to the pupil's present capability. A positive school experience is sometimes completely new for some adolescents. School provides an essential part of the unit's treatment in being a link between psychiatric and psychological treatment and the necessary acquisition of skills essential for survival in the adult world. The teacher is usually able to start off with a positive comment about application if not academic achievement, which can also be a new experience for some.

The teacher then enquires about the week on the ward and whether the set goal has been met. The adolescent may still affect disinterest, and other staff members may offer their view on progress. On the other hand a positive review of goals achieved offers another opportunity for overt praise from all quarters. The young person may also be praised for sticking with difficult therapy sessions or issues, or some other positive or helpful aspect of behaviour. The staff do try and find some positive that can be commented upon, as the effect of praise is immense in this population. It is a group of people who can unfortunately be totally unaccustomed to positive comment. This may explain the strong and seductive appeal of an apparently uncritically accepting peer group, so beloved of the adolescent.

Most patients will be spending the weekend or part of it at home if they are well enough or circumstances allow it. Those remaining on the unit face a certain amount of choice and planning of their weekend. Enquiries about the forthcoming weekend can bring its range of replies but it is usually clear if there is a particularly difficult weekend ahead. Thus everyone is hopefully 'in the know' and support can be offered in the form of extra staff time, telephone contact over the weekend or early return to the unit. All staff members play their part in these discussions. Finally the group is wished a good weekend and the meeting finishes on time.

Conclusions

The introduction of the above group format to our adolescent inpatient acute unit has been successful. The format demands and supports participation, and the rationale for all meetings are evident. The whole supports and is supported by the opportunities to reinforce unit rules and expectations. Life on the unit is given limits and boundaries and the underlying basic assumption is that patients and staff are engaged in the task of helping the individual recover relative health and autonomy; to move from relative dependence on the unit to the prospect of more developmentally appropriate independent functioning in the community. The adolescent and staff feel themselves to be part of an ongoing process of experience and communication within the unit. It is very encouraging to witness a young person making more appropriate use of the meetings as they progress with their treatment on the unit. Very often the position of YP Chair will be assumed, or discharged very credibly, by a more 'senior' member of the adolescent group. All the more surprising when one remembers the challenging and tolerance of negativity which went before. One is continually surprised by how well even the most verbally challenged adolescent does when supported in assuming the role of Chair or minute taker. It speaks of how easy it is to overlook developmental potential in some young people. The Start and End the Week meetings do what they say. They bracket the week, providing a structure for the unit's work. They also serve the general purpose of observation and evaluation, for staff and young people. The role of the school gains a wider unit appreciation, and the groups require multidisciplinary input from all levels of the team.

I would wish to return to Tom Main's idea of a therapeutic community first espoused in his 1946 paper, 'The hospital as a therapeutic institution' (Main, 1989). His ideas grew from a wish to challenge a basic assumption that hospital authority knew best and that patients were helpless. His community at the Cassel Hospital subjected everything to scrutiny and continued monitoring, promoting self-modification. Main regarded therapeutic thinking as 'informed common sense', and discussion as necessary for health and ordinary life as an important agent of therapy. The self contained therapeutic community was born, with groups at its centre to promote the necessary self examination from which change would come. The model has been the inspiration and structure for specialised child and adolescent therapeutic communities such as Pepper Harrow and the Cotswold Community in this country. Also inpatient units and other psychiatric and psychological services who wish to make their practice less authoritarian and more user–led have utilised the model of participative group based approaches. Therapeutic communities have evolved and been developed by particular user's needs, such as drug and alcohol problems and offender based programmes. Mostly these approaches have added in an organizing structure based around users perceived needs. This was very much behind our efforts to improve the experience of our community group for the adolescents and in addition maximise its therapeutic, teaching and communicative potential.

Foulkes and Anthony (1957), make some interesting comments on group techniques for young people in residential units. They see groups in these settings as providing an 'equalising experience' helping to decrease dichotomies between staff and the young person, with a corresponding reduction in unnecessary authoritarianism. By their nature they can provide the young person with a wide range of educational experience and objects, and act to increase 'discrimination of response'. Opportunities for assessment and early location of disturbance are seen as an advantage of the continual attention to the group's 'collective unconscious'. They are optimistic this may be changed to a 'rational collective consciousness' by the group experience. They stress the importance of the realistic handling of complaints and conflicts with staff remaining honest and straightforward. Tolerance of all feelings, in both young people and staff is essential. A wonderfully concise passage states that unilateral receiving is not healthy for young people, unilateral giving not healthy for the adult and that 'the establishment of a reciprocal relationship is as good an ending to short term therapy as any'.

Yalom (1985), in a chapter on Specialized Therapy Groups, speaks of the demands of some specialised inpatient groups. It is important to assess the clinical situation, being ready to accommodate such variables as turnover (in staff and patients) and heterogeneity of presentation. He sees the formulation of achievable goals for the therapists and patients as crucial. Some basic goals, also echoed in our unit groups, are positive engagement in the therapeutic process, problem spotting, decreased isolation, being helpful to others, the reinforcement of 'talking helps' and the alleviation of hospital related anxiety. Most of these are met in our groups. Our main aims were to increase young person participation and develop social and communication skills. Yalom is very clear on the necessity to modify normal group technique. He stresses the need for greater activity, support and structure within a limited time frame, with an emphasis on here and now issues. He gives an example of a group that is encouraged to develop and review a self determined agenda around issues of communication. However he also warns against excessive therapist control, which risks decreasing spontaneity and the development of autonomy.

In keeping with the original thought about the unit being a 'good enough' unit, there have been times when the groups have slipped into authoritarian mode but also times when the groups have usefully encouraged autonomy and growth. This last is very gratifying but is not necessarily exclusively the function of a particular group format. Rather it is the result of the steady determination of a clinical team to survive the vicissitudes of adolescent unit life. This allows us to remain engaged in an ongoing process and not become too distracted by apparent success or failure. Lastly the resilience, determination and untapped resources of our adolescents needs acknowledging. These factors are made all the more potent when the adolescents begin to interact meaningfully with each other and are taking their own responsibility for their actions and treatment.

References

Bion, W.A., (1967) 'Theory of Thinking' In *Second Thoughts*. London: Maresfield Library (reprinted 1993).

Foulkes, S.H. and Anthony, E.J. (1957) *Group Psychotherapy*. London: Maresfield Library (reprinted 1990).

Main,T. (1989) *The Ailment and other psychoanalytic essays*. London: Free Association Books

Segal, H., (1973) *Introduction to the Works of Melanie Klein*. London: Hogarth Press

Winnicot, D.W. (1960) Ego distortion in terms of true and false self. In *The Maturational Process and the Facilitating Environment*. London: Hogarth Press.

Winnicot, D.W. (1971) Death and Murder in the adolescent process; Contemporary concepts of adolescent development. In *Playing and Reality*. London: Tavistock Publications (reprinted Harmondsworth: Penguin Books 1980).

Yalom, I.D. (1985), *The Theory and Practice of Group Psychotherapy*. New York: Basic Books.

18
Moving groupwork into the day hospital setting

Isaura Manso Neto

Introduction

The psychoanalyst, Frieda Fromm-Reichman, who had great experience in the treatment of schizophrenia, stated in 1958 (Schermer & Pines, 1999): 'a decade was needed to understand the patient; a decade to learn how to enter into a relationship with the patient, and still a third decade to learn how to incorporate group psychotherapy and community therapy into the therapeutic arsenal of these patients'. Over 31 years our therapeutic team have been carrying out the last task outlined by Fromm-Reichman, and this is the subject of this chapter.

A meta-analysis of 18 investigations published between 1957 and 1997 found that psychiatric day hospitals with partial hospitalisation were an effective alternative to inpatient treatment (Horvitz-Lennon et al., 2001). These authors concluded, 'The outcomes of partial hospitalisation patients in these studies were no different from those of inpatients.' They also found that patients and families were more satisfied with this type of provision. Bateman and Fonagy (1999) studied treatment of borderline personality disorder and concluded that partial hospitalisation was effective in relation to decreased suicidality, self-harm, readmission and depression when compared to controls. In 2005, the World Health Organisation (WHO) suggested that partial hospitalisation was a cost-effective alternative to full hospitalisation (Marshall, 2005).

In this chapter I will describe the psychiatric day hospital of the Santa Maria Hospital in Lisbon, where I have been working since its foundation as resident in Psychiatry and as director for the last eleven years. I will describe the objectives, the treatment methods, the patient and staff groups, and the therapeutic elements. I will explore in greater detail the three times a week group psychotherapy and the fortnightly multi-family therapy group. I will conclude by referring to outcome data over the period the unit has been operating.

Background: the Day Hospital of the Psychiatric Service of the Hospital de Santa Maria in Lisbon

The day hospital was set up in 1977 by a group of psychiatrists with group analytic training who were working in the psychiatric department. The aim was to reorganise the existing day hospital into a dynamic facilitating environment (Winnicott, 1965) using a psychoanalytic and group analytic framework (Dinis & al., 1978). As well as treating patients, the unit provides training placements for psychiatrists, child psychiatrists, psychologists, nurses and medical students. Group therapy is the dominant form of therapeutic action.

Patient population

The patients suffer from different disorders and different personality organisations. They show extreme fragility, little cohesion of personality, chronic low self-esteem and disorganised superego functioning. We view these problems as arising from difficulties in very early formative relationships that have resulted in narcissistic deficiencies creating an insufficiently developed sense of self and separation anxiety. Patients' sense of themselves and others is fragmented, and a range of primitive defence mechanisms can be seen, including splitting (idealization and denigration), projection, and projective identification. These patients have difficulty in mentalising (Bateman & Fonagy, 2004) and consequently cannot conceptualise their internal and relational conflicts. They therefore disinvest in themselves and their relationships, leading to profound social difficulties.

Between 1977 and 2008, 1012 patients have passed through the unit. The current average length of day hospital stay is eight months. This day hospital is an alternative to an inpatient psychiatric unit. The only exclusion criteria are severe learning disability, dementia, severe confusional states and severe agitation. The focus is on younger acutely unwell patients with an average age of 30 although the age range is between 18 and 65. Young people between ages 13 and 17 were also admitted until 2001, when specialist adolescent units were created. The sources of patient referrals are shown in Table 1. The unit's capacity and proportions of different diagnoses have varied over time but the approximate proportions of the different diagnoses seen are shown in Table 2. The employment status of patients is shown in Table 3.

Table 1
Referral source (%)

Outpatient departments	48
Psychiatric inpatient dept	22
Medical / surgical wards	5
Accident and Emergency	5
Other	20

Table 2
Proportions of patients with different diagnoses between 1977 and 2008 (ICD – 10 diagnostic criteria)

	Range (%)
Schizophrenia, schizotypal and delusional disorders	26 - 38
Mood (affective) disorders	40 - 50
Neurotic, stress related and somatoform disorders	15 - 20
Behavioural syndromes associated with physiological disturbances and physical factors	4 - 10
Disorders of adult personality and behaviour	40 - 50
Multiple diagnoses	50 - 60

Table 3
Employment status

	Range (%)
Unemployed	21 - 30
Employed	28 - 36
Student	20 - 25

The staff team

The senior staff team at present consists of two psychiatrists, two psychologists and a nurse, each of whom have a psychoanalytic or group analytic training. These constitute the central nucleus of the staff team. There are in addition between two and five trainees from the four core professions including psychiatrists, child psychiatrists, psychologists and nurses, as well as 100 medical students in the last five years. The functioning of the staff team as a group is highly significant. Although it is not a therapeutic group, the way the group functions has similarities with the way a group analytic group functions (Neto & Centeno, 2005). Junior staff members find this group functioning of great importance in their learning and development (Neto et al,

2008). Furthermore, despite the fact that it is not a therapeutic group, since in staff meetings there are no interventions of an interpretative nature explicitly directed to the trainees, the group favours questioning and stimulates curiosity by presenting different perspectives of the same observed reality. The atmosphere is one of freedom, spontaneity and mutual respect, promoting 'psychic development and growth' in trainees as revealed in their responses to a survey about the impact of this day hospital on their training (Neto et al, 2008).

The team leader and senior staff essentially have the function of listening, facilitating discussing, elaborating and synthesising complex information. Teamwork implies a constant confrontation with difference. After exploration, decisions are largely reached by consensus rather than being hierarchically imposed and are based on a profound respect for the opinions of each member. They are often reached on the basis of new views, which are convincing to everyone because of their clarity. These characteristics of the staff group create a pleasure in learning and contribute to the personal growth of the trainees beyond their original expectations (Abercrombie, 1974).

The nature of the team's pattern resides in the personalities of its members as well as in the team's knowledge, culture and cohesiveness. We aim to promote an empathic attitude, to understand patients' communications, and to increase insight. Authenticity is important in the treatment of any form of psychiatric problems but especially so with severe psychotic patients (Neto, 2002; Resnick, 2005). Reliability, continuity, and capacity for integration are the key staff attributes. We convey the unit's culture and tradition to new members through shoulder-to-shoulder work, training and supervision.

The objective of our pattern is twofold:

1. Create an institutional matrix in which it is possible to act on the 'personal group matrices (Leal, 1983) of the patients in order to promote cure or symptom reduction, restore the personality's equilibrium as far as possible, or still, introduce more profound alterations in the psychic structures that enable qualitative modifications, which will be pursued in other therapeutic settings in the community.
2. Provide undergraduate and postgraduate training.

Therapeutic activities

Direct patient work

This comprises the admission interview, group analytic therapy, family interventions (family interviews, parents group, parents psychotherapy, multifamily group), individual psychotherapy, medication group, mind-body intervention therapy (gymnastics, dance), recreational and creative activities, daily living activities, the social skills group, theatre group, cinematherapy, and a news discussion group. I will describe some of these and the group analytic therapy and family groups in more detail.

Admission interviews

A two-hour admission interview is carried out by a senior staff member with the patient and family members, in the presence of the whole staff team, followed by a staff discussion of diagnosis, psychodynamic formulation and planning. This is a crucial moment for the establishment of the therapeutic alliance with patients and their families.

Group analytic psychotherapy

This takes place three times a week, each session lasting for 90 minutes. The whole patient and staff group are present and a senior staff member conducts the sessions, thus providing continuity. Given an average stay of eight months, these groups can be described as 'slow-open' (Foulkes & Anthony, 1957). Following Neto (1989, 2001), and Neto and Centeno, (2005) the objectives are:

1. For patients to experience and express their feelings in relation to each other, to staff and to the institution, thereby promoting mentalisation (Bateman & Fonagy, 2004) and the working-through. These are initially experienced in relation to the group matrix and are later extrapolated to relationships outside the hospital.
2. Guilt and shame play a key role in many patients' difficulties, and these are reduced by patients discovering that others suffer from these feelings and similarities emerging between clusters of members in the group. Belonging to a group creates a 'structuring fellowship', which Patrick de Maré (1991) named 'Koinonia'. He describes an atmosphere of friendliness as opposed to individual friendships, of spiritual and humanising participation where people can speak, hear, see, and think freely. Togetherness and friendliness creates a pooling of resources that stimulates each participant's personal resources.

Example 1:

L., a 21-year-old man with a borderline personality, was complaining of feeling lonely. He said that he could not tell the doctor about the horrible ideas that were constantly assailing him. The *group conductor* said he was not alone, and it seemed like he was afraid that we would not understand if he were to say more about what he felt and thought.

L. looked at each person in silence, then said that he would try. He then described his fear of having sexual intercourse with his mother: 'She does everything else for me. If I ask her for this too, she might agree. My mother used to caress me and I felt she desired me sexually.'

Some older female patients indignantly remarked that L. was confused. They said that he was unwell and had misinterpreted his mother's normal affection. They spoke about their relationships with their own children.

A *co-therapist* remarked that incest does sometimes happen. The *female patients* maintained their position, saying, 'Those people are ill!'

The *group conductor* said as children, boys usually want to be like their father and girls want to be like their mother: 'Perhaps, we can all remember being alone with our father or with our mother, and wanting to be more capable and interesting than the parent who wasn't there. Whereas, in fact, reality was that this other parent was the grown-up who we most needed and admired.'

Several patients responded with their associations:

S. (young woman): 'I once told my mother to go away. I told her that she was useless and that my father and I could live together happily without her' (she smiled.)

L.: 'Once when I was very small I put the latch on the door to keep my father out. I never told my mother!'

Some patients reacted with relief whilst others became tense.

L.: 'That's it - these are fantasies that I have! It doesn't mean that they will come true, they are just in my head.' He pauses: 'I feel relieved. Saying all this in front of this many people is just a huge relief. There are days that I feel so well when I'm here in the group.'

Salomon Resnick (2005) points out: 'Such misunderstandings, in which affection becomes confused with erotic feelings, play an important role in the pathological development of children and perhaps in the emergence of a psychosis.' During 31 years in the unit we have learned that such misunderstandings are prevalent in our patients and their parents:

+ The activation of mirroring (Foulkes & Anthony, 1957; Pines, 1983; Neto, 2002). This involves patients hearing others talking about experiences that they themselves have had. This stimulates structuring identifications which refer to the development of a stronger sense of identity and hence the development of ambitions, ideals, self-esteem and autonomy. Once worked through, the 'malignant mirroring' (Zinkin, 1983) that arises when the patients operate largely using projection and pathological projective identification is corrected.

+ Increased awareness of previously unconscious aggressive feelings and some expression of these feelings. This can often occur more easily in the group than in individual sessions where the idealisation of the therapist and fear of retaliation inhibits the expression of hostility. The identification of aggressiveness and eventual interpretation by another group member or a group conductor can be easier to hear in the group.

+ The expression of love and hate without destroying or being destroyed, which can be of great relief (Neto, 1999a).

+ The transformation of symptoms and behaviour into words expressing conscious feelings and ideas (Cortesão, 1989). This leads to a gradual abandonment of the language of symptoms to express the formative experiences, which have been enacted in the group.

There follows three examples of interchanges in the group where patients were able to explore and express hitherto unconscious feelings.

Example 2:

In this example the importance of the patients' answers and actions towards each other can be seen. The patients responded empathically and rationally to each other, showing that they had internalised the containing function previously carried out by the staff:

R., a patient with paranoid schizophrenia enters the group and starts showing muscle spasms in his legs (a potential side-effect of certain antipsychotic medications) twisting his neck and arching his spine. Another young patient, *C.*, also suffering from schizophrenia, says, 'R.! Look at me. Put your feet on the floor and the pain will go away. Keep looking at me!' *R.* responded by trying to straighten his body and there was a silence, laden with emotion. *C.* continued: 'I sometimes feel like giving up the treatment and going back to normal life.'

R.: 'Everyone is looking at me. They want to hurt me. I must leave behind my hatred, pride and excessive ambition.'

C.: 'We all have to go through treatment, take our medication and come to this group. But you are stronger than me.' She speaks of her own suspicious thoughts: 'Even now I feel I am under surveillance and I'm being controlled.'

R.: 'The problem is my spirit. This treatment should be spiritual, not medical.'

Female patient, *H.:* 'I used to hate everyone. I'm still suspicious about their feelings, but now I know that my problems have a psychological cause and not a spiritual one. Now I feel I've got more people on my side.'

There is a pause, and then the *main conductor* says: 'We are all on your side R.'

The session ends with the *group* saying goodbye to the trainee nurses, to whom we were all very attached. *R.* showed that he was finally capable of mentalising and expressing the separation anxieties which we felt he had expressed earlier with his physical symptoms. Attentive and tranquil, *R.* says that he will be sorry he will not see the trainees next day.

Example 3:

Some of the patients had mounted an insurrection against some of the rules of the unit. In this context, several patients had been describing their anger towards their parents for what they did to them in their childhoods.

M., who is suffering from agoraphobia: 'I was annoyed but I felt I had to cover it up. I didn't want anyone to know when I was feeling low.' He complains about a recent phone call from his father; 'He only makes demands on me. He never understands me', and he also complains about his mother who is so inconsistent. *Several others* complain about their parents' lack of understanding in the past and present.

Two psychotic patients try to defend themselves against feeling rejected by their parents by displacing their anger onto staff for not supplying free coffee, and by getting angry with each other.

G., who had been suffering from anorexia and was near to discharge, said, 'You probably feel misunderstood but you think that being understood means being given what you need. We need money, but perhaps, it is more important to feel that we are loved.'

Example 4:

All the nurses were absent from the unit. A complaint arose about the poor quality of food which was variously described as tasteless, unspiced, cold etc, a theme that regularly crops up when patients feel frustrated and deprived.

After a time the *group conductor* interprets that the complaints are caused by anger at being abandoned by the nurses, who are maternal figures. This enabled the *patients* to start talking about their experiences of abandonment.

At times, the aggressive feelings expressed by members of the group towards the institution and the staff group enables the nature of individuals' internal object relations to be seen with great clarity. This especially occurs around holidays, long week-ends, discharges, and when new members join the unit.

Group analytic techniques and concepts

Individual patients and groups of patients communicate their experiences in the group on several different levels (Cortesão, 1974). These experiences are either expressed spontaneously or staff draw attention to what is going on when they feel that tensions reflecting unconscious feelings are being ignored. Some of these unconscious feelings can be difficult to mobilise, because patients resist this process of allowing their unconscious feelings, memories and conflicts, to become conscious. The therapists aim to help patients to mentalise their feelings and conflicts, in other words step back and think about them. This is done by reframing verbal and non-verbal communications to take into account hidden meanings. Members of the group are encouraged to share their opinions about other patients who are largely communicating non-verbally, and to say what these intense expressions could reflect about these patients' earlier experiences. The therapists occasionally make transference and extra-transference interpretations (Thomä & Kächele, 1989; Wallerstein, 1995) about the origins of patient's difficulties but only when this is not too intrusive. At times we offer interpretations of dreams, after hearing the dreamer's own associations and those of other group members (Neto, 2006). When acting-out becomes too destructive we draw the patients' attention to the reality, in the form of the unit's rules. This commonly happens when there are several borderline patients on the unit. In general, the group therapist takes a more active stance than in classical group analysis, preventing long persecutory silences. Therapists must also be particularly sensitive to the dangers and impact of painful narcissistic wounds and not leave patients without recognising them in their suffering, commenting, verbalizing empathically on what has taken place.

The parents group and the multifamily group

Most of our patients come from dysfunctional families characterised by symbiotic attachment patterns (Searles, 1966) and poor differentiation between generations. Separation and individuation are a source of anguish and so are evaded. The parents do not treat the children as separate individuals but rather as extensions of themselves, becoming as Kohut (1984) puts it, their parents' 'self-objects'. Neto (1997) describes children also becoming 'displacement objects' of relational figures with whom they had established 'pathological and pathogenic interdependencies' (Badaracco, 1986, 1990), most commonly these figures being their parents. Communication within such families is often of the paradoxical or double-bind variety, obstructing the ability of the children to develop a strong sense of self and to develop their own resourcefulness. As so many of our patients are highly dependent on their parents, family work is a vital component of the work. Without it, there is a danger of parents undermining the treatment (Neto, 1997).

For work with parents to be successful, the parents need to feel understood. Where possible we attempt to reduce some of the more pathological patterns of relationships operating within the family. We do this by avoiding being judgemental, blaming or morally superior, and instead view difficulties as passed down through earlier generations.

We have run parents groups and worked with individual families for several years (Neto, 1996). In 2001, we started a multi-family psychoanalytic group for patients and their parents using Jorge Garcia Badaracco's model (Bararacco, 2000). The group allows us to quickly and clearly identify parents' unhelpful patterns of relating to their children. We commonly find a lack of empathy, paradoxical communication, and hidden or expressed conflict between the parental couples (Centeno et al, 2001). Badaracco (1986) refers to these various aspects as patients' 'psychological heritage', which we have found to be an apt phrase. The recurrent themes which spontaneously occur are dependency-autonomy, separation difficulties, parent-children conflict, issues of control, and conflict between the parents (Neto & Centeno, 2003).

Parents typically start by complaining about their children. They compare them unfavourably to themselves, stressing the efforts that they have taken on their children's behalf. There is little acknowledgement of any responsibility for their children's problems; they are healthy whilst their children are ill. At this stage, the patients remain largely silent whilst the parents sympathise with each other. To move things on, the group conductors actively intervene to help the patients express their views. Over time, themes emerge in the descriptions of several families, and in the safe environment of the group a capacity to think and communicate becomes possible. Mirroring enables individuals to see and understand the psychological defences that are operating. The revelation of similarities, differences, and contradictions progressively help create new 'cross-identifications' (Balduz & Atienza, 2003; Godinho & al, 2006) between parents and patients in different families. This leads to a route out of symbiotic relations towards psychic change. Similarities, differences, and contradictions can be revelatory and the parents can become more aware of their children's real difficulties. Accusation and devaluation lessen and are replaced by more tolerant attitudes. The parents can start to recognise previously denied conflicts and this can be transformational. Reparative emotional experiences can take place in the group and this enables patients to start expressing themselves more freely and creatively. It is not uncommon for intense anger and rage to be expressed, but gradually it becomes possible to bear the guilt at what has been done in the past, and both parents and children are increasingly able to empathise with each other.

Other family interventions

In certain moments in patients' development, individual family sessions can be helpful. The patients' individual therapist is present as well some other members of the team. The therapist functions as an auxiliary ego, protecting the patient from excessive hostility and trying to prevent the repetition of the usual patterns of communication, and promoting its transformation. Sometimes family members request individual help and can be referred on for outpatient group psychotherapy or individual work.

In the course of the family interventions, we attempt to facilitate parents' own abilities to mentalise about themselves and their children. Progressively, patterns of interactions become less rigid. They become aware of their own aggressiveness and are often able to see its origin in their own backgrounds. Destructive projective functioning is reduced (Neto, 1997).

In the course of these interventions, by means of the parents' empathic listening, we attempt to facilitate their narcissistic restructuring, which will lead to the enhancement of their ability to mentalise and fantasize about themselves and about their ill children, thus recovering or stimulating the alpha function (Bion, 1959). Progressively, the behaviour and the interactions that they establish become less rigid and more thinkable. The aggressiveness also becomes more conscious and its origins understood - the oppressive and repressed past – the disturbed relation with their own progenitors. Progressively, the denied projective functioning that is violently pathogenic and destructive is lessened and lost (Neto, 1997).

Weekly individual psychotherapy

Every patient is seen for one hour of individual psychotherapy with the aim of promoting mentalisation, verbalisation, developing an ability to connect current here-and-now events with past experiences, identifying relational patterns and pathological behaviour, and strengthening of the patient's ego resources to allow the development of healthier relationships. The therapists receive supervision on each individual session, discussed below.

Weekly medication group

This group is conducted by a senior psychiatrist and attended by all patients, doctors and nurses. The doctors use the group to prescribe medication and monitor compliance and side-effects. The free discussion and sharing of common problems associated with medication allows embarrassing or anxiety provoking themes to be broached. These are mainly of a sexual nature, as well as weight management. The discussion decreases associated fears, guilt and shame and promotes a more informed and participatory involvement in the management of the medication by patients.

Staff supervision and reflection

These are the spaces where, in the absence of patients, staff can share information and concerns, reflect on their counter-transference reactions to patients, and synthesise information about patients from different contexts in order to develop formulations. These reflective spaces aid the continuity of staff members' interest and investment in their patients, as well as the continuous training of the staff. We have tried to make these settings in which one can develop the capacity to learn with pleasure (Szcecsödy, 1997).

Weekly clinical meeting

The weekly clinical meeting is at least two hours and usually four hours whenever we have our maximum capacity of 22 patients. Each patient is discussed but with more time spent on those for whom there are particular problems. The objective is to enable a differentiated and coherent therapeutic approach to each patient. We reflect on the institutional realities of the unit, and try to understand and eventually solve the problems relating to each patient as they arise. These inevitably concern counter-transference responses. Usually the nurses begin by relaying the concrete difficulties that have occurred that week that have not been cleared up through informal conversations or in the therapeutic groups. The opinions of all staff are heard, regardless of how much direct contact with the patient they have had. Usually the problems centre on the patient's psychopathology, or the staff's reactions to the patient, or both. Generally the difficulties and the conflicts can be cleared up in a satisfactory manner by understanding what is going on in terms of the patient's mental functioning and by the clarifying how this relates to staff's reactions to them.

Debrief and supervision of group psychotherapy and multi-family groups

Each psychotherapeutic group and multifamily group is followed by a 40-minute staff discussion. Hochman (1986), in a paper about the relations between psychoanalysis and institutional psychotherapy, emphasises the importance of therapists containing patients' experiences by processing them to transform them into something meaningful, and then communicating their understandings back to the patients. That they are also important for staff, can be seen in the anticipatory pleasure of the discussion with colleagues about what has been happening in the sessions. A written register is made of the main phenomena consciously communicated and our ideas about hidden or unconscious processes. In this way we try to deepen our understanding of each patient and their family, as well as tracking their development and evaluating the impact of the staffs' individual therapeutic work. The staff discussion is one of the team's 'detoxifying' tools (Neto, 2001; Neto & Centeno, 2005). The atmosphere of free expression, humour, and the sharing of fantasies, which would be anti-therapeutic if expressed elsewhere favours the relief of tension

Supervision

Supervision is an immediate need for those who work in mental health. It is all the more pressing whenever the patients are more disturbed, and when the psychotherapist is more inexperienced or struggling (Neto, 1999b). Supervision is not treatment, however, it is a means of growth for the psychotherapist, facilitated by the supervisor's attitude, which should essentially be that of teaching how to think (Grinberg, 1997), consider other perspectives on the patient and the countertransference, in such a manner that induces creativity and autonomy in the therapist. In addition to the individual supervision of each session of individual therapy we have a two-hour weekly supervision group for staff in training to share experiences.

Co-therapy

We consider the working of the team as co-therapy and this constitutes one of the advantages of working in an institution, with direct benefits for the patients and trainees. Co-therapy provides a triangular situation that enables the patient to escape pathogenic relationships. Co-therapy of the groups also facilitates a degree of supervisory control. By bringing out diverse contributions and perspectives, more correct and complete interventions and interpretations are engendered. There is also a reduction of the counter-transferential burden on one therapist. Co-therapy offers a space for psychic detoxification that facilitates the return to the patient, with greater knowledge and greater affective availability.

Trainees' experiences of the unit

The findings of a survey of pre- and post-graduate trainees on placement from adult and child psychiatry, nursing and psychology backgrounds over three decades were that trainees of each discipline rated the experience highly (Neto & al, 2008). Group psychotherapy was the most valued activity followed by the multi-family group and team meetings.

Outcome data

Over the 31 years of the unit's operation we have carried out several follow-up studies. Space does not allow these to be described in detail, but the results are encouraging. These include high rates of remission of symptoms and improved social and employment functioning (Fialho, 2007). Relapse rates for eating disorders were low at 2-15 year follow-up (Godinho et al, 1994). There is good outcome for the treatment of schizophreniform disorders (Neto et al, 1997) and personality disorders (Neto et al, 2000).

Summary and conclusions

Over the 31 years of its operation a total of 1012 patients have passed through the unit. Our clinical experiences and outcome data show that the unit performs as an effective environment for the treatment of severe and acute patients. It is a viable alternative to full hospitalisation as well as providing therapeutic training for a range of professions. The psychoanalytic and group analytic model is at the heart of the approach. We ensure that patients' and their families' experiences are predominantly positive and these are often transformative. Compliance is good and dropout rates are low. There are statistically significant improvements in symptom-reduction, social functioning and occupational re-adaptation. We find low mortality rates both during hospitalisation and on follow-up. We would like to especially emphasize the importance of the multifamily group as an aid to early diagnosis and formulation, and the benefits of working with patients and families together. This also promotes treatment compliance as well as post-discharge adaptation. Together, these various elements allow us to treat severely unwell patients in the relatively short period of eight months. The success of the unit in its task of training the next generation of mental health professionals results from the team's cohesiveness, the clarity of its model, and the culture of group discussion. Our experience has enabled us to combat early incapacitation and prolonged sick leave. This has made us question the commonly held belief that psychiatric patients' problems are inevitably chronic and recurrent. Furthermore, we believe that through narcissistic restructuring, and transformation of the object relations, the likelihood of future relapse is reduced and positive mental health is engendered, thereby breaking the transmission of mental health problems to future generations.

References

Abercrombie, M.L.J. (1974). *Aims and Techniques of Group Teaching.* Society for Research into Higher Education Ltd, 3rd Edition, Guildford: University of Surrey.

Badaracco, J.G. (1986). Identification and its vicissitudes in the psychoses. The importance of the concept of the 'Maddening Object'. *International Journal of Psycho-Analysis,* 67: 133-146.

Badaracco, J.G. (1990). *Comunidad Terapéutica Psicoanalítica de Estrutura multifamiliar.* Madrid: Tipublicaciones.

Badaracco, J.G. (2000). *Psicoanálisis Multifamiliar, Los Otros en Nosotros y el Descubrimiento del sí Mismo.* Buenos Aires: Paidós.

Balduz, J. M. and Atienza, J. L. (2003) - El grupo multifamiliar: un espacio sociomental, Avances en Salud Mental Relacional, 2, no.1 *in* Coderch, J. (1995) -Psicoanálisis-Fundamentos y teoría de la técnica. Barcelona: Editorial Herder

Bateman, A. and Fonagy, P. (1999). Effectiveness of partial hospitalization in the treatment of borderline personality disorder: a randomized controlled trial. *American Journal of Psychiatry*, 156: 1563-1569.

Bateman, A. and Fonagy, P. (2004). *Psychotherapy for Borderline Personality Disorders: Mentalisation- based treatment.* New York: Oxford University Press

Centeno, M.J., Neto, I.M. and Fialho, T. (2001). A Multifamiliar Group at a Psychiatric Day Hospital – a Groupanalytic Experience. *Regional Mediterranean Conference of the International Association of Group Psychotherapy - 'New Integration, Partnerships and Applications'.* Workshop. Croatia, Zadar, 28th – 1st de September de 2001.

Cortesão, E.L. (1974). Transference neurosis and the groupanalytic process. *Group-Analysis*, 7, 20-22.

Cortesão, E.L. (1989). *Grupanálise – Teoria e Técnica.* Lisboa: Fundação Calouste Gulbenkian.

de Maré, P., Piper, R. and Thompson, S (1991). Koinonia, In *Koinonia – from Hate, through Dialogue, to Culture in the Large Group.* London: Karnac.

Dinis, C.V., França De Sousa, J., Ferro, S., Sampaio, D. Cardoso, G. and Fazenda, I.,(1978). Hospital de Dia de Santa Maria entre Maio de1977 e Outubro de 1978. *VII Congresso Mundial de Psiquiatria Social.* Lisbon: Conference paper.

Fialho, T. (2007). O Hospital de Dia do Hospital de Santa Maria entre 2001 e 2006. *V Encontro Nacional de Hospitais de Dia*, Lisboa, Hospital de Júlio de Matos, 19 de Abril 2007 . Lisbon: conference paper.

Foulkes, S.H. and Anthony E.J. (1957). *Group-Analytic Psychotherapy – The Psychoanalytic Approach.* Harmondsworth: Penguin.

Godinho, P., Neto, I.M., Ferro, S., Camilo, E., Carvalho, G., Dinis, C. V. and de Sousa, J.F.(1994). The outcome of anorexia nervosa after day hospital treatment (some trends). *Simpósio Regional Europeu da World Psychiatric Association (W.P.A.).* Poster. Estoril, 10 a 14 de Julho de 1994. Estoril: poster presentation.

Godinho, P., Centeno, M.J., Fialho, T. and Neto, I.M. (2006). The multifamily group as a magnetic resonance of Psychiatry: Observing, treating and training. *15th International Symposium for the Psychotherapy of Schizophrenia and other Psychosis.* Madrid, 11-16 June. Madrid: conference paper.

Grinberg, L. (1997). On Transference and Countertransference and the Technique of Supervision, In *Supervision and its Vicissitudes,*: B. Martindale, M. Morner, R., M.E.C. & J.P.Vidit (Eds.) EFPP Clinical Monograph Series – London : Karnac.

Hochman, J. (1986). Un Point de Vue sur les Rapports de La Psychanalyse et de la Thérapie institutionelle d'aujourd'hui. *Confrontations Psychiatriques, n.* 26, 65-77.

Horvitz-Lennon, M., Normand, S-L.T., Gaccione, M.A. & Frank, R.G. (2001) Partial versus full hospitalization for adults in psychiatric distress: A systematic review of the published literature (1957-1997). *American Journal of Psychiatry 158*, 5, 676-685.

ICD -10 (1992) International Classification Diseases – Classification of Mental and Behavioural disorders), Geneva: WHO, PG.364.

Kohut, H. (1984). How does analysis cure? In P. Stepansky and A. Goldberg (eds.), *Kohut's Legacy: Contributions to Self Psychology*. Chicago and London: University of Chicago Press.

Leal, M. R. M (1983). Why group analysis works? In Malcolm Pines (Ed.) '*The Evolution of Group Analysis*, London: Jessica Kingsley.

Marshall, M. (2005). *How effective are different types of day care services for people with severe mental disorders*. Copenhagen, WHO Regional Office for Europe (Health Evidence Network report; http://www.euro.who.int/Document/E87317.pdf accessed May 2009.

Neto, I.M. (1989). Grupanálise e Instituição, *I Encontro Nacional de Grupanálise*. Lisboa, Maio de 1989. Lisbon: conference paper.

Neto, I.M. (1996). Empathic failure: one of the most destructive forms of mental functioning. *10th. European symposium in Group Analysis 'Destruction and Desire'*. Copenhagen: conference paper.

Neto, I.M. (1997). Inter and Transgenerational Transmission of Psychopathology, *12th International Symposium for the Psychotherapy of Schizophrenia and other Psychosis (ISPS)*. London: conference paper.

Neto, I.M. (1999a). The Freedom and the Capacity to say NO and its healing potential, *II EFPP European Conference on Group Psychoanalytic Psychotherapy*. Barcelona, 28 - 29- 30 de Mayo de 1999. Barcleona: conference paper.

Neto, I.M. (1999b). A Supervisão – Outra Visão Sobre Os Pacientes, O Grupanalista e o Supervisor – Um Caminho Para O Inconsciente, *V Encontro Luso-Brasileiro de Grupanálise e Psicoterapia Analítica de Grupo/X Congresso Brasileiro de Grupanálise e de Psicoterapia Analítica de Grup*. Rio de Janeiro, 12-14 de Novembro de 1999. Rio de Janiero: conference paper.

Neto, I.M. (2001). Groups in the Institution: Where? When? To Whom? Why? How? *Regional Mediterranean Conference of the International Association of Group Psychotherapy*. Croácia, Zadar, 29 de Agosto a 1 de Setembro de 2001. Zadar: conference paper.

Neto, I.M. (2002). To see and be seen: one of the 'added values' of Group Analysis. *12 th. European Symposium in Group Analysis 'The Economy of the group: The emergence of relational goods in society, mind and brain'*. Bologna: conference paper.

Neto, I.M. (2006). The Clinical Applications of Dreams, *2º Mestrado em Ciências do Sono 'How and Why we dream'*. Workshop. ISPA. Lisbon 28 de Abril 2006. Lisbon: conference paper.

Neto, I.M., Casado, E., Abreu, M., Barbosa, A. and Dinis, C. (1997). Psychotherapeutic approach and follow-up of Schizophrenic Psychosis in a Psychiatric day Hospital of a general Hospital, *12th. International Symposium for the Psychotherapy of Schizophrenia and other Psychosis (ISPS)*. Poster. London.

Neto, I.M., Casado, E., Barbosa, A. and Dinis, C. (2000). Schizophrenia and Personality Disorders, a Comparative Follow-up Study. *13th International Symposium for the*

Psychotherapy of Schizophrenia and other Psychosis (ISPS). Poster. Norway, Stavanger, 5-8th July 2000.

Neto, I.M. and Centeno, M.J. (2003). Crossing Generations, Through An Institutional Psychoanalytical Group Psychotherapy – A Multifamiliar Group Psychotherapy, *15th International Congress of the IAGP, 'Crossroads of Culture: Where Groups Converge'.* Workshop. Istanbul, August 2003. Istanbul: conference paper.

Neto, I.M. and Centeno, M. J. (2005). Group analysis within a Psychiatric Day Hospital- To Treat Patients and Train the Team/Treating and Training. *13th European Symposium in Group Analysis, 'Between Matrix And Manuals Contemporary Challenges In Group Analysis'.* Workshop. Norway, Molde, 8-13 August.

Neto ,I.M., Fialho,T., Godinho, P. and Centeno, M. J. (2008). Treating and Training - a 30 Years experience of a Team with a group-analytic frame-work. *Jane Abercrombie Prize 2008* award, attributed by GAS- London. 14th. Symp. Group Analysis, Dublin, August 2008. Dublin: conference paper.

Pines, M. (1983). Reflexions on mirroring. *Group Analysis, 15,* supplement: 1-32.

Resnick, S. (2005). *Glacial Times: A Journey Through the World of Madness.* London: Routledge.

Searles, H.F., (1966). *Collected Papers on Schizophrenia and Related Subjects,* Ed. London: Hogarth, International Universities Press.

Schermer,V.L.and Pines, M. (1999). Introduction: Reality and Relationship in 'Psyche's Web'. In *Group Psychotherapy of the Psychoses: Concepts, Interventions and Contexts.* Victor L. Schermer and Malcolm Pines (Eds.). London: Jessica Kingsley.

Szecsödy, I. (1997). (How) is learning possible in supervision? In *Supervision and its Vicissitudes, EFPP Clinical Monograph Series.* Eds. Brian Martindale, Margareta Mörner, Maria Eugenia Cid Rodríguez, Jean-Pierre Vidit. Chapter seven: 101-116.

Thomä, H., Kächele, H. (1989) Transferencia como repetición. In *Teoria y práctica del psicoanálisis – I – Fundamentos.* Barcelona: Herder.

Wallerstein, R. S.(1995). The transference, Transference Interpretation and the Transference Neurosis. In chapter three, *The Talking Cures: Psychoanalyses and the Psychotherapies.* New Haven and London: Yale University Press.

Winnicott, D.W. (1965) *The Maturational Process and the Facilitating Environment.* London: Karnac.

Zinkin, L. (1983) 'Malignant mirroring'. *Group Analysis,* 16:113-26.

About the contributors

Jerome Carson, BA(Hons), MSc., PhD, C. Psychol., is Consultant Clinical Psychologist. Jerome works in a community mental health team which is part of the South London and Maudsley NHS Foundation Trust. He has spent his entire career in the adult mental health field. He has co-edited three books, written one self-help guide, and over 100 journal papers or book chapters. His current interests are in recovery and positive psychology. He is on the editorial board of the journal *Groupwork.* E-Mail: Jerome.Carson@slam.nhs.uk

Debora Diamond, PsychD, Psychotherapeutic and Counselling Psychology Consultant, Counselling Psychologist, Joint Lead of Acute Care and Recovery Services at Plymouth Teaching Primary Care Trust. Debora is a trained supervisor and practitioner of CBT for psychosis and works in a Low Secure Male Recovery Unit, a female only open unit and on an inpatient ward. Her special interests are groupwork, treatment of severe and enduring mental illness and complex trauma, particularly in relation to those labelled with a personality disorder. E-Mail: Debora. Diamond@plymouth.nhs.uk

Richard Duggins, BA (Hons), MBBS, MMedSci, MRCPsych, NEAPP, is Consultant Psychiatrist in Psychotherapy who works in the Regional Department of Psychotherapy in Newcastle upon Tyne. Richard is qualified as a psychoanalytic psychotherapist as well as a general adult psychiatrist, and has previously worked in acute wards, a therapeutic community, a high secure hospital and community mental health teams. He has published three chapters and two journal papers. His special interests are creating therapeutic environments, and tackling psychological stress in health professionals. He is a member of the National Advisory Group for Doctors' Health. E-Mail: richard.duggins@ntw.nhs.uk

Chris Evans, MRCPsych, MSc, Mem.Inst.GroupAnalysis, is a Medical Psychotherapist in the Nottinghamshire Personality Disorder and Development Network. He holds a personal chair at Nottingham University and responsibilities as Clinical Director for Psychological Therapies and Trust Research Governance Lead.

He has 25 years psychotherapy experience, group analytic and systemic trainings, authored over 140 publications including over 80 peer-reviewed papers but is particularly proud to be a parent of the CORE outcome measures project (www.coreims. co.uk) and the Art Therapy Practice Network (http://www.baat.org/atprn.html) and to be still involved in both projects which aim to bridge the researcher/practitioner gap. E-Mail: chris@psyctc.org

Leonard Fagin, Méd (Arg) FRCPsych., is Consultant Adult Psychiatrist and Honorary Senior Lecturer. After a 34 year career in the NHS, working in in-patient and community settings, Dr Fagin is currently associated with the Anna Freud Centre and Haringey Social Services dealing with parental mental health issues, and with London Metropolitan University dealing with student mental health problems, as well as privately offering psychiatric support to psychotherapists. He is a Lord Chancellor's Medical Visitor and a Second Opinion Appointed Doctor for the Mental Health Act Commission. Leonard has authored or co-edited three books, and over 100 articles and book chapters. He has lectured widely in the UK and abroad. E-Mail: lfagin@ blueyonder.co.uk

Alistair L. Grandison, MB.Ch.B., MSc, MRCPsych, is an Associate Specialist in Psychiatry and has worked for twelve years for South London and Maudsley NHS Trust on John Dickson Ward, which is an acute admission ward at Guy's Hospital. E-Mail: Alistair.Grandison@slam.nhs.uk

Susan Grey, BA, MPhil, PhD. C.Psychol. is Consultant Clinical Psychologist at King's College and the Maudsley Hospital, London. Susan works partly in a community adult mental health team and partly on a research team investigating therapeutic interventions in acute psychiatric wards. She has worked in various areas of adult mental health, and published papers on topics including, anxiety, addictions, and service development. She was previously editor of the Journal of Mental Health. Current interests include cognitive bias in anxiety and treatment for psychosis. E-Mail: S.Grey@iop.kcl.ac.uk

Dylan Griffiths, MB,BS, MRCPsych (London), is a Consultant Adolescent Psychiatrist at The Priory, Ticehurst House. He is also a supervisor and lecturer for the Lincoln Centre for Psychotherapy. Dylan worked as a consultant in Child and Adolescent Psychiatry since 1983 - initially in a community Child and Adolescent Mental Health Service. For the last thirteen years he has worked in adolescent inpatient care while continuing outpatient work. He qualified as a psychoanalyst in 1991 and conducts a separate psychoanalytic practice. He has a commitment to applying a psychoanalytic frame of reference in his practice and a special interest in borderline and psychotic presentations. E-Mail: dylan.griffiths@btopenworld.com

Katja Hajek, PhD, AFBPsS, is Consultant Clinical Psychologist and Psychology Lead for Adult Acute Inpatient wards in Lambeth; part of the South London and Maudsley NHS Foundation Trust. She has run inpatient groups for over fifteen years and has trained and supervised other staff in running interpersonal groups. Katja has contributed to teaching group therapy on the Institute of Psychiatry clinical psychology doctoral training course. She has also devised and run training courses for inpatient staff in SLAM. Her main interests are inpatient group therapy and staff training. E-Mail: katja.hajek@slam.nhs.uk

Bob Harris, Cert Ed., Mem.Inst.GroupAnalysis, is an Independent Consultant Group Analyst and Psychotherapist. For over twenty years Bob has been working in the NHS and a wide variety of therapeutic environments as consultant, clinical supervisor, clinician and trainer. He has held a number of professional positions,including Director of Programmes at the Institute of Group Analysis,London; Group analyst at the London School of Economics and is Clinical Supervisor and trainer at Denbridge House NHS Eating Disorders Unit. He is currently Clinical Supervisor to Newham Arts Therapy Service, City and Hackney Alcohol Service and the Drug and Alcohol Foundation. He is Consultant and trainer to Personality Disorder services and is a regular conference speaker and writer. He has a special interest in group work with psychosis and severe sychopathologies and currently teaches on the Russian training in Group Analysis in St Petersburg.
E-Mail: Bob.1000@yahoo.com

Torben Heinskou, M.D., is Group Analytic Psychotherapist (Institute of Group Analysis) and Consultant Psychiatrist. He is the Head of Outpatient Clinic of the Psychotherapeutic Center Stolpegaard, Gentofte, Mental Health Services, The Capital Region, Denmark. Torben has been working in adult and adolescent mental health throughout his career. He has co-edited two books and has written numerous papers and book chapters as well as setting up many educational activities in psychotherapy, milieu therapy and organizational psychology. He is on the board of Institute of Group Analysis, Copenhagen. E-Mail: tohe@dadlnet.dk

Frank Holloway, FRCPsych, is Consultant Psychiatrist and Clinical Director at Croydon Integrated Adult Mental Health Service. Frank has been a Consultant Adult Psychiatrist since 1987. He has co-edited two books and has published numerous chapters and papers, mainly in the areas of mental health services research, rehabilitation and mental health policy. He is on the Editorial Boards of the International Journal of Social Psychiatry and the Psychiatric Bulletin and a member of the International Advisory Board of the British Journal of Psychiatry. He is the immediate past chair of the Faculty of Rehabilitation and Social Psychiatry of the Royal College of Psychiatrists. Frank.Holloway@iop.kcl.ac.uk

Nick Huband, PhD, RMN, Dip Couns., is Clinical Research Fellow at Nottinghamshire Healthcare NHS Trust and holds an honorary position at the University of Nottingham, UK. He has over thirteen years experience working in community mental health settings. Special interests include self-injury and research into outcomes of psychological interventions. E-Mail: nick.huband@nottingham.ac.uk

Adam Jefford, Bsc, Msc, R.M.N., Group analyst (Goldsmiths training, UKCP accredited), is Clinical Service Manager for the Intensive Psychological Treatment Service (IPTS), and the Co-ordinated Psychological Treatment Service (CPTS) based at Guy's Hospital. Previously, Adam was the manager of an adult acute psychiatric ward with a therapeutic group programme for 10 years. Subsequently he has set up and managed the IPTS day therapeutic community programmes. Adam has special interests in therapeutic groups in NHS settings, Therapeutic Communities and personality disorder.
E-mail: adam.jefford@slam.nhs.uk

Steven Livingstone, M.A. (Hons), D.Clin.Psy., is Clinical Psychologist at the Institute of Psychiatry and South London & Maudsley NHS. Steven is currently involved in the DOORWAY project at the Institute of Psychiatry, the aim of which is to improve psychological therapies in an inpatient setting. He takes part in the practice of inpatient group therapy and has trained other mental health professionals in the delivery of psychological therapies, mainly CBT-based groupwork. E-Mail: steven.livingstone@iop.kcl.ac.uk

Oded Manor, BA(Jerusalem),PhD(LSE),PGDip Applied Soc. Sc. and CQSW (Goldsmiths), Dip. Couns. Skills (SWLC), is an Independent Groupwork Consultant. Before retiring, he was Principal Lecturer in Social Work at Middlesex University, London, after having served as Senior Practitioner for Group and Family Work in the field. Oded has published four books, numerous papers and book chapters. Previously the editor of the journal Groupwork, he is currently the editor of the book series Groupwork Monographs. Oded has a special interest in applications of the systems approach and, over nearly forty years, has lectured extensively in various parts of the world. E-Mail: oded.manor@btopenworld.com

Ronan McIvor, MB BCh BAO, MRCPsych, is a Consultant Psychiatrist in Forensic Mental Health at the South London & Maudsley NHS Foundation Trust. He has extensive experience in treating patients in community and inpatient settings, and a long-standing interest in psychological reactions to trauma and group processes. An Honorary Senior Lectureship at King's College London School of Medicine, and an Honorary Lectureship at the Division of Psychological Medicine, Institute of Psychiatry, reflect his continuing interest in research and teaching. He has published extensively on aspects of mental health provision, biological aspects of mental illness and stalking behaviour. E-Mail: ronan.mcivor@slam.nhs.uk

Jack Nathan, B.Sc, CQSW, M.Sc, Ass. Mem. LCP, Mem. BPC, is Consultant Psychotherapist at the Maudsley Psychotherapy Service and Self-Harm Out-Patients' Service (SHOPS), and a Senior Lecturer in Social Work at the Institute of Psychiatry. Jack originally trained as a social worker and had been a Social Work Team Manager at the Maudsley Hospital before he went on to train as a psychoanalytic psychotherapist at the London Centre for Psychotherapy. His interests and publications have centred on developing psychoanalytically-based treatments for self-harmers and borderline personality disorders as well group therapy with patients with psychosis. He has also written extensively on making psychoanalytic ideas available to social workers in their everyday practice. E-Mail: Jack.Nathan@slam.nhs.uk

Isaura Manso Neto, MD, is Consultant Psychiatrist and Head of the Day Hospital at the Psychiatric Department of Hospital de Santa Maria, in Lisbon. She has been practicing in Public Psychiatric Hospitals and in private practice, as well as teaching and supervising other professionals. Isaura has published numerous papers. She is a Training and Supervising Member of the Portuguese Society of Groupanalysis. In 2008 she was awarded the Jane Abercrombie Prize from the Group Analytic Society in London where she is currently a member of the Management Committee. Isaura has special interests in psychoanalytic understanding and psychotherapy of mental health difficulties, transgenerational transmission of psychopathology and outcome studies. E-Mail: isauramansoneto@gmail.com

Tom O'Reilly, RMN, SRN, Dip Psychodynamic Psychotherapy (Liverpool), South Trent Training in Dynamic Psychotherapy, MA Consultation to the Organisation, Psychoanalytic Approaches. Tom is a Consultant Adult Psychotherapist in Nottinghamshire Healthcare NHS Trust. He works in Nottingham Psychotherapy Unit and Nottinghamshire Personality Disorder and Development Network where he is the Therapeutic Community Team Leader. Tom has worked across a range of psychiatric services including inpatient wards and day service provision. His present interests include developing services for patients with personality disorder and the application of psychoanalytic thinking to organisations. E-Mail: Tom.O'Reilly@nottshc.nhs.uk

Eleanor Overton, BA (Hons) works as Clinical Informatics Project Lead for Nottinghamshire Healthcare NHS Trust. She is particularly interested in early withdrawal from services and is currently undertaking a study of the views of referrers and service users of Nottinghamshire Personality Disorder and Development Network. She is studying towards an MA in Counselling Practice with the University of Nottingham. E-Mail: Eleanor.Overton@nottshc.nhs.uk

Wil Pennycook MA, Mem.Inst.GroupAnalysis is Consultant Psychotherapist and Group Analyst at the Maudsley Psychotherapy Service, where she is the lead clinician for Group Psychotherapy, and part of senior management. She has experience in conducting and supervising inpatient groups in both acute and forensic settings, and has also facilitated staff groups in both settings. Currently, Wil facilitates a staff group of the DSPD ward at the Bethlem Royal Hospital, and as part of her work with the MPS, co-conducts an out-patient group for patients with severe and enduring mental illness. Wil is also co-leading a research project using Mentalisation Based Treatment with patients with Borderline Personality Disorder.
Email: wil.pennycook@slam.nhs.uk

Bhupinderjit Pharwaha, BSc(Hons), currently works in Primary Care Mental Health in London. She has been involved in groupwork for over five years and has published two other papers with her colleagues on inpatient group work. In addition to groupwork she is interested in mental health resilience, recovery and mental health inequalities. Email: pinder.pharwaha@nhs.net

Jonathan Radcliffe is a Consultant Clinical Psychologist working in adult mental health in Lewisham, in the South London and Maudsley NHS Foundation Trust. He is lead psychologist for the Lewisham adult wards. He has run a weekly psychodynamic ward group for ten years and supervises colleagues in running ward groups. He trained as a psychoanalytic psychotherapist at the Lincoln Centre, London, and has a private practice. Before joining the NHS he worked as a primary school teacher and then an educational psychologist. E-Mail: jonathanradcliffe@sky.com

Ian Simpson, BA (Hons), PGCE, Mem.Inst.GroupAnalysis, ACAT is a Group Analyst and a Consultant Adult Psychotherapist. He is Head of Psychotherapy at St Thomas' Hospital, London, which is part of the South London & Maudsley NHS Foundation Trust. He has worked in the NHS for over 20 years and is particularly interested in contextual and process issues around staff welfare, support and containment within mental health organisations and in working with personality disorder. E-Mail: Ian.Simpson@slam.nhs.uk

Roger Smith, B.Sc.(Hons), M.Phil., D.Clin.Psychol., C.Psychol., is in private practice as a therapist and supervisor. His last NHS post was that of Head of AMH psychological therapy for an inner-city borough. Over the last forty years Roger has been involved in many areas of psychology as therapist, researcher, and trainer. He published several co-authored papers and has a special interest in the history of psychotherapy. E-Mail: smith1815@netscape.net

Til Wykes, BSc, MPhil, DPhil, FBPS, AcSS, is Professor of Clinical Psychology and Rehabilitation at the Institute of Psychiatry, King's College London and the first Director of the NIHR Mental Health Research Network. She has been involved in the development of novel psychological treatments and their evaluation for more than twenty years. She has been a pioneer in the involvement of mental health service users in research. Til founded and is now co-director of the Service User Research Enterprise at King's College London. She is also editor of the *Journal of Mental Health.* E-Mail: T.Wykes@iop.kcl.ac.uk

Index

F

G

H

I

CPSIA information can be obtained at www.ICGtesting.com
Printed in the USA
LVOW110336180113

316232LV00008B/144/P

9 781861 771148